Pascal Chabrot • Louis Boyer
Editors

Embolization

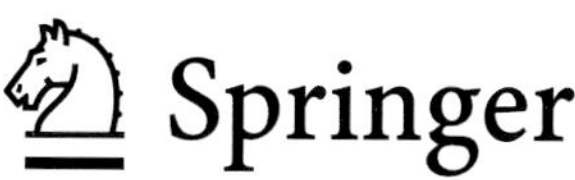

Editors
Pascal Chabrot, MD, PhD
Department of Radiology
University Hospital of Clermont-Ferrand
Clermont-Ferrand
France

Louis Boyer, MD, PhD
Department of Radiology
University Hospital of Clermont-Ferrand
Clermont-Ferrand
France

ISBN 978-1-4471-5791-5 ISBN 978-1-4471-5182-1 (eBook)
DOI 10.1007/978-1-4471-5182-1
Springer London Heidelberg New York Dordrecht

Softcover re-print of the Hardcover 1st edition 2014

Printed on acid-free paper

Springer is part of Springer Science+Business Media (www.springer.com)

Embolization

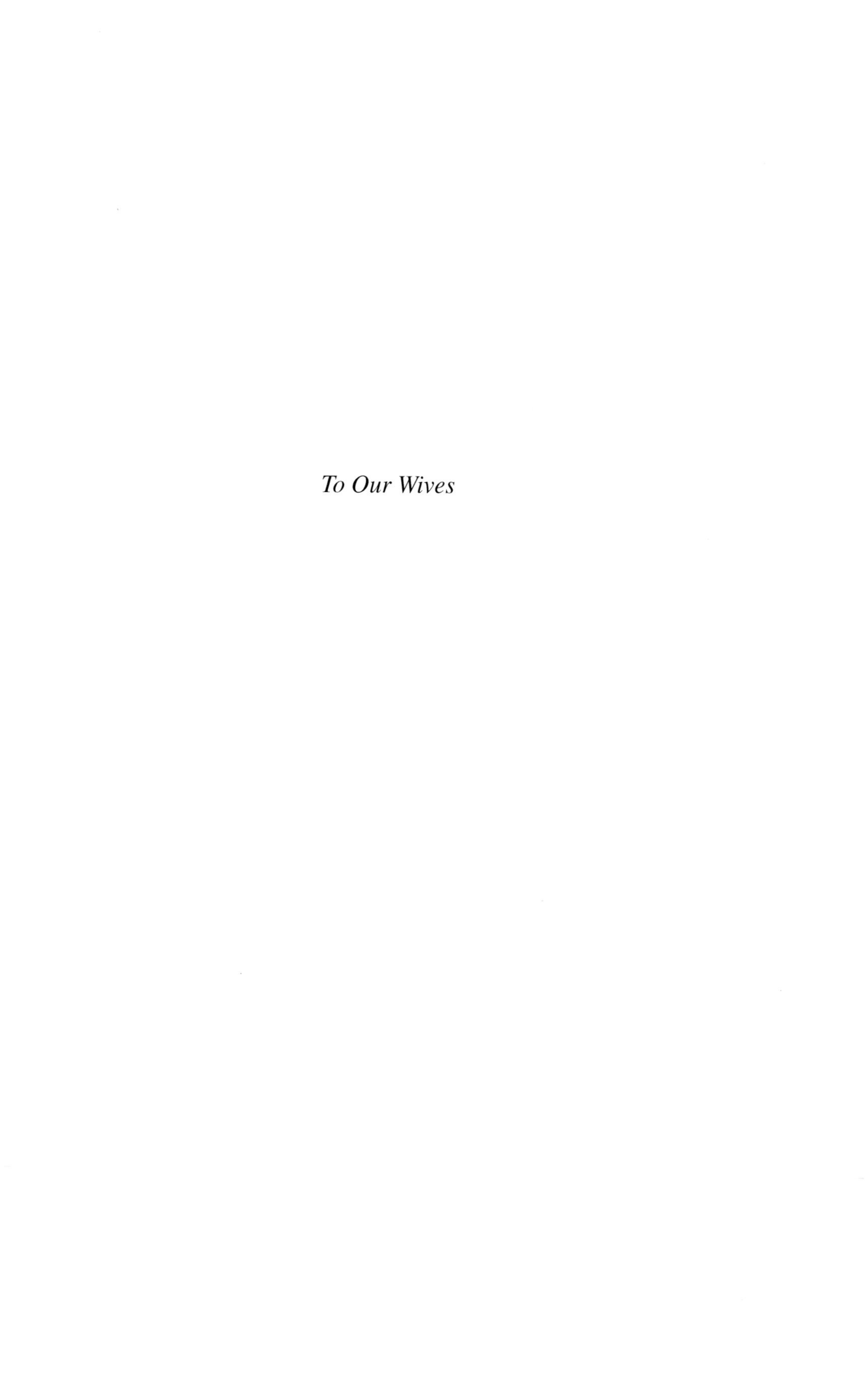

To Our Wives

Foreword

Interventional radiology emerged in the 1960s, with Charles Dotter's report of the first percutaneous angioplasty. As it quickly appeared that an endovascular catheter "could replace a scalpel," interventional radiology soon became a valuable alternative to surgical management.

The first embolizations were realized in the 1970s: neuroradiological embolizations carried out in France by R. Djindjian and hemostasis embolizations to treat GI tract hemorrhages by J. Rosch in the United States and to treat hemoptysis by J. Remy in France.

Embolization has since become one of the pillars of interventional radiology, and over the years considerable improvements have been made concerning catheters as well as occlusion agents.

The indications of interventional radiology are constantly broadening: the most remote anatomical areas are today within our range and a wider number of clinical conditions are nowadays treated. Embolization allows not only vessel occlusion but also in situ administration of various therapeutic agents, particularly drugs. In addition, it is no longer only restricted to symptomatic indications (e.g., hemostasis embolization) but also more and more as a curative technique in many fields.

Specific training is required to acquire the mandatory anatomical, clinical, and technical prerequisites for the realization of embolization. The radiologist is the ideal candidate for this training as he has the essential background required. It is a public health issue to train young interventional radiologists, to ensure a sufficient number of operators likely to support this activity.

It is essential to maintain the attractiveness of this discipline among the young radiologists and to ensure their training with inventive pedagogic methods so as to compensate for the lesser know-how in endovascular navigation due to the blossoming of the vascular cross-sectional imaging.

This book proposed by my friend Louis Boyer and his colleagues is a valuable tool for the promotion and the development of embolization. This team's experience in diagnostic and interventional vascular radiology, which was initiated by Professor Pierre Viallet, one of the pioneers of vascular radiology in France, makes

Clermont-Ferrand one of the most important French centers of interventional radiology and embolization.

This handbook which reviews and summarizes the key points of various embolization techniques and their indications will be particularly useful as a learning tool for young radiologists. It can also be used by more experienced interventional radiologists for a quick "refresher lesson" on a specific procedure.

I am convinced that all interventional radiologists should have this handy, practical daily reference tool, and I sincerely wish it has a great success.

Francis Joffre
President of the Interventional Radiology Federation
of the French Society of Radiology
Toulouse, France

Preface

The development of the embolization techniques, especially in oncology, led us to propose this practical handy book as a teaching aid for the training of young interventional radiologists which is now promoted in France as in the rest of Europe.

The innovations in catheterization techniques and embolization agents have considerably contributed to the development of endovascular occlusion techniques in arterial and venous trunks as much as distal parenchymal capillary beds. Mini invasive therapies, endovascular embolization, and chemo-embolization now constitute major therapeutic alternatives in various fields: on a purely palliative or on a curative basis in oncology, traumatology, functional diseases, for the treatment of benign tumors, or when dealing with postoperative complications.

Very in-depth and detailed books describing these techniques are ready available for the specialists. Our ambition here is to provide a basic handbook for the young vascular radiologists in training and a checklist for the more experienced vascular radiologists by providing for each indication a synthetic approach of the technique and of the expected results of constantly increasing embolization procedures in widening indications.

The first part of this book relates to the toolbox (the materials) and the procedure techniques as well as the physiopathological requirements for carrying out embolization; the second part is an analytical description of the main situations and anatomo-clinical strategies.

This book therefore does not have the ambition to appear in academic libraries, but rather to be a readily available memory aid for clinical interventional radiologists, accessible in the multidisciplinary staff rooms and in angiography suites.

We express our sincere thanks and our friendship:

- To our teacher and boss Professor Jean François Viallet
- To all the coauthors
- To Danielle Sol for preparing the manuscript

- To Matthieu Dondey and Agaïcha Alfidja for their help in translating the French version of the book into English
- To Mickaël Fontarensky for the preparation of the illustrations
- To all our team members for the years of joint work, which have enabled us to develop our experience and to gather our radio-clinical cases

Clermont-Ferrand, France

Louis Boyer, MD, PhD
Pascal Chabrot, MD, PhD

Contents

Contributors

Armand Abergel, MD, PhD Department of Hepatogastroenterology, University Hospital of Clermont-Ferrand, Clermont-Ferrand, France

Amr Abdel Kerim, MD Department of Radiology, University of Alexandria, Alexandria, Egypt

Agaïcha Alfidja Lankoande, MD Department of Radiology, University Hospital of Clermont-Ferrand, Clermont-Ferrand, France

Jean-Michel Bartoli Department of Radiology, Assistance Publiqúe, Hôpitaux de Marseille, Marseille, France

Romain Bellini, MD Department of Radiology, Jean Perrin Cancer Centre, Clermont-Ferrand, France

Stéphane Boisgard, MD, PhD Department of Orthopedic Surgery, University Hospital of Clermont-Ferrand, Clermont-Ferrand, France

Philippe Bourlet, MD Department of Radiology, Riom Hospital, University Hospital of Clermont-Ferrand, Clermont-Ferrand, France

Louis Boyer, MD, PhD Department of Radiology, University Hospital of Clermont-Ferrand, Clermont-Ferrand, France

Isabelle Brazzalotto, MD Department of Anesthesia, University Hospital of Clermont-Ferrand, Clermont-Ferrand, France

Emmanuel Buc, MD, PhD Department of Abdominal Surgery, University Hospital of Clermont-Ferrand, Clermont-Ferrand, France

Pierre Cassagneau Department of Radiology, Assistance Publiqúe, Hôpitaux de Marseille, Marseille, France

Lucie Cassagnes, MD Department of Radiology, University Hospital of Clermont-Ferrand, Clermont-Ferrand, France

Pascal Chabrot, MD, PhD Department of Radiology, University Hospital of Clermont-Ferrand, Clermont-Ferrand, France

Rami Chemali, MD Department of Radiology, Saint Georges Hospital, Beyrouth, Lebanon

Frédéric Cohen Department of Radiology, Assistance Publiqúe, Hôpitaux de Marseille, Marseille, France

Bruno De Fraissinette, MD Department of Radiology, Clinique La Chataigneraie, Beaumont, USA

Department of RadiologyUniversity Hospital of Clermont-Ferrand, Clermont-Ferrand, France

Florian Desmots Department of Radiology, Assistance Publiqúe, Hôpitaux de Marseille, Marseille, France

Abdoulaye Ndoye Diop, MD Department of Radiology, University Hospital, Dakar, Senegal

José Dubois, MD, MSc Department of Radiology, University Hospital Sainte Justine, Montréal, QC, Canada

Eric Dumousset, MD Department of Radiology, University Hospital of Clermont-Ferrand, Clermont-Ferrand, France

Le Thanh Dung, MD Department of Radiology, Viet Duc University Hospital, Hanoï, Hanoï, Viet Nam

Grégory Favrolt, MD Department of Radiology, Clinique de Fontaine, Dijon, France

Mickaël Fontarensky Department of Radiology, University Hospital of Clermont-Ferrand, Clermont-Ferrand, France

Cristi Gageanu, MD Department of Radiology, Issoire Hospital, University Hospital of Clermont-Ferrand, Clermont-Ferrand, France

Gérald Gahide, MD, PhD Department of Radiology, Sherbrooke University Hospital, Sherbrooke, QC, Canada

Denis Gallot, MD, PhD Department of Obstetrics and Gynecology, University Hospital of Clermont-Ferrand, Clermont-Ferrand, France

Jean-Marc Garcier, MD, PhD Department of Anatomy and Radiology, University Hospital of Clermont-Ferrand, Clermont-Ferrand, France

Hatem Gobara, MD Department of Radiology, Riom Hospital, University Hospital of Clermont-Ferrand, Clermont-Ferrand, France

Rémy Guillon, MD Department of Radiology, Clinique Saint Roch, Montpellier, France

Laurent Guy, MD, PhD Department of Urology, University Hospital of Clermont-Ferrand, Clermont-Ferrand, France

Alexis Jacquier Department of Radiology, Assistance Publiqúe, Hôpitaux de Marseille, Marseille, France

Antoine Maubon, MD, PhD Department of Radiology, University Hospital of Limoges, Limoges, France

Nathalie Mazet, MD Department of Radiology, CMC Beau Soleil, Montpellier, France

Guy Moulin Department of Radiology, Assistance Publiqúe, Hôpitaux de Marseille, Marseille, France

Cyril Muller Department of Radiology, Assistance Publiqúe, Hôpitaux de Marseille, Marseille, France

Pierre Perreault, MD Department of Radiology, University of Montreal Hospital Center, Montreal, QC, Canada

Antoine Petermann, MD Department of Radiology, University Hospital of Clermont-Ferrand, Clermont-Ferrand, France

Denis Pezet, MD, PhD Department of Abdominal Surgery, University Hospital of Clermont-Ferrand, Clermont-Ferrand, France

Laurent Poincloux, MD Department of Gastroenterology, University Hospital of Clermont-Ferrand, Clermont-Ferrand, France

Anne Ravel, MD Department of Radiology, University Hospital of Clermont-Ferrand, Clermont-Ferrand, France

Antoine Roche, MD Department of Radiology, University Hospital of Clermont-Ferrand, Clermont-Ferrand, France

Gilles Soulez, MD, MSc Department of Radiology, University Hospital Notre Dame, Montréal, QC, Canada

Eric Therasse Department of Radiology, Hôtel-Dieu – University of Montréal, Centre Hospitalier de l'Université de Montréal (CHUM), Montréal, QC, Canada

Arthur Varoquaux Department of Radiology, Assistance Publiqúe, Hôpitaux de Marseille, Marseille, France

Marie-Aude Vaz Tourret, MD Department of Radiology, University Hospital of Clermont-Ferrand, Clermont-Ferrand, France

Hélène Vernhet, MD, PhD Department of Radiology, University Hospital of Montpellier, Montpellier, France

Vincent Vidal, MD, PhD Department of Radiology, Assistance Publiqúe, Hôpitaux de Marseille, Marseille, France

Tan Duc Vo, MD Department of Radiology, Medical Sciences University, Ho Chi Minh Ville, Viet Nam

Part I
Technical Bases

Chapter 1
The Toolbox: Catheterization Devices and Embolization Agents

Pascal Chabrot, Vincent Vidal, and Louis Boyer

Innovations in occlusion agents and catheterization devices, as well as the broadening of their indications, make embolization procedures nowadays valuable therapeutic means for the treatment of various degenerative, congenital, traumatic, or tumor diseases.

Technical skills for the use of a large range of materials must be acquired in order to implement embolization, which can sometimes be indicated in emergency situations. The most challenging decision in practice is to choose the appropriate agent for different specific indications.

We shall not insist on the technical requirements for the angiographic unit which should ideally provide 3D and CT-like (CArm CT) acquisitions and include an automatic injector: the image quality obviously conditions the safety of the procedure, whether it is performed on large vessels or through microcatheterization.

The goal of this chapter is to present the specific characteristics of various embolization agents and vascular access devices as well as the specificities of selective catheterization for these indications. We limited ourselves to the most commonly used occlusion agents.

1.1 Occlusion Agents

Since the first embolization using an autologous clot to treat a gastric ulcer reported by Rösch, Dotter, and Brown [1], embolization agents have rapidly diversified: at first, thrombogenic materials used in situations other than their initial indications

P. Chabrot, MD, PhD (✉) • L. Boyer, MD, PhD
Department of Radiology, University Hospital of Clermont-Ferrand, Clermont-Ferrand, France
e-mail: pchabrot@chu-clermontferrand.fr; lboyer@chu-clermontferrand.fr

V. Vidal, MD, PhD
Department of Radiology, Assistance Publiqùe - Hôpitaux de Marseille, Marseille, France

P. Chabrot, L. Boyer (eds.), *Embolization*,
DOI 10.1007/978-1-4471-5182-1_1, © Springer-Verlag London 2014

Table 1.1 Agents according to the target and the duration of occlusion

	Small vessels	Large vessels and cavities
Temporary	Absorbable gelatin sponge: Gelfoam	Absorbable gelatin sponge (torpedo)
Permanent	Particles	Coils
	Biological glues	Plugs (AVP)
	Onyx	Thrombin
	Sclerosing agents	

(contrast agents, suture thread, guide wire's external filaments, etc.) and, secondarily, more specific agents.

Some agents cause a mechanical obstruction which induces the formation of a thrombus; some cause an inflammatory reaction in and around the vessel; sclerosing agents cause the destruction of the endothelium.

Temporary agents must be distinguished from permanent ones on one hand and those targeting large vessels from those intended for the small vessels (Table 1.1).

The choice of an embolic agent depends on the anatomy of the target, the desired interaction with the surrounding parenchyma, and the sustainability of the desired occlusion. The following questions must be answered first:

1. Is the desired occlusion a temporary or a permanent one?
2. At what level on the vascular tree: truncal or distal parenchymal?
3. Does one wish to preserve the viability of the downstream tissues?

The balance between safety and effectiveness must be systematically analyzed. Finally, the cost is another parameter that must be taken into account.

Autologous clots (for which the lysis is too rapid to obtain a clinical success), larguable balloons (which are at risk of migrating when deflated), and heated contrast agents (which caused severe pain) are today very seldom used.

Guide wire fragments or joining silk threads (2–0 or 3–0) have been sometimes used, especially for aneurysms or voluminous false aneurysms. Although their low cost is an advantage, they cannot however be used alone as it is difficult to position them and then control their landing; repositioning them is also very complicated. We do not use them.

1.1.1 Absorbable Gelatin Sponge (Gelfoam)

(a) Technical Characteristics

Absorbable gelatin sponge is derived from purified porcine gelatin (Gelfoam®, Pharmacia & Upjohn; Gelita-Spon®, Gelita Medical; Curaspon®, CuraMedical, etc.).

It ensures a temporary occlusion obtained through a mechanical obstruction and platelet adhesion. It is reabsorbed in 3–4 weeks, allowing a recanalization from 3 weeks to 3 months post-procedure: it is thus largely used in preoperative settings or to treat hemorrhages (trauma, GI hemorrhages, postpartum hemorrhages, etc.). Downstream *ad integrum* restitution can be expected once homeostasis is obtained. It can also be used as a complement of permanent agents (e.g., coils).

The other advantages are its usability and low cost.

(b) Instructions for Use

Available in pledgets of 1 or 10 mm in thickness, in precut cubes of 2 or 4 mm, in cylinders, in particles, or as a powder, it can be injected after dilution or in fragments. Dilution is carried out in a saline and water-soluble iodine contrast agent (ICM), using 3-way feeding taps and two Luer-Lock syringes. The desired viscosity is obtained according to the size of the manually cut fragments and the mixing procedures. By using small-size diluted fragments, the injection can take place through a 2.7 French microcatheter.

Tips and Tricks

- First use fragments of increasing size to ensure a distal embolization.
- A "torpedo" can allow a temporary proximal embolization: 3 mm wide by 10–15 mm long strip, rolled up and then inserted in a Luer-Lock syringe and vigorously injected through a diagnostic catheter (minimum 4 Fr).
- Gelatin sponge can complete a coil or plug occlusion, in order to obtain hemostasis, especially in case of coagulation disorders.

Pitfalls

- The powder form is the easiest to prepare, providing quickly homogeneous mixtures, but it gives very distal embolizations. In our team we have observed complications of embolization with powders in the treatment of postpartum hemorrhages such as necrosis and endometritis and have since abandoned their use when carrying out temporary embolizations.
- Air is often contained in the contrast-gelatin mixture and should not be interpreted on the CT scan as a sign of post-procedure infection.

(c) Future Developments

Several manufacturers are trying to develop absorbable microspheres (some of which are made of gelatin), of various sizes and absorption times.

1.1.2 Microparticles

Initially used to treat arteriovenous malformations, vascular traumatisms, and tumors [2, 3], particles allow distal parenchymal devascularization. They can be injected into the flow through a catheter or a microcatheter. They are characterized by their size, composition, and coating; the latter two determine their elasticity, rigidity, and aggregation ability as well as their interaction with adjacent parenchyma (inflammatory reaction of variable intensity).

Table 1.2 Characteristics of available microparticles

Particles	Composition	Diameters (μm)	Presentation	Color
PVA Foam®	PVA particles	90–2,800	1 ml bottle	No
Bead Block®	PVA spheres	100–1,200	1 or 2 ml syringe	Colored
Contour®	PVA particles	45–1,180	1 or 2 ml bottle	No
Contour SE®	PVA spheres	100–1,200	1 or 2 ml syringe	No
Embosphere®	Tris-acryl spheres	40–900	Bottle or syringe	No
Embogold®	Tris-acryl spheres	40–1,200	1 or 2 ml syringe	Colored
Embozen®	Hydrogel	40–1,300	1 or 2 ml syringe	Colored

Occlusion occurs through a mechanical obstruction, a stasis thrombus, and an inflammatory reaction. This occlusion of the distal capillary bed can induce tissue ischemia and necrosis.

(a) Technical Characteristics

- Composition
  Historically the particles were derived from polyvinyl alcohol (PVA) surgical hemostatic sponges. Depending on the way they were cut, they produced elements of variable and irregular forms. The aggregation of these particles was important, making the assessment of the injected aggregates difficult and leading to more proximal embolizations than those planned [2].
  The first evolution concerned the calibration of these particles (Contour®, Boston Scientific) so as to obtain a range of particles of various sizes by increments 200 μ (calibrated particles). Then spherical particles appeared, made of PVA (Contour SE®, Boston Scientific; Bead Block®, Terumo Biocompatible) and of tris-acryl (Embosphère® and Medical Embogold®, Biosphere), characterized by a lower adhesion factor enabling more distal embolizations.
  More recently, hydrogel spheres with a fixed gauge have been developed (the variation being less than 5 % of the nominal gauge), covered with a polymer (Polyzen-F) limiting their aggregation (Embozen®, CeloNova) (Table 1.2).
- Elasticity, Rigidity
  The *elasticity* is the capacity of the particle to return to its initial form after a deformation such as an injection through a microcatheter. The *rigidity* is the capacity of the sphere to preserve its form in spite of a compression.
  The rigidity and the elasticity of the PVA particles (Contour SE®) are more limited than those of the tris-acryl (Embosphere®), which results in a more distal embolization of the deformed PVA particles, more particularly when injected through a microcatheter. Thus, to establish an equivalent embolization level, the caliber of the tris-acryl must be lower than that of the PVA [4, 5]. In the same way, in order to obtain an equivalent occlusion level, the diameter of hydrogel-polyzene spheres chosen must be higher than that of tris-acryl particles.

- Interactions with the Adjacent Parenchyma
  The intensity of the inflammatory response which conditions the occurrence of a post-embolization syndrome varies according to the extension of the necrosis, the nature, and the size of the particles. Particles of less than 300 μ result in a much more significant inflammation. Over 500 μ, the size is no longer a determining factor [3]. After embolization using PVA, an acute inflammatory reaction mediated by polynuclear neutrophils is observed (more marked with particles than with spheres), which gradually gives way to a predominantly giant cells reaction. With tris-acryl spheres, the initial inflammation is limited, then giving way to a more intense delayed lymphocytic reaction [4].

  The composition of the microspheres allows their combination with other therapeutic agents (cytotoxics, anti-inflammatory drugs). These loaded particles allow a targeted and progressive delivery of the associated agent. Various drug-fixing methods are used: *ionic link* between a positively charged particle and the negative doxorubicin (cd. Bead®, biocompatible Terumo), passive *hydrophilic link* between ibuprofen and Bead Block, or *a combination of both* (Hepasphere®). The fixation capacities and the release kinetics depend on the particles and the associated agents. Microparticles can also be loaded with isotopes (yttrium 90), thus allowing a selective in situ radiation therapy.

(b) Instructions for Use (Table 1.3)
Before injection, the particles are diluted with a saline and ICM, according to ratios specified by the manufacturer (generally isovolume saline/ICM), in order to obtain a homogeneous suspension. To limit the risk of aggregation, dilutions are more important with the smaller particles (100–500 μ) (diluted up to 100× their volume) than with the larger ones (up to ×10) [2]. Prefilled syringes facilitate this operation, which can be carried out with a 3-way tap and a standard Luer-Lock syringe. The mixture can be obtained with the prefilled syringe and a 10 ml syringe, but the injections during embolization are generally carried out using syringes of 1 or 3 ml (Medallion® Merit), given that they take place in microcatheters.

The initial particle diameter is selected according to the topography but also to the nature of the target: for a tumor embolization, the size of the tumor, its vascularization, and the risk of intra-tumoral arteriovenous shunts must be taken into account. In this indication, very-small-caliber particles would more readily induce necrosis by occluding the most distal vessels. Particles of progressively increasing diameter are then selected, to the "end point" which is sometimes difficult to establish: the most commonly used criterion is a reflux or an off-target embolization. Initially the goal of embolization with PVA was to obtain a complete exclusion of the embolized segment. Today with calibrated particles, the aim is to slow down the flow and obtain the "dead-tree" pattern.

In order to maintain the patency of the microcatheter, an arterial purge with saline (via a Y valve) must be carried out.

Table 1.3 Recommended diameter of the catheter internal lumen (according to the manufacturers' instruction notice)

Particles (μ)	45–120	100–300	300–500	500–700	700–900	900–1,200	1,300
PVA foam	0.018″				0.044″		
Contour®				2.4 Fr	2.7 Fr	4 Fr	
Contour SE®		0.021″			0.024″	0.035″	
Embosphere	0.008″	0.013″	0.018″	0.023″	0.027″	0.035″	
Embogold®	0.008″	0.013″	0.018″	0.023″	0.027″	0.035″	
Embozen®	0.004″	0.013″	0.018″	0.023″	0.027″	0.0 35″	0.038″
Bead Block®		0.010″	0.014″	0.021″	0.023″	0.035″	

Table 1.4 Dilution of the microparticles

Particles	500 μ	>500 μ
Dilution	×100 to ×1,000	×10
ICM/saline	50/50 % adapted to the volume and the radio opacity If particles float = too much ICM	

Tips and Tricks

- The use of microparticles requires a rigorous management of the tools (syringes, catheters, cups, etc.), to avoid unexpected injections. The methods vary according to the centers, but in all cases the embolization material (syringes and cups) must be clearly identified. Some particles are naturally colored.
- To obtain a homogeneous suspension, the ICM/saline ratio is variable, but generally if the particles float in the mixture, then the quantity of ICM is excessive. However, the choice of a heterogeneous suspension can be deliberate, so as to progressively inject the required quantity of particles.
- Control angiography (after having rinsed the microcatheter) depicts flow redistribution in the collateral networks, which are in some cases only secondarily unmasked. These ICM injections must be carried out with limited pressure, so as not to cause any reflux.
- To benefit from the blood flow, the carrier catheter can sometimes be withdrawn, leaving only the microcatheter in place and thus authorizing a better washing by the arterial flow.
- The last angiographic control must be carried out after a delay of 3–5 mn, to ensure a stabilized end point (Table 1.4).

Pitfalls

- Catheter obstruction frequently occurs when particles are not sufficiently diluted or if the catheter is not regularly rinsed.
- Microspheres of small caliber should not be used in the presence of arterio-venous shunts.
- A hyperpressure injection exposes to endothelium damage, to off-target reflux, and to the opening of anastomoses which can also induce off-target embolization; it can also deform the Embospheres (tris-acryl).

- The occurrence of a vasospasm distal to the microcatheter can artificially limit the volume of the target and lead to an early revascularization. A careful catheterization, the comparison with images obtained on global injections, and sometimes an injection of vasodilator are helpful in overcoming this limit.

(c) Future Prospects
A challenging indication of loaded particles could be the implantation of cells such as hepatic transplantation of small Langerhans islets by percutaneous catheterization of the portal vein to treat some cases of type I diabetes patients.

Little is known about the particle-tissue interactions. This embolization agent constitutes a foreign body which induces an inflammatory reaction which up until now has undoubtedly been underestimated. It causes the release of mediators, leads to a vascular wall remodeling, and results into an extravascular migration and a stimulated angiogenesis. It evolves into intolerance (chronic inflammation, immunity), modifies the environment of the absorbable materials, and lastly can limit the diffusion of the drugs carried by the loaded particles. The histological assessment can only be carried out at a late stage: progress in molecular biology will undoubtedly allow an earlier evaluation of these intolerance phenomena and bring about an evolution in the embolization agents, particularly loaded particles.

1.1.3 Liquid Agents

1.1.3.1 Biological Glues

(a) Technical Characteristics
Biological glues were initially used to embolize cerebral arteriovenous malformations.

The polyethylene glycol and the aldehydes used in surgery have only very rare endovascular applications [5]. To embolize, cyanoacrylates (Trufill®, Cordis; Histoacryl® Braun; Glubran2®, GEM; Neuracryl, Prohold Technologies) are predominantly used. They are made up of an ethylene molecule coupled with a cyanogen group and an ester. Depending on the associated ester, several agents were initially proposed (isobutyl, n-butyl, 2-hexyl cyanoacrylate); the occurrence of sarcomas in animals resulted in abandoning the isobutyl group. The contact of ionic substances (saline, water, plasma, blood cells, epithelium) initiates the polymerization, starting from the ethylene groups, by releasing heat energy. An inflammatory reaction accompanies the polymerization. The length of the hydrocarbon chain proportionally increases the speed of the polymerization and decreases the importance of the exothermic reaction and the cellular toxicity. Thus, Glubran®, compared to Histoacryl®, polymerizes more slowly, is less painful with the injection, and causes a less marked inflammatory reaction [6]. In spite of a Glubran exothermic reaction which is less marked (<45°), the reduction of the pain remains limited [7].

It should be noted that complete absorptions, which possibly leads to recanalizations, have been described.

To facilitate their visibility, the glues can be mixed with metallic powders (tantalum or tungsten) or with radiopaque oils (Lipiodol®, Guerbet or Ethiodol®, Savage Laboratories) [8]. These radiopaque oils also contribute to slowing down the speed of the polymerization in a linear way. In vitro, polymerization speeds with a glue/Lipiodol ratio between 1:1 and 1:4 spread over 1 and 4 s.

The injection causes an acute inflammatory response of the vessel and the perivascular tissues, evolving into a chronic organized granuloma within a month. The embolization can be permanent if it fills the entire arterial volume. Colonization by neocapillaries within the embolized vessels has been described [5, 6].

(b) Instructions for Use

To carry out the embolization, the microcatheter should to be positioned as close as possible to the target (less than 1 cm). The correct positioning is verified by a control angiogram. The microcatheter is led via a diagnostic catheter or a delivery/carrier catheter: they ensure the stability of the catheterization and allow a fast withdrawal of the microcatheter after injection of the glue; they must be rinsed continuously (purge). Gloves must be changed when preparing the glue. The volume, the speed of the injection, and the viscosity (glue/Lipiodol ratio) are adapted according to a prior test injection (supposed volume of glue = volume of injected ICM – dead volume of the catheter). The microcatheter is then rinsed by a nonionic solution (dextrose or glucose 5 %); the physiological saline solution is contraindicated because it initiates polymerization. This volume is then pushed by the dextrose serum or 5 % glucose solution, through a lateral path in a three-way tap via a 3 ml Luer-Lock syringe. The glue injection is performed through the tap, distally with the help of an 1 ml Luer-Lock syringe. A high flow rate exposes the patient to a reflux, while slow one induces a fragmented embolization. The lateral way allows the dextrose injection to be given by a 3 ml Luer-Lock syringe. The volume of the glue is often lower than the evaluated ICM volume, and in vivo polymerization occurs more rapidly in vitro [9]. After the injection of the desired volume, the catheter is either removed using an aspiration or carefully rinsed using dextrose according to the evaluated flow established at the time of the test injection.

Tips and Tricks

- Procedure is generally safer with a microcatheter, even when catheterization is easily carried out.
- The use of coated hydrophilic microcatheters facilitates the injection by limiting friction within the catheter [10].
- The viscosity can be increased by adding glacial acetic acid [11].
- In complex indications such as tumor embolizations, where the evaluation of the adequate volume is difficult, the embolization can be carried out using the “sandwich” technique, by repeated injections of a low volume of nBCA-Lipiodol mixture, separated by serum glucose injections [12].

Table 1.5 Examples of DMSO-compatible[a] microcatheters

Catheter	External diameter (Fr) (proximal/distal)	Internal lumen (″v)	Length (cm)
Cantata® (Cook)	2.5	0.021	100–150
	2.8	0.025	
Progreat® (Terumo)	2.4	0.022	130–150
	2.7	0.025	110–130
Progreat Ω®	2.8	0.027	130
Rebar ™ 18 (eV3)	2.8/2.3	0.021	135–158
Rebar ™ 27	2.8	0.027	135–150
Renegade Hi-Flo® (Boston Scientific)	3/2.8	0.027	105–150

[a]A wider range is available for smaller diameters, rarely used in peripheral embolization

- In order to limit the risk of a retrograde embolization, it is necessary to (1) inject slowly, in order to prevent a reflux; (2) withdraw the catheter in time by maintaining an aspiration; and (3) avoid rinsing the dead volume.

Pitfalls

- With an antegrade embolization, the principal risks are the obstruction of the internal lumen, the clogging up of the distal end of the catheter, and the mobilization of proximal fragments in contact with the catheter.
- Because of polymerization in contact with blood and a physiological saline solution, the internal lumen and the end of the catheter must thoroughly be rinsed by a dextrose serum or a glucose solution.

1.1.3.2 Ethylene Vinyl Alcohol (EVA)

(a) Technical Characteristics
Ethylene vinyl alcohol (*Onyx*®, eV3) is a copolymer which forms a nonadhesive solution when associated with dimethyl sulfoxide (DMSO); this solution progressively polymerizes when it is in contact with ionic materials and blood. Various concentrations of EVA are available (Onyx 18, 20, 34), with a gradually increasing viscosity. It is more easily monitored with fluoroscopy by the adjunction of tantalum powder.

Onyx solidifies, from the periphery towards the center, gradually forming a cast of the vessel (aneurysm, AVM, etc.).

(b) Instructions for Use
Onyx is prepared in advance by a recomposition of the solution (solvent and powder), then mixed for 20 min in a centrifuge dedicated for this purpose. In this form, the solution is stable for 15–20 min and can be injected into a microcatheter compatible with the DMSO (Table 1.5). The catheter is slowly rinsed with DMSO; the volume used corresponds to the dead volume of the catheter (specified by the manufacturer). After disconnecting the syringe, the end of the catheter is rinsed so as to limit air bubbles at the DMSO-Onyx interface.

Onyx is then slowly injected. This second phase must be carried out slowly (<0.5 ml/min), because it initially corresponds to the injection of the DMSO. A rapid injection of the solution exposes to a systemic toxicity. The pulmonary elimination of the DMSO induces a specific a rotten apple breath.

Once in contact with blood, the polymerization is carried out gradually, from the periphery towards the center. A sheath develops around Onyx during its injection, allowing its containment. Onyx is not adhesive; therefore, it is possible to limit its reflux by producing a first "stopper" at the distal end of the catheter. Once this stopper has solidified, the injection can be renewed safely.

This technique can be used to carry out proximal occlusions.

To treat AVM or tumor neovascularizations, the injection can be pursued before solidification, thus allowing the filling of the nidus, the efferents, and the collateral networks.

Tips and Tricks

- Control angiogram can be improved by the use of a "negative roadmap" (image subtraction fluoroscopy). After the activation of the road-map function, the first fluoroscopy showing the injected Onyx is used as a mask: the following injections will then appear, after subtraction of the previously injected Onyx.
- To avoid vasospasm, the injection must be given slowly (0.5 ml/min).
- To limit the volume of the DMSO, the catheters are not rinsed but changed for each injection site.
- Extraction procedures using thromboaspiration [13] or thrombectomy devices [14] have been reported to treat Onyx off-target occlusions or embolizations depending on their topography and consequences.

Pitfalls

- Once onyx has been injected, the guide wire should not be reintroduced into the microcatheter, because of a theoretical risk of expulsion of microemboli.
- Preoperative "burns" have been described when using electric bistouries or electrocoagulation in patients previously treated with Onyx [15].
- Even if Onyx does not have any adhesive property, a limited fragment can remain attached to the catheter's distal end. It is usually an extension of an intracatheter residue.

1.1.3.3 Sclerosing Agents

Sclerosing agents include absolute alcohol and detergents. Hypertonic saline and glycerol are currently no longer used for embolization. The mechanisms are variable (endothelial cell membrane impairment, surface protein alteration, destruction of the extracellular matrix), but these agents all have a common principle: destruction of the endothelium, which is responsible for the vascular occlusion. This destruction is more or less intense and can extend to the surrounding tissues. The intensity of the reaction is determined by the concentration of the agent and its contact time. The use of detergents is limited, due to the direct and systemic toxicities and to the difficulties in controlling their diffusion.

Absolute Alcohol

(a) Technical Characteristics
Absolute alcohol or ethanol has a high direct toxicity on the endothelium, which induces a thrombosis and a rapid transmural necrosis extending to the surrounding tissues. This property is largely used in endovascular or percutaneous tumor destruction, but the effects on the surrounding tissues are all the more marked.

(b) Instructions for Use
Alcohol, which is radiotransparent, can be mixed with and ICM (20–30 % ICM) or with Lipiodol, so as to allow its visualization under fluoroscopic control. Its injection is painful; therefore, it is frequently carried out under a general anesthesia particularly in children. Systemic toxicity (hemolysis, renal toxicity, and pulmonary arterial vasoconstriction) is frequent observed when alcohol is administered beyond a volume of 1 ml/kg of body weight [8]. To prevent this risk of locoregional and general complications, a great technical mastery is required. When treating large vascular malformations, an invasive monitoring of the pulmonary pressure is recommended due to the high risk of severe pulmonary arterial hypertension (PAHT), even if there is no consensus on its utility [16]. The injections are fractioned and slowly carried out: not more than 0.1 ml/kg per injection, every 10 min, without exceeding a total volume of 1 ml/kg [16].

Tips and Tricks

- Systemic diffusion must be limited as much as possible when an injection in a closed system is not possible (i.e., alcoholization of a cyst): the reduction of flow can be obtained by limiting the upstream flow (injection downstream of an occlusion balloon) or the exit flow. Some have proposed the creation of a "closed" system, by aspirating the venous return during the intra-arterial injection of alcohol to treat kidney tumors.
- ICM injection downstream of an inflated occlusion balloon allows an assessment of the flow and the volume needed to obtain tumor exclusion. The injection must be slow, and the balloon will be deflated a few minutes after the last injection, after an aspiration.
- Invasive monitoring of the pulmonary blood pressure is necessary for the alcoholization of voluminous lesions. When a PAHT occurs (increase of 50 % of the initial pressure, or an increase higher than 10 mmHg), injection must be immediately stopped. Intravenous injection of sildenafil (Viagra®) has been described as being effective for the initial management of PAHT [17].

- Anti-inflammatory drugs are frequently prescribed in the immediate aftermath of major visceral alcoholization.

Pitfalls

- Alcohol injection exposes to a risk of cutaneous necrosis during the treatment of superficial arteriovenous malformations and to a risk of neurological complication when the treatment takes place near large nervous trunks.

Detergents

(a) Technical Characteristics

Sodium tetradecyl sulfate (STS), Aetoxisclerol, and ethanolamine oleate are the three main detergents. They interact with the blood and the endothelium and induce a vascular occlusion and a perivascular fibrosis [18, 19]. These detergents require an extended contact time with the endothelium; they are used to occlude slow flow lesions. Compared to alcohol, the inflammatory reaction and the tissue destruction are less marked, but the fibrous reaction is more intense.

STS (Sotradecol®, AngioDynamics; Trombovar®, Kreussler Co.) is a synthetic fatty acid largely used since the 1940s to treat lower limb venous valvular incompetence.

Available in dilutions of 1 and 3 %, the useful concentrations vary from 0.1 to 3 %, based on the volume and the flow of the lesion. The maximum volumes recommended are 4 ml of STS 3 % and 10 ml of STS 1 %.

Cutaneous necrosis has been observed with therapeutic concentrations in the case of extravascular injections (0.5 ml of STS 1 %). Hyperpigmentation has been frequently reported but seems to be related to inappropriate concentration levels. Rare hemolytic and allergic complications have also been described.

Aetoxisclerol or *polidocanol* is a urethane polymer initially used as a local anesthetic and since the 1960s as a sclerosing agent to treat medium to large-size telangiectasia and varicose veins. The useful concentrations vary from 0.3 to 3 %, depending on the size and the flow of the target vessels. The recommended maximum dose is approximately 2 mg/kg of body weight (10–20 ml of solution at 3 %).

Hyperpigmentation and hemolysis are less frequent than with the other sclerosing agents.

In vitro Aetoxisclerol appears to have a lower sclerosing effect than the other detergents, without any difference in its effectiveness (but there is a lack of comparative study) ([20], [21]).

Ethanolamine oleate (*Neosclerol®*, *Ethamolin®*) is an unsaturated thrombogenic fatty acid largely used for sclerotherapy of esophageal varices. The recommended maximum dose is 0.4 ml/kg.

It causes little local toxicity. But the general complications (hemolysis and renal toxicity) are the same than with the other detergents. Furthermore, pulmonary cardiogenic shock, edemas, and DIC have also been reported.

(b) Instructions for Use

The detergents can be used as liquid and as foam, which increases the surface and the contact time with the endothelium.

- *Liquid*

  Usually injected via direct puncture, as in venous malformations, the detergent is associated with a hypo-osmolar ICM or with Lipiodol (dilution detergent/contrast agent: 1/1 or 2/1). A preliminary ICM injection confirms the intravascular positioning of the needle and allows an evaluation of the flow and of the volume of the lesion which is to be excluded. The injection is done under fluoroscopic control, by direct visualization [21] or by negative controls during the emptying of contrast agent from the lesion's area [22]. The flow must be carefully controlled so as to avoid any extravasations.
- *Foam*

  The quantity of sclerosant is largely reduced. Various techniques have been described [23]; Tessari's method is to mix 1 volume of sclerosing agent with 1–5 volumes of air, using 2 Luer-Lock syringes and a 3-way tap [24]. After 20–30 to-and-fro motions between the two syringes, a homogeneous mixture is obtained which is easily detected as it has a hyper-echoic aspect on ultrasound. The fluoroscopic control can be indirectly carried out using the negative-contrast technique: a progressive emptying of a venous segment previously opacified [22]. An alternative method is to associate a nonionic ICM in equal quantities to the sclerosing agent (sclerosing agent/air/ICM: 1/5/1) allowing a direct visualization.

  Foam has been largely used for the sclerosis of varicose veins, venous malformations, or GI varices and more recently to treat the pelvic venous congestion and varicoceles [22] and more rarely for portal embolizations [25].

Tips and Tricks

- These agents should be used in slow flow. Contact times can be increased by simultaneous compression, tourniquets, or preliminary occlusion by coils, as done for varicocele exclusion.
- When direct puncture scleroses are carried out, once the lesion is completely filled, the needle is left in place a few minutes to facilitate necrosis and to avoid reflux.

Pitfalls

- The risk of off-target embolization is a major concern: it can be avoided by a complete diagnostic angiogram and repeated angiography per procedure controls to verify the intravascular positioning and unmask aberrant drainage; hyperpressure injections are forbidden.
- When treating superficial venous malformations with ultrasound-guided injections, foam gradually masks the residual zones. Therefore, these treatments must be carried out in multiple sessions.

1.1.4 *Mechanical Agents*

1.1.4.1 Coils

(a) Technical Characteristics

Coils are spires which are delivered by a selective diagnostic catheter with a distal hole or by a microcatheter, in vessels of more than 2 mm. Most of them have synthetic fibers braided on the metallic frame, thus facilitating thrombosis.

They are used to occlude arterial trunks, aneurysms, or cavities. They were initially used for proximal embolizations (renal, hepatic, and splenic arteries or internal iliac arteries [2, 3]). Downstream occlusion is obtained by a mechanical occlusion of the vessel or aneurysm, associated with a thrombogenic effect: the coils help in slowing down the flow and make vascular occlusion possible while avoiding downstream necrosis.

Coils are characterized by their composition, their coating, their shape, their dimensions (length, expansion diameter), and the modality of their release.

- *Composition and coating*: They can be made out of steel, platinum, or alloy. Stainless steel coils (Stainless Steel® Cook) are more radiopaque and present a higher radial force but cause important MRI artifacts and are thus not compatible with MRI according to the manufacturer's recommendations.

  Platinum coils are more flexible. The use of superalloy (Iconel®) gives the MReye® Cook coils a higher radial force than platinum, and they are nonetheless MRI compatible.

  Azur® Terumo coils are covered with a hydrogel polymer, which increases their expansion by a factor of 4 or 5 in an aqueous environment.
- *Shape*: Coils are available in different plane shapes (linear, J form, circular, cloverlike, etc.) and sometimes complex 3D shapes providing a genuine framework adapted to the filling of vessels or vascular cavities (aneurysmal sac, false aneurysm, etc.) by packing.
- *Dimensions*: In addition to the size of the catheter lumen (microcatheter or selective catheter), the coils are characterized by their length and their expansion diameter. The choice of coil length depends on the size of the target. The diameter is adapted to the target vessel: oversizing which should be greater for veins (130–150 %) than for the arteries (120 %) is necessary to develop a higher radial force and a better stability. Oversizing exposes to the risk of inadequate deployment in small-caliber vessels. The choice of the coil size is a key factor for the result of embolization.
- *Deployment methods*: The coils are delivered through a catheter or a microcatheter with a distal hole. Multi-perforated catheters are proscribed: the coil could escape by a side hole.

The deployment mechanism can be simple: coils pushed by guide wire, or flushed with saline using a Luer-Lock syringe (1–3 cc) (with a random precision release), or more complex and controlled release by a mechanical device (tenon and mortise system) (IDC®, Cook, etc.), or by a piezoelectric mechanism

Table 1.6 Characteristics of the available coils (according to the instruction manuals)

Coils	Material	Fibers	Deployment	Introduction diameter (″)	Catheter/guide wire	Diameter (mm)	Length (cm)
Spirale®	Platinum	/	Pushed	0.010″	1.9 Fr/0.014	2–10	5–15
Balt				0.018″	2.1 Fr/0.018	2–11	2.5–15
				0.037″	5 Fr/0.038	5–16	3–30
Spirale®	Platinum	Fibered	Pushed	0.015″	3 Fr/0.021	2–9	2.5–10
Balt				0.032″	5 Fr/0.038	4–10	5–10
GDC® Boston Scientific	Platinum	Bare	Controlled	0.018″		5–20	15–30
IDC® Boston Scientific	Platinum	Bare	Controlled	0.018″	<0.027″		
IDC®	Platinum	Fibered	Controlled	0.018″	<0.027	3–14	2.3–30
Boston Scientific				0.035″		3 to 20	4–40
Nester®	Platinum	Fibered	Pushed	0.018″		2–10	3–14
Cook				0.035″		4–20	7–20
Tornado®	Platinum	Fibered	Pushed	0.018″	<0.027″/0.018	3–10	2–14
Cook				0.035″	4 Fr/0.035	4–10	2.6–12.5
Stainless Steel®	Metal	Fibered		0.035″		2–8	2–5
Cook				0.038″		2–15	3–15
				0.052″		15–20	15
MReye®	Iconel®	Fibered	Pushed	0.035″	4 Fr/0.035	3–20	2–15
Cook				0.038″	5 Fr/0.038	3–25	2–15
MReye® *Flipper* Cook	Iconel®	Fibered	Controlled	0.041″	5 Fr	3–8	3–12
Axium® eV3	Platinum		Controlled	0.015″		2–25	2–50
Azur®	Platinum	Hydrogel	Pushed	0.018″	2.4 Fr/0.018	4–10	2–14
Terumo				0.035″	4 Fr/0.035	4–15	4–14
Azur® Terumo	Platinum	Hydrogel	Controlled	0.018″	2.7 Fr/0.018	4–20	10–20

using an external device (Azure®, Terumo; Axium®, eV3, GDC®, Boston Scientific, etc.).

The controlled-release coils have the advantages of a very precise and readjustable deployment but within a limited time delay for the fiber coils and hydrocoils, which can be trapped in the catheter after their expansion. Another important drawback is their price (Table 1.6).

(b) Instructions for Use

The coils are pushed with a straight-tipped guide. We prefer Teflon-coated guides to hydrophilic ones which can penetrate into the spires and disturb their deployment.

The deployment of the first and the last coils represents the essential steps of the embolization: the first coil can be deployed according to the anchor and the knitting technique or based on a previously deployed support. Each one of these methods aims to obtain the densest possible filling (coils of decreasing size), after deployment and stabilization of the first coil. Throughout the deployment, the catheter is carefully rinsed (continuous purge), so as to facilitate the progression of the material.

The *anchor technique* is possible only if there is a side branch that can be sacrificed upstream the target vessel. The first coil is released a few millimeters into this branch, before withdrawing the catheter for additional coil release into the target artery. The initial coil must be stabilized before completing the occlusion with additional coils.

The *knitting technique* uses the radial force of the first coil to establish an implantation base for the remaining spires. A back and forth movement of the catheter during coil release enables it to acquire its spiral form.

The *packing technique* aims to fill the aneurysmal sac while respecting the parent vessel. The initial choice could be a 3D coil which allows the filling of the sac while preserving the neck.

The aneurysm neck protection techniques initially described in neuroradiology may sometimes be necessary: temporary inflation of a balloon in front of the neck [26], or a bare stent previously positioned, through the mesh of which the coils will be deployed.

In some large vessels, the stabilization of the first coil can only be obtained after the deployment of an anchoring system. In these situations, we prefer today using occlusion plugs whenever it is possible. The development of 0.035 caliber controlled-release coils (IDC®, Boston Scientific, Balt) could be an alternative.

In small vessels, once the target has been reached with a microcatheter, flushing the coils with saline is a time-saving method.

The protection of the deployment can be ensured by the upstream inflation of an occlusion balloon: this is especially interesting in high-flow vessels. The safety of the coilsv also depends on the ability to retrieve them by various endovascular methods, in case of accidental migration.

Tips and Tricks

- In order to ensure the correct functioning of the fixing device, we verify the mechanically detachable coils by extruding them by a few millimeters on the preparation table, to make sure that their recapture is satisfactory.
- If embolization exposes to a risk of distal migration, then one can initially use controlled deployment coil, followed by pushed coils.
- The choice of the size of the coils depends on:
  - The size of the target vessel: if the coil is too small, there is a risk of migration; if the coil is excessively oversized, it remains linear. Embolization with saline-flushed coils through microcatheters allows very distal occlusions of small arteries for which the use of liquid agents is not possible.

  - The volume to be excluded: it is better to use long lengths for large volumes.
  - The platinum coils have less radial force than that of metallic ones which were initially used: their oversizing is thus recommended for the first coils (about 20 % for the arteries and 30–40 % for the veins).

- The progression in the last millimeters of IDC® coils must be carefully carried out so as not to move the pack with the deployment guide, which is more rigid than the coil itself.
- Use the roadmap established without ICM, showing the first coils in place, in order to place the following ones.
- The control injections must be carried out carefully, so as not to move the coils already deployed.
- At the end of the procedure, Gelfoam fragments can quickly complete the occlusion.

Pitfalls

- When choosing a coil, its diameter *after deployment* must be considered.
- The addition of additives (fibered coils or hydrogel) reduces the thrombosis delay: the recapture of long coils then increases the risk of an occlusion of the catheter if the time for the coil detachment is prolonged.
- If the internal microcatheter lumen is too wide, coil deployment can be disturbed:

  - With the pushed micro-coils, the diameter should not exceed 0.027, to the guide wire gliding beside the coil instead of pushing it. If the catheterization is stable and the risk of migration controlled, the coil can be flushed by a screw syringe.
  - With mechanically controlled deployment micro-coils, the diameter should not exceed 0.027, to prevent the disunion of the tenon-mortise device in the catheter.

- Sometimes the mechanically controlled deployment coils remain attached to their deployment guide, even outside the microcatheter: rotation of the guide wire can facilitate their detachment. If a resistance is encountered, it is recommended to rotate and not to pull the guide wire (which could stretch and ultimately break it).
- The deployment guide wire can sometimes cling to the pack of coils: rotating the guide wire allows its careful detachment and withdrawal while avoiding coil displacement.
- Recanalization through the coils is a classical phenomenon: to prevent it, the initial pack must be very dense, even if an occlusion is very quickly obtained during the procedure.

1.1.4.2 Plugs

Initially used for the closure of atrial septum or ductus arteriosus, Amplatzer® vascular plugs (AVP) (AGA medical) are also able to occlude large-size vessels as well as high-flow arteriovenous communications: by using only one device, the risks related to its deployment are reduced as well as the costs of the procedure. They constitute an obstacle in the blood flow which gradually brings about the thrombosis of the plug and the exclusion of the downstream vessel.

(a) Technical Characteristics

The plugs are made of an expansible nitinol lattice work which is screwed to the guide wire's extremity.

Four generations of AVP have been available in Europe; the first 3 versions required guiding catheters of large calibers:

- AVP 1: composed of a cylindrical piece, available in 4–16 mm by 2 mm levels, requires internal lumen from 4 to 6 Fr.
- AVP 2: available up to 22 mm, is composed of two disks (proximal and distal) placed on one side and the other of the central cylinder; it contains three times more nitinol mesh (2–3 layers): its occlusion capacity is higher, allowing faster thrombosis times and occlusion of larger size vessels. But it requires a longer vessel segment to be implanted. Four to seven French microcatheter introducer sheaths are required.
- AVP 3: is also composed of two disks and a cylinder, but its form is elliptic. It is intended for complex morphology vessels; internal lumen required is 4–7 Fr. Compared to AVP 1, AVPs 2 and 3 authorize a faster occlusion, with an extension for larger vessels (AVP 2) or sinuous ones (AVP 3).
- AVP 4: of biconical shape, available from 4 to 8 mm, it is also composed of two layers of nitinol, permitting an occlusion capacity close to that of the AVP 2. Its advantage is its possible delivery from a 4–5 Fr catheter with a 0.038 in. non-hydrophilic internal lumen (Imager II 5 Fr, Boston Scientific; Tempo and Tempo Aqua 4 Fr, Cordis; Impress 5 Fr, Merit), allowing it to be used in small vessels.

(b) Instructions for Use

The diameter of the device is chosen depending on the vessel sizing, keeping in account an oversizing greater than with coils: 30–50 % for the arteries and 50 % for the veins.

For the AVPs 1 and 2, the deployment is generally carried out via a guiding catheter which will be led just beyond the landing zone. The "pullback" technique is used for the deployment: the catheter is withdrawn on the guide wire, which is maintained still. A control injection using the lateral path of the guiding catheter confirms the good positioning of the AVP.

With the AVP 4, the pullback procedure is produced after positioning the diagnostic catheter (0.038) just a little beyond the target.

The release of the plug is achieved by unscrewing the guide (1/4 of a turn anticlockwise). An occlusion is obtained after a variable time, seldom less than 5–7 min in medium-sized vessels.

Table 1.7 Recommended internal lumen according to the diameter of the AVP (in mm)

	Delivery catheter: internal diameter			
	4 Fr	5 Fr	6 Fr	7 Fr
AVP I	4–8 mm	10–12 mm	14–16 mm	
AVP II	3–8 mm	10–12 mm	14–16 mm	18–22 mm[a]
AVP III	/	4–8 mm	/	14–16 mm
	Diagnostic catheter: external diameter			
AVP IV	4–8 mm	4 Fr	Tempo® and Tempo Aqua® (Cordis)	
		5 Fr	Imager II® (Boston Scientific)	
			Impress® (Merit)	

[a]Out of recommendation, plugs of 18 and 20 mm have been delivered by a 6F Destination (Terumo) introducer sheath

The occlusion does not only rely upon a mechanical obstruction of the device: it requires a thrombosis of the nitinol cage. For larger devices, or when confronted with moderate coagulation disorder, a Gelfoam injection can accelerate the occlusion process. The plug can also be used like a support in order to implant complementary coils.

In fact, the AVP 3 is very rarely used to treat vascular diseases: its main indications are paravalvular leaks (Table 1.7).

Tips and Tricks

- For a harmonious release, withdraw the catheter on the guide wire instead of pushing the guide wire into the catheter.
- The post-procedure control injection must take place 10 mn after the delivery, as the thrombosis is slowly progressive.
- Anticoagulants/antiplatelets: no particular recommendation.

Pitfalls

- In 2011, the AVP 3 was not refunded by health insurance in France, and the AVPs 3 and 4 were not available in the USA.
- The lateral way of the introducer of the AVPs 2 and 4 may only be used for rinsing the device: they do not allow any opacification; with the AVP 4, it is possible to carry out an injection via a guiding catheter.
- In the event of severe hemostasis disorders, the occlusion can be significantly slowed down.
- The heavily calcified landing zones can prevent a correct apposition of the plug on the vascular wall, contributing to persistent leaks.
- Compared to the AVP 1, the AVPs 2 and 4 require a longer landing zone: this length must be clearly measured before the implantation, because the length of the device in the sheath does not represent its final length. It is sometimes difficult to clearly assess the shortening for the biggest AVP, and the "jump" phenomenon at the time of the deployment is even more important. The analysis of the landing zone before and during the deployment is mandatory.

1.1.5 Thrombin

Initially, thrombin was used in local application so as to accelerate hemostasis during surgical interventions or to reduce the occurrence of hematoma among patients treated with anticoagulants (portacath or pacemaker). Thrombin has also been used to exclude iatrogenic femoral false aneurysm complicating catheterization.

(a) Technical Characteristics

Thrombin may be of human origin or derived from bovine prothrombin (D-Stat® Flowable Hemostat, Vascular Solutions). It induces an acceleration of platelet aggregation. Once activated, it authorizes the conversion of fibrinogen into fibrin, which initiates the formation of a platelet plug. Its action is not inhibited in vitro by heparin.

Hypersensibility reactions have been reported. The bovine thrombin injection may induce antibodies with a crossed action on the factor V and which can lead to its deficit; these injections must thus be limited.

The intravascular injection is contraindicated, exposing the patient to the risk of disseminated coagulation disorders.

Thrombin is used via direct percutaneous injection in order to accelerate the thrombosis of puncture site to treat false aneurysms. It is also interesting in case of endoleaks after stent grafting, via percutaneous intra-saccular and extra-prosthetic injection.

(b) Instructions for Use

The thrombin powder is reconstituted by softly mixing it with the diluent (calcium chloride). A collagen solution is often associated so as to encourage the formation of a matrix support which assists in the platelet aggregation. But this association limits the echogenicity of the solution, making the echo-guided procedures more difficult.

Tips and Tricks

- The medical assessment before the percutaneous exclusion must be meticulous: in case of a femoral false aneurysm including a clinical workup but also an ultrasound exploration depicting precisely its neck and helping in the differential diagnosis with arteriovenous fistula which would contraindicate the injection; in case of endoleaks around a stent graft: CT.
- To limit the embolic risks in case of unfavorable neck, some authors have proposed to inflate an intra-arterial balloon occluding the neck, prior to percutaneous injection which is thus secured.

Pitfalls

- Coagulation occurs suddenly but after a variable time; the injection must thus be progressive and sequential.

1.2 Catheterization Devices

1.2.1 Introducer Sheaths and Catheters

In spite of the improvement of the introducer sheaths profile and the development of the microcatheters, it is sometimes necessary to stabilize the approach by using a guiding catheter or a long introducer sheath, which contributes to a better support for selective catheterization and authorize opacifications via a lateral way. The choice of the material will be made according to the internal lumen, the length, the shape, and the needed rigidity. The crossing of the aortoiliac bifurcation presenting an acute angle can require to use an "armed" introducer sheath so as to limit the risk of bending, even more so for limited calibers. In general, these devices must be purged via their lateral path or by a Y valve, in order to limit the risk of thrombosis of the dead volume.

The external diameter is expressed in French (Fr) (1 Fr = 0.33 mm) and the internal diameter in inches (0.1″=2.5 mm). Depending on the coating, differences in internal diameter might exist while external diameter is equivalent.

The majority of the embolizations can be carried out using 4 or 5 Fr introducer sheaths.

1.2.2 Selective Catheters

The initial catheterization generally requires a selective catheter, chosen for its shape, after having checked internal lumen and length compatibilities. Some catheters are intended for a specific application (Yashiro®, Terumo, for the complex celiac trunk; Spermatic®, Merit, for the spermatic veins via a femoral access; etc.); others are of more universal use (Cobra C2, Terumo; Mikaelsson®, Merit).

Depending upon the occlusion agent, the catheterization will be more or less selective and possibly prolonged by the use of a microcatheter. The hydrophilic catheters, often more flexible, allow more distal catheterization but are less stable.

In Table 1.8, examples of the catheters that are frequently used in our group depending on the arteries are given. But great variations are possible from one operator to another.

1.2.3 Microcatheters

Microcatheters permit an optimized access to some targets and facilitate the realization of supra-selective or flow-guided embolizations.

Table 1.8 Catheter daily used in our group

Vessels	First intention	Second line
Pulmonary	Pigtail	
Bronchial A	Mikaelsson	Bronchial
Celiac trunk	Mikaelsson	Cobra/Yashiro
Superior mesenteric A	Cobra C2	Mikaelsson
Renal A	Cobra C2	Mikaelsson, DRC
Inferior mesenteric A	Mikaelsson (4 Fr)	Simmons/Cobra
Internal iliac A: crossover	Cobra C2	
Internal iliac A: ipsilateral cath	Simmons	
Epigastric A: ipsilateral cath	Bolia	
Epigastric A: contralateral cath	Mikaelsson (4 Fr)	

The choice of the catheter depends on its internal diameter, length, flexibility, coating (hydrophilic or stiff), and its compatibility with the occlusion agent used (glue, chemotherapy, DMSO and Onyx®, etc.). For most of the catheters available, the caliber is regularly decreasing from the baseplate to the distal end, in order to obtain a compromise between the push and distal flexibility. A distal radiopaque marker is useful to control the position of the catheter and that of the delivered agent. The flexible distal end can generally be pre-shaped. More rigid catheters are available: 45°, 90°, or double curve (Maestro®, Medical Merit). Some catheters have a distal end which can break off (Apollo®, eV3; Sonic®, Balt) should catheter entrapment occur during embolization with glue. Initial manipulations are limited with microcatheters preloaded with their guide wires (Progreat Ω®, Terumo; Renegade HiFlow®, Boston Scientific).

1.2.4 Guide Wires

The choice of the guide wires depends firstly on the diameter (from 0.014 to 0.038 in.) and the length (from 150 to 300 cm), which must be adapted to the materials and to the target. On one hand, *catheterization guide wires* are used to facilitate catheterization of tortuous vessels; generally hydrophilic, their distal end is pre-shaped or adjustable (45°, 90°, double curve), and on the other hand, *exchange guide wires* are used to change catheters; they are more rigid, and their length must allow the exchange of the material and must therefore have a length which is at least equal to two times the length of the exchanged catheter.

Various coatings improve the distal sliding (hydrophilic coating) and the proximal push (PTFE coating), whereas the central body (central hypotube) improves movement transmission at the distal end and strengthens the support and the resistance to bending. Visibility of the distal end may be improved by associating a gold spiral or by incorporating tungsten salts.

1.3 Closure Devices

Arterial closure devices provide a correct hemostasis at the puncture site and decrease the duration of bed rest and the hospitalization stay [27]. Their use must be well founded as there is no evidence of a significant reduction of post-catheterization complications when compared to manual compression, particularly for introducer sheaths lower or equal to 5 Fr: 5 % hematoma, 4 % persistence of bleeding at puncture site, 0.3 % local arterial complication, and 0.6 % requiring surgery in the meta-analysis of Biancari based on 7,538 patients [27]; marginal reduction of the complication rate in the meta-analysis of Das [28], which excluded cardiac catheterizations, coronary angiographies, non-femoral accesses, and introducer sheaths of more than 8 F; and the complication rates among the non-comparative series (3,662 patients) of Das's review varied from 3.1 to 11.4 %. However, these closure devices can be of a great help, even with limited introduction diameters, in case of severe coagulopathy or in polytraumatized patients when a compression bandage is difficult to implement.

Their implantation requires an angiographic series centered on the puncture site, so as to exclude any anatomical contraindication (insufficient caliber, inadequate entrance site, wall calcification, etc.).

Various principles are used (suture, clip, collagen, procoagulant agent, etc.), letting or not letting in place endovascular material.

According to the manufacturer's instructions, closure devices can be used to close accesses up to 10 Fr, but complementary techniques have been described to

Table 1.9 Characteristics of the arterial closure devices

	Mechanism		Arteriotomy caliber	
	Intra-arterial	Extra-arterial	Theoretical	Described
Angioseal® St Medical Jude	Resorbable anchor	Collagen	10 Fr	8 Fr
Cardiva Catalyst® Cardiva Medical [29]	Protamin sulfate[a] Disk coated[b]	/	7 Fr	
Exoseal® Cordis	/	Plug PGA[c]	7 Fr	
Fish® Morris Innovative	Balloon[b]	Collagen porcine derivatives	7 Fr	
Mynx® AccessClosure	Balloon[b]	Hydrogel	7 Fr	
Perclose® Abbott Vascular	Sutures		10 Fr	24 Fr
Starclose® Abbott Vascular	Nitinol clip		6 Fr	8 Fr

[a]20–120 s of application before a 5 mn manual compression
[b]The device has been withdrawn
[c]Polyglycolic acid (PGA) (non-collagen absorbable in 60–90 days)

extend this to higher sizes: by using the double-guided technique as described by Azmoon, an 8 Fr Angioseal® enables the closure of a 10 Fr access; by using the "preclose" technique, accesses up to 24 Fr were closed by Prostar® after aortic endoprosthesis (Table 1.9).

References

1. Rosch J, Dotter CT, Brown MJ. Selective arterial embolization. A new method for control of acute gastrointestinal bleeding. Radiology. 1972;102(2):303–6.
2. Laurent A. Microspheres and nonspherical particles for embolization. Tech Vasc Interv Radiol. 2007;10(4):248–56.
3. Stampfl S, et al. Inflammation and recanalization of four different spherical embolization agents in the porcine kidney model. J Vasc Interv Radiol. 2008;19(4):577–86.
4. Siskin GP, et al. Pathologic evaluation of a spherical polyvinyl alcohol embolic agent in a porcine renal model. J Vasc Interv Radiol. 2003;14(1):89–98.
5. Vidal V, et al. Effectiveness of endovascular embolization with a collagen-based embolic agent (Marsembol) in an animal model. J Vasc Interv Radiol. 2010;21(9):1419–23.
6. Levrier O, et al. Efficacy and low vascular toxicity of embolization with radical versus anionic polymerization of n-butyl-2-cyanoacrylate (NBCA). An experimental study in the swine. J Neuroradiol. 2003;30(2):95–102.
7. Heye S, Maleux G, Wilms G. Pain experience during internal spermatic vein embolization for varicocele: comparison of two cyanoacrylate glues. Eur Radiol. 2006;16(1):132–6.
8. Cromwell LD, Kerber CW. Modification of cyanoacrylate for therapeutic embolization: preliminary experience. AJR Am J Roentgenol. 1979;132(5):799–801.
9. Widlus DM, et al. In vivo evaluation of iophendylate-cyanoacrylate mixtures. Radiology. 1992;185(1):269–73.
10. Mathis JM, et al. Hydrophilic coatings diminish adhesion of glue to catheter: an in vitro simulation of NBCA embolization. AJNR Am J Neuroradiol. 1997;18(6):1087–91.
11. Lieber BB, et al. Acute and chronic swine rete arteriovenous malformation models: effect of ethiodol and glacial acetic acid on penetration, dispersion, and injection force of N-butyl 2-cyanoacrylate. AJNR Am J Neuroradiol. 2005;26(7):1707–14.
12. Rossi G, et al. Selective embolization with N-butyl cyanoacrylate for metastatic bone disease. J Vasc Interv Radiol. 2011;22(4):462–70.
13. Duymus M, et al. Easy retrieval of escaping Onyx fragment with percutaneous manual aspiration. Cardiovasc Intervent Radiol. 2011;34(3):661–3.
14. Michael SG, et al. Revascularization of Onyx induced intra-operative occlusion of vertebrobasilar artery using the Merci device. Neurocrit Care. 2010;12(2):269–71.
15. Schirmer CM, Zerris V, Malek AM. Electrocautery-induced ignition of spark showers and self-sustained combustion of onyx ethylene-vinyl alcohol copolymer. Neurosurgery. 2006; 59(4 Suppl 2):ONS413–8.
16. Mitchell SE, Shah AM, Schwengel D. Pulmonary artery pressure changes during ethanol embolization procedures to treat vascular malformations: can cardiovascular collapse be predicted? J Vasc Interv Radiol. 2006;17(2 Pt 1):253–62.
17. Sidi A, et al. Treatment of ethanol-induced acute pulmonary hypertension and right ventricular dysfunction in pigs, by sildenafil analogue (UK343-664) or nitroglycerin. Ann Card Anaesth. 2008;11(2):97–104.
18. Griffin DJ, et al. Chemical ablation of the canine kidney using sodium tetradecyl sulfate (Sotradecol). A histopathologic study. Invest Radiol. 1986;21(3):217–20.
19. Mac Gowan WA, et al. The local effects of intra-arterial injections of sodium tetradecyl sulphate (S.T.D) 3 per cent. An experimental study. Br J Surg. 1972;59(2):101–4.

20. Duffy DM. Sclerosants: a comparative review. Dermatol Surg. 2010;36 Suppl 2:1010–25.
21. Tan KT, et al. Percutaneous sodium tetradecyl sulfate sclerotherapy for peripheral venous vascular malformations: a single-center experience. J Vasc Interv Radiol. 2007;18(3):343–51.
22. Reiner E, et al. Initial experience with 3% sodium tetradecyl sulfate foam and fibered coils for management of adolescent varicocele. J Vasc Interv Radiol. 2008;19(2 Pt 1):207–10.
23. Wollmann JC. The history of sclerosing foams. Dermatol Surg. 2004;30(5):694–703. discussion 703.
24. Tessari L, Cavezzi A, Frullini A. Preliminary experience with a new sclerosing foam in the treatment of varicose veins. Dermatol Surg. 2001;27(1):58–60.
25. Chung SH, et al. Foam sclerotherapy using polidocanol (Aethoxysklerol) for preoperative portal vein embolization in 16 patients. Cardiovasc Intervent Radiol. 2011;34(6):1236–43.
26. Moret J, et al. Reconstruction technic in the treatment of wide-neck intracranial aneurysms. Long-term angiographic and clinical results. Apropos of 56 cases. J Neuroradiol. 1997;24(1):30–44.
27. Biancari F, et al. Meta-analysis of randomized trials on the efficacy of vascular closure devices after diagnostic angiography and angioplasty. Am Heart J. 2010;159(4):518–31.
28. Das R, Ahmed K, Athanasiou T, Morgan RA, Belli AM. Arterial closure devices versus manual compression for femoral haemostasis in interventional radiological procedures : a systematic review and meta-analysis. Cardiovasc Intervent Radiol. 2011;34:723–38.
29. Doyle BJ, et al. Initial experience with the Cardiva Boomerang vascular closure device in diagnostic catheterization. Catheter Cardiovasc Interv. 2007;69(2):203–8.

Suggested Reading

Abada H, Golzarian J. Gelatine sponge particles: handling characteristics for endovascular use. Tech Vasc Interv Radiol. 2007;10:257–60.

Das R, Ahmed K, Athanasiou T, Morgan RA, Belli AM. Arterial closure devices versus manual compression for femoral haemostasis in interventional radiological procedures : a systematic review and meta-analysis. Cardiovasc Intervent Radiol. 2011;34:723–38.

Duffy DM. Sclerosants: a comparative review. Dermatol Surg. 2010;36 Suppl 2:1010–25.

Laurent A. Microspheres and nonspherical particles for embolization. Tech Vasc Interv Radiol. 2007;10(4):248–56.

Pollak J, White R. The use of cyanoacrylate adhesives in peripheral embolization. J Vasc Interv Radiol. 2001;12(8):907–13.

Chapter 2
Vascular Occlusions and Parenchymal Embolizations: Principles

Pascal Chabrot, Isabelle Brazzalotto, and Louis Boyer

Several occlusion agents were presented in the Chap. 1. We shall specify now the principles common to all the procedures: initial assessment and indications, choice of the occlusion agents, sedation and anesthesia, antibiotic prophylaxis, and follow-up.

2.1 Initial Assessment: Prerequisite and Indication of the Procedure

Prior to an embolization procedure, the initial morphological assessment will detail the following:

- *The Lesion*
  - The origin of the bleeding is sometimes depicted by CT, appearing as a blush (extravasation of ICM on the arterial phase and increasing on the late phase). In other situations, a hypertrophy of the afferent vessels or a parenchymal devascularization can be observed.
  - The angio-architecture.
  - The afferents vessels: anastomotic network or terminal circulation.
  - Accessibility.
- *The Extension of the Underlying Clinical Condition*
  - In a traumatic setting, associated lesions are frequent, sometimes requiring the embolization of several sites.
  - In atheromatous disease, the extent of the lesions must be specified.

P. Chabrot, MD, PhD (✉) • L. Boyer, MD, PhD
Department of Radiology, University Hospital of Clermont-Ferrand, Clermont-Ferrand, France
e-mail: pchabrot@chu-clermontferrand.fr; lboyer@chu-clermontferrand.fr

I. Brazzalotto, MD
Department of Anesthesia, University Hospital of Clermont-Ferrand, Clermont-Ferrand, France

P. Chabrot, L. Boyer (eds.), *Embolization*,
DOI 10.1007/978-1-4471-5182-1_2, © Springer-Verlag London 2014

Table 2.1 Vascular lesions as depicted by multiphase angioCT

	Without injection	Arterial phase	Parenchymal phase
Extravasation blush	Hematic hyperdensity	Extravascular contrast	Extension of the leak with persisting hyperattenuation
False aneurysm	Isodense	Contrast-enhanced outpouching without a delimiting wall	Persistent enhancement of the well-circumscribed outpouching
Arteriovenous fistula	Isodense	Early venous opacification	Washout

- In oncologic indications, the number, the volume, and the topography of metastases can have a direct impact on some procedures. Palliative embolizations can be carried out as a symptomatic treatment, whatever the tumor stage is.
- Assessment of the underlying systemic disease must be carried out before symptomatic treatment of their vascular localizations.
- In case of malformative diseases, constitutional abnormalities are usually associated and must be looked for.

• *The General Assessment*
A part from emergency situations, a global patient assessment must be carried out to identify an infectious state, a renal dysfunction, coagulation disorders, and an allergic or immunodeficient background. Programmed parenchymal embolization is generally contraindicated in case of an active infection, even more so should a bacteremia exist.

• *The Conditions for Endovascular Navigation*
The choice of the materials (puncture needle, introducer sheath, catheters and micro-catheters, occlusion agents) is conditioned by the puncture site, the access path which must be direct as possible and foreseeable catheterization difficulties.

The morphological evaluation is generally carried out with CT, ideally including at least three helical acquisitions (without, then with ICM injection at the arterial, venous, and even sometimes late phases). A blush or an extravasation is depicted as an arterial enhancement that extends on the venous phase. In case of a false aneurysm, the arterial enhancement remains circumscribed even in the later phase. In case of an arteriovenous fistula, an early washout is observed (Table 2.1). In the specific case of arteriovenous anomalies, assessment and follow-up are carried out with Doppler ultrasound and MRI.

During arteriography, initial global injections allow the cartography of the afferent supplying vessels. Distal selective injections depict a low-flow extravasation or unmask one hidden by a vasospasm. High frame rate (6 frames/s) might be necessary so as not to ignore transient bleeding or to evaluate more precisely the hemodynamic features of arteriovenous communications.

• If the morphological assessment is the radiologist's responsibility, the embolization indication, however, as a rule, must be decided by a multidisciplinary team among which anesthesiologists, medical specialists, surgeons, oncologists, and radiotherapists, within a formalized framework (multidisciplinary meetings) or in an emergency setting. This multi-team decision as well as the other therapeutic alternatives should be reported in the medical file.

2.2 Embolization Techniques

The embolization target (truncal or parenchymal), the vessel size and the flow rate, the vascularization type (end artery or anastomotic), the catheterization pathway, and the occlusion type (permanent or temporary) are the parameters which condition the choice of the access (puncture site, catheters) and the choice of the occlusion agent. Three questions must thus be answered:

1. What type of occlusion: a temporary or a permanent one?
2. What is the target of occlusion: vascular truncal (vessels depicted on angiography) or distal parenchymal (vessels undepicted by angiography)
3. How much parenchyma should be preserved? (The more distal is the embolization, the greater the risk of ischemia.)

When choosing an occlusion agent, it is necessary to put into the balance its safety with its effectiveness. The cost is also an essential parameter.

2.2.1 *Truncal Embolizations*

They are carried out to divert blood flow or to treat a vascular lesion (aneurysm, vascular injury, etc.). No matter what the initial clinical condition is, two situations are distinguished:

- Preservation of the parent vessel patency (aneurysm, arterial rupture, etc.).
- Vascular occlusion is the possibility of occluding the concerned segment (Table 2.2).

In the first case, in order to preserve the parent vessel, according to the target size and its accessibility, a covered endoprosthesis can be used (endobypass), or a filling of the vascular cavity can be carried out (aneurysmal sac or false aneurysm).

Larguable balloons are no longer used and have been replaced by coils which can be deployed safely by using remodeling techniques should the collar be difficult to treat; the collar can thus be protected by a balloon or a stent during the coil delivery. In addition, in high-flow vessels, a balloon can be inflated upstream, thus reducing the flow and securing coils release. More recently, the use of Onyx® has been reported to treat visceral aneurysms.

In the second case, to exclude a vascular segment, a distal and proximal "sandwich" occlusion is the ideal solution in order to prevent a reinjection by anastomotic networks. When it is not possible to cross the lesion, liquid agents (glues, Onyx®) can in some cases be used, after assessing the risks of out of target embolization. In

Table 2.2 Truncal embolization strategy

Vessel to be preserved: access?	Vessel to be excluded: caliber, flow, downstream parenchyma?
Covered stent	Gelfoam
	Coils
Packing	Plugs
	Liquid agents

case of end arteries, a proximal embolization may be carried out. Occlusion agents are selected according to the caliber of the vessel and the type of embolization (permanent or temporary):

- Absorbable gelatin sponge (Gelfoam) is very frequently used in a trauma context, allowing a temporary hemostasis, even in vessels of medium size. Vessel recanalization is generally observed 3 weeks post-procedure.
- Coils ensure a mechanical occlusion. Their profile allows both distal and proximal occlusions.
- AV plugs have considerably simplified the occlusion procedure for large vessels, with a controlled release, even in case of high flow.

A temporary upstream inflation of an occlusion balloon, before the delivery of embolic agent, can simplify the procedure by reducing the flow. In the event of arteriovenous communication, a balloon brought through the venous system can also be inflated downstream.

2.2.2 *Parenchymal Embolizations*

The goal here is to devascularize a tumor, a traumatic or hyperfunctioning tissue, in order to obtain hemostasis, ischemia, or tumor necrosis, to divert blood flow or to deliver cytotoxic drugs or radioactive particles. But whatever the aim, the main principles of embolization are common:

- Preliminary assessment of the blood flow, afferent vessels and collaterals, and careful iterative reevaluations during embolization.
- Choice of the occlusion agent accordingly to the need or not to preserve downstream tissues.
- Additional proximal occlusion should be carried out only in specific cases (Table 2.3).

2.2.2.1 Evaluation of Flow, Afferent Vessels, and Collateral Networks

A comprehensive assessment of the afferent vessels is a prerequisite: non-bronchial systemic arteries in case of hemoptysis, diaphragmatic or parietal arteries and hepatic tumors, polar renal arteries for kidney trauma, etc.

Table 2.3 Parenchymal embolization strategy

Initial assessment	Material	Associated measures
Afferent vessels	Gelfoam	Non-systematic proximal embolization
Collaterals	Particles	Protection of the collateral network
Flow	Glues	Analgesics and/or anti-inflammatory drugs
Access	Alcohol	

During embolization, this vascular reevaluation should be carried out whenever there is the slightest doubt, as vascular redistributions can unexpectedly occur.

In some indications (radio-embolization, chemoembolization, etc.), it can be necessary to carry out a truncal occlusion of the collateral network (i.e., gastroduodenal artery) to preserve the downstream parenchyma and to avoid off-target embolization.

When using particles or cyanoacrylate, the flow is a decisive factor in the progression of the occlusion agent. It will sometimes be necessary to withdraw the diagnostic catheter or the carrier catheter/sheath, to carry out a free-flow injection via a micro-catheter.

2.2.2.2 Choice of a Distal Embolization Agent

Particles, biological glues, sclerosing agents, and alcohol can be used. Particles are preferred when one wishes to avoid a complete downstream necrosis (uterine fibroids, hemoptysis, GI tract hemorrhages, etc.). Their diameter must be adapted to the target. Because of the intra-tumor shunts, particle diameters inferior to 300 μm are rarely used. The risk of parenchymal ischemia is inversely proportional to the size of the particles. Apart from tumor embolization, the size of the particles is usually gradually increased, in order to complete with a proximal exclusion.

Glues, alcohol, and sclerosing agents can be used to obtain tissue necrosis (superselective tumor embolization, etc.). Pure alcohol exposes to the risk of necrosis of adjacent and distal tissues. Systemic diffusion is its main pitfall, which makes it difficult to administer precisely.

Glues ensure exclusion of some distal targets, but their use requires considerable skill. Their association with Lipiodol enables the modulation of their viscosity.

2.2.2.3 Associated Proximal Occlusions

In inflammatory diseases or tumors, the reoccurrence of hemorrhages is possible: a prior proximal occlusion precludes other embolizations. So the proximal occlusion is in theory performed in specific situations (preoperative embolization, hemostasis embolization in traumatic context, etc.).

2.3 Adjuvant Medications

Vasoactive drugs, pro-thrombotic agents, and antiangiogenic agents have been proposed to complete and/or extend the duration of vascular occlusions.

In practice, their use remains limited. In specific chapters of this book, we shall describe the elective indications for each targeted zone (GI tract and postpartum hemorrhages, etc.).

Similarly we shall discuss the complementary prescription of hormones, growth factor inhibitors, and antimitotic agents.

Anti-inflammatory drugs will be detailed in the following paragraph (sedation).

2.4 Anesthesia and Sedation

If most of the simple procedures can be carried out under local anesthesia or conscious sedation, the use of major sedation or of general anesthesia is sometimes necessary. The collaboration with anesthesiologists is particularly helpful for the management of vulnerable patients with comorbidities: from our point of view, this collaboration is mandatory. Patient management is determined by initial clinical status, foreseeable pain, procedure duration, and required patient positioning. Ideally the clinical evaluation carried out during a pre-procedure consultation is standardized according to the scale of the American Society of Anesthesiology (Table 2.4).

2.4.1 Local Anesthesia

Local anesthesia is generally obtained with an injection of 5–20 ml of local anesthetics with an amide bond in its molecular structure (lidocaine (Xylocaine®), mepivacaine (Carbocaine®)). The onset of action is obtained rapidly with lidocaine (2–5 min) and lasts from 60 to 90 min. The association of adrenalin decreases the cutaneous absorption by a vasoconstriction effect. In adults, the maximum injection dose by local infiltration is lidocaine (200 mg), and lidocaine + adrenalin (500 mg). In 30 months and older children, the maximum amount must not exceed 5 mg/kg. The intravascular injection can lead to an overdose: seizures, respiratory depression, and cardiac arrhythmias. Atropine (0.02 mg/kg) can be used to treat bradycardia, and benzodiazepines (diazepam (Valium®) 0.1–0.2 mg/kg, midazolam (Hypnovel®) 0.05–0.1 mg/kg) to treat seizures (Table 2.5).

Allergies to local anesthetics with an amide bond are very rare. Should an anaphylactic reaction occur, then patient must undergo an allergologic work-up. It can be prevented with slow and fractionated injections.

Table 2.4 ASA physical status classification system

I: A normal healthy patient
II: A patient with mild systemic disease without functional limitation
III: A patient with systemic disease and functional limitation
IV: A patient with severe systemic disease that is a constant threat to life
V: A moribund patient who is not expected to survive without the operation
VI: A declared brain-dead patient whose organs are being removed for donor purposes

Table 2.5 Dosage and delay times of common local anesthetics

	Concentration (%:mg)	D max (mg)	Time delay (min)	Duration (min)
Lidocaine	0.5 %: 100 mg	200	2–5	60–90
Lidocaine + adrenalin	1 %: 200 mg	500	2–5	60–90
Carbocaine	2 %: 400 mg	200	10–30	60–90

2.4.2 Locoregional Anesthesia

Plexus blocks are proven to be useful in interventional radiology, especially when treating hemodialysis fistulas. They are not usually indicated for embolizations.

2.4.3 Sedation and General Anesthesia

Sedation is obtained by intravenous administration of association of morphinic, analgesics, and sedatives causing amnesia:

- Diazanalgesia: morphine (i.e., sufentanil (Sufenta®)) and benzodiazepine (i.e., midazolam (Hypnovel®))
- Neuroleptanalgesia: morphine (i.e., sufentanil (Sufenta®)) and a neuroleptic (i.e., droperidol (Droleptan®)) (Table 2.6)

A constant monitoring of the vital parameters is necessary (and particularly respiratory rate, oxygen saturation, capnography), due to the risk of respiratory depression.

These patients are unable to understand the explanations given immediately after the procedure: therefore, recommendations must be given to them a few hours later.

The intravenous general anesthesia associates a hypnotic (propofol, etomidate) and a morphinic (sufentanil), plus sometimes a benzodiazepine and, if it is necessary, a curare. It can be complemented with anesthetic gases (nitrogen protoxide, halogenated volatile anesthetics). It requires monitoring and a permanent control of the hemodynamic parameters and of either the mechanical or the spontaneous ventilation.

Sufentanil (Sufenta®) is a synthetic morphine derivative, pure agonist, with an analgesic action 1,000 times more powerful than morphine and ten times more than fentanyl. The dose is 0.1–2 μg/kg at the induction depending on associated drugs. Its onset of action delay is 20 s, and the duration of action varies from 20 to 30 min

Table 2.6 Dosage and kinetics of diazanalgesia and its antagonists

	Class	Dosage	Delay time duration	Risks
Midazolam (Hypnovel®)	BZD	0.5–3 mg/doses from 0.5 to 1 mg	2–5 min 1–4 h	Respiratory
Flumazenil (Anexate®)	BZD antagonist	0.2 mg by direct IV injections every 60 s (± perfusion: 0.1–0.4 mg/h)		Return sedation
Sufentanil (Sufenta®)	Morphinic	0.1–2 μg/kg	20 s 20–30 min	Bradycardia Respiratory
Naloxone (Narcan®)	Morphinic antagonist	1–2 μg/kg by direct IV injections every 3 min (± perfusion: 10–20 μg/kg/h)	2–5 min 1–4 h	

and can be prolonged in case of an accumulation phenomenon. The adverse effects are those related to morphine, particularly respiratory depression (risk of apnea), bradycardia, nausea, and peri-nasal itching. Its competitive antagonist is the *naloxone* (Narcan®), used to counteract overdoses: 1–2 μg/kg, to be repeated every 3 min by direct IV injection. A 10–20 μg/kg/h infusion might be necessary for the morphinics having prolonged duration effects.

The *midazolam* (Hypnovel®) is a hypnotic, sedative, and anticonvulsive medication, of the benzodiazepines group. Its onset of action delay and half-life are short, respectively, 1–2 min and 1–4 h. To obtain a moderate sedation, 0.5–3 mg is administered in fractions of 0.5–1 mg. The main adverse effect is a respiratory depression. A paradoxical reaction (confusion, agitation) is sometimes observed. Its selective antagonist is *flumazenil* (Anexate®): an injection of 0.2 mg repeated every 60 s, up to a maximum dose of 2 mg. The half-life of flumazenil is shorter than that of benzodiazepines; the risk of sedation wear off thus makes a close monitoring mandatory.

Droperidol (Droleptan®) is an antiemetic and antipsychotic neuroleptic, used as a complement to sedation, with a dose of 0.02–0.03 mg/kg and an onset of action delay of 1.5–3 h; the risk is an extrapyramidal syndrome.

Propofol (Diprivan®) is an intravenous hypnotic anesthetic agent, commonly used as an induction agent (0.5–2.5 mg/kg) and to maintain anesthesia. Its action duration is short: 5–10 min. It causes a dose-dependent reduction of the blood pressure and a respiratory depression.

Etomidate (Hypnomidate®, Lipuro®) is a hypnotic intravenous anesthetic agent. Its onset of action delay is 30 s, with a duration time of 3–10 min. It can give myoclonia and abnormal movements. It is a valuable induction agent for patients who are in a precarious state or hemodynamically unstable (0.2–0.4 mg/kg).

2.4.4 Pain Control

Truncal embolization rarely induces significant post-embolization pain. On the other hand, post-embolization pain of varying intensity is systematically observed with parenchymal embolizations. Its management must be adapted to its intensity (visual analog scale); it can be anticipated in some procedures (uterine fibroid embolization, renal or splenic parenchymal embolizations, etc.), thus facilitating its management.

As soon as induction phase begins, an association of paracetamol (Perfalgan®: 1 g/6 h), nefopam (Acupan®: 120 mg/24 h, preferably in continuous flow), and non-steroid anti-inflammatory drug (Profenid®: 100 mg/8h, in the absence of contraindication) is administered. It is then supplemented as soon as the embolization is performed by a morphine titration (initially a bolus of 2–3 mg then through a patient-controlled analgesia pump (PCA)), sometimes associated with other drugs (droperidol, ketamine, clonidine).

Pain control and follow-up should be continued beyond the angiographic room and requires a collaboration of the in- and outpatient care team. The prescription of analgesics must be reported on the monitoring sheet and transferred with the patient.

2.5 Antibiotic Prophylaxis

These general considerations have been drawn from 2010 official guidelines of the Society of International Radiology (SIR), the Société Française d'Anesthésie et Réanimation (SFAR) to which the Société Française de Radiologie (SFR) considerably contributed. In each chapter of the second part of this book, we will describe the practices that are usually carried out by our team for specific indications.

The morbidity of nosocomial infections and their cost makes the prevention of post-embolization infections crucial. Publication data concerning infectious complications in interventional radiology is rather abundant, but it is mainly retrospective data. There are no randomized trials on antibiotic prophylaxis in intervention radiology, whereas prospective clinical results are available for prophylaxis and surgery. The rationale and the guidelines available in interventional radiology (guidelines of the SIR and the SFAR) are based on the approach of the antibiotic prophylaxis in surgery.

Antibiotic prophylaxis must be discussed during the preoperative consultation. Its administration must begin before the intervention, within 30 min upon arrival in the angio suite, and effective tissue concentrations must be maintained throughout the procedure. The duration of the prescription must be short: for many procedures, a single preoperative injection is to be preferred and prescriptions lasting more than 48 h must be avoided. The choice of antibiotics and their dosing must be carefully adapted to individual factors (e.g., comorbidities, associated medications), local factors (e.g., antibiotic resistance), as well as the evolving innovations.

In 2010, the SIR recommended an antibiotic prophylactic therapy targeting pathogenic germs of the skin before carrying out *embolization of tumors and/or solid organs, including the liver, kidney, and spleen, aiming or at risk of parenchymal infarction, as it may result in a significant necrosis of potentially infected tissues*. The antibiotic prescription should be adapted to the clinical setting, the aim of embolization, the target organ, and the likelihood of additional associated pathogens.

A routine antibiotic prophylaxis is on the other hand controversial for hemostasis vascular or parenchymal bleedings embolizations and in trauma patients.

Literature regarding the use of antibiotic prophylaxis for *chemoembolization* is very limited, and its efficacy has not been proven, even if severe infectious complications can occur. Nevertheless, many operators routinely administer an antibiotic prophylaxis versus the skin flora and for gram-negative enteric organisms. Histories of sphincterotomy, surgery, or biliary duct drainage are risk factors for abscess formation: the risk of post-embolization infection is reduced by associating a bowel preparation the night before and a gram positive, gram negative, and aerobic and anaerobic organisms antibiotic coverage.

In the French guidelines of the SFAR, no antibiotic prophylaxis is recommended before carrying out hepatic chemoembolization.

Even fewer reports exist concerning the infectious complications of radio-embolization.

Uterine Artery Embolizations: The infectious risk is considered as low; skin flora organisms are often the main cause (*Staphylococcus*, *Streptococcus*).

The role of an antibiotic prophylaxis before a uterine embolization has been largely debated. A joint working group associating the Royal Colleges of Radiology and of Obstetrics and Gynecology in the UK does not recommend an antibiotic prophylaxis treatment. The French SFAR recommendations are identical.

Nevertheless pre-procedure administration of 1 g of cefazolin is frequently prescribed.

Even if there is no official consensus, particular attention must be given in case of a history of hydrosalpinx (doxycycline 100 mg, twice per day, 7 days before the procedure) (SIR).

Antibiotic prophylaxis and embolizations and chemo-embolizations: the SIR guidelines

Procedures	Clean; clean-contaminated (bilio-digestive surgery)
Organisms	*Staphylococcus aureus*, *Streptococcus*, Corynebacterium with or without GI flora (in patients: without intact sphincter of Oddi, after bilio-enteric surgery)
Routine antibiotic prophylaxis recommended	*Recommended, if high likelihood of infarction*
1st-choice antibiotic	No consensus
Common antibiotic choices	1 - 3 g of ampicillin/sulbactam IV (*hepatic chemoembolization*) 2 - 1 g cefazolin + 500 mg metronidazole IV (*hepatic chemoembolization*) 3 - 2 g ampicillin IV + and 1,5 mg/kg gentamicin (*hepatic chemoembolization*) 4 - 1 g ceftriax 1 IV (*hepatic chemoembolization or splenic or renal embolizations*) 5 - If penicillin allergic: vancomycin or clindamycin + aminoglycoside
Special consideration	Tazobactam/piperacillin, digestive preparation,in the event of *hepatic chemoembolization with impaired sphincter of Oddi (sphincterotomy, biliary drainage, bilio-enteric anastomosis)*
Level of evidence	4, 7, 8

Antibiotic prophylaxis and uterine artery embolization: SIR guidelines

Procedures	Clean; clean-contaminated
Organisms	*Staphylococcus aureus*, *Staphylococcus epidermidis*, *Streptococcus*, with or without *E. coli*
Routine antibiotic prophylaxis recommended	*Recommended*
1st-choice molecule	No consensus
Common antibiotics choices	1 - 1 g of cefazolin IV 2 - 900 mg of clindamycin IV + gentamicin 1.5 mg/kg 3 - 2 g of ampicillin IV 4 - 1.5–3 g ampicillin/sulbactam IV 5 - If penicillin allergic: vancomycin can be used
Special consideration: *previous hydrosalpynx*	Doxycycline 100 mg, two times per day, 7 days before
Levels of evidence	4, 5, 8
NB: evidence level 4	Historic, non-randomized, cohort, or case–control studies
Level 5	Case series: compiled patients but without control group
Level 7	Extrapolations from existing data collected for other purposes, theoretical analyses
Level 8	Rational conjecture (common sense); common practices accepted before evidence-based guidelines

2.6 Post-procedural Follow-Up

Post-embolization follow-up must be planned and described in the procedure report. Planned imaging controls (CT, MRI, or Doppler ultrasound) are necessary for most of the indications. Compared to coils, plugs have the advantage of generating fewer artifacts on CT, thus facilitating the follow-up. The development of dual-energy CT acquisitions would help in limiting these artifacts.

In the absence of a downstream infarction, parenchymal embolizations frequently induce a moderate inflammatory syndrome which is clinically asymptomatic. Significant post-embolization syndrome however occurs after parenchymal embolizations requiring an appropriate pain management at an early stage (stage II or III) associated with anti-inflammatory drugs (cf., paragraphs 2–3): it will be detailed in the following chapters, for each embolization target.

Suggested Reading

Bratby MJ, Lehmann ED, Bottomley J, et al. Endovascular embolization of visceral artery aneurysms with ethylene-vinyl alcohol (Onyx): a case series. Cardiovasc Intervent Radiol. 2006;29(6):1125–8.

Knape JT, Adriaensen H, van Aken H, et al. Guidelines for sedation and/or analgesia by non-anaesthesiology doctors. Eur J Anaesthesiol. 2007;24(7):563–7.

Loffroy R, Rao P, Ota S, et al. Packing technique for endovascular coil embolisation of peripheral arterial pseudo-aneurysms with preservation of the parent artery: safety, efficacy and outcomes. Eur J Vasc Endovasc Surg. 2010;40(2):209–15.

Martin C coordonnateur. Antibioprophylaxie en radiologie et médecine interventionnelle. In Antibioprophylaxie en chirurgie et médecine interventionnelle (patients adultes). Actualisation 2010, conférence de consensus de la SFAR (avec la collaboration de 14 sociétés savantes, dont la Société Française de Radiologie).

Muller-Wille R, Heiss P, Herold T, et al. Endovascular treatment of acute arterial hemorrhage in trauma patients using ethylene vinyl alcohol copolymer (Onyx). Cardiovasc Intervent Radiol. 2012;35(1):65–75.

Owens CA, Yaghmai B, Aletich V, et al. Coil embolization of a wide-neck splenic artery aneurysm using a remodeling technique. AJR Am J Roentgenol. 2002;179(5):1327–9.

Uchiyama D, Koganemaru M, Abe T, et al. Coil embolization of splenic artery aneurysm with preservation of the parent artery using a neck remodeling technique. J Vasc Interv Radiol. 2007;18(3):447–50.

Venkatesan AM, Kundu S, Sacks D, et al. Practice guideline for adult antibiotic prophylaxis during vascular and interventional radiology procedures: standards of practice for the Society of Interventional Radiology. J Vasc Interv Radiol. 2010;21:1611–30.

Part II
Situations and Strategies

Chapter 3
Hemorrhages of the ENT Area

Arthur Varoquaux, Pierre Cassagneau, Vincent Vidal, Alexis Jacquier, Frédéric Cohen, Cyril Muller, Florian Desmots, Jean-Michel Bartoli, and Guy Moulin

Arterial embolization is the treatment of choice for refractory epistaxes and can be indicated in hemorrhages of the ENT area. When carried out by trained radiologists, it proves to be an efficient method that presents little risk of complications.

Hemorrhages of the ENT area are of different nature and etiology. Their management should be considered according to specific clinical context.

Interventional radiology is not indicated in the treatment of hemorrhages of venous origin. Endovascular or percutaneous embolization treatment of vascular malformations will not be treated in this chapter.

Several types of arterial hemorrhages of the ENT sphere can be distinguished:

- Hemorrhages of nasal origin (epistaxes). They can be idiopathic or symptomatic.
- Other hemorrhages:
  - Hemorrhages due to ENT cancers, pre- or postoperative by hemostasis disorders, or secondary bleeding specifically after a laryngectomy or a tonsillectomy
  - Devascularization of hypervascular tumors (paragangliomas and nasopharyngeal fibromas) by preoperative embolization
  - Carotid rupture, due to a progressive tumor, or post-radiotherapy, or trauma

In some cases, these hemorrhages are cataclysmic and require extreme emergency care. In all cases, close collaboration with the ENT surgery department, the presence of an anesthetist, and at least a sedation are determining factors in the improvement of care and therefore in the success of the embolization. Every patient and/or family is to be given true, clear, and appropriate information.

A. Varoquaux (✉) • P. Cassagneau • V. Vidal • A. Jacquier
F. Cohen • C. Muller • F. Desmots • J.-M. Bartoli • G. Moulin
Department of Radiology,
Assistance Publiqùe - Hôpitaux de Marseille, Marseille, France
e-mail: arthur.varoquaux@ap-hm.fr

P. Chabrot, L. Boyer (eds.), *Embolization*,
DOI 10.1007/978-1-4471-5182-1_3,

3.1 Epistaxes

3.1.1 Background

With a prevalence of around 60 % among the adult population, epistaxis is the most frequent acute pathology in ENT clinical practice. Its natural evolution leads to spontaneous recovery in a majority of cases. For Small [1], only 6 % of epistaxes require medical supervision. However, some epistaxes can be lethal if they are not treated.

Etiologies can be divided into two subgroups: an idiopathic group and a "symptomatic" group, in which the epistaxis is a symptom of an underlying pathology.

More than 70 % of epistaxes are "idiopathic" [2]. Known risk factors are high blood pressure, hypercholesterolemia, smoking, ethylism, NSAIDs (mainly aspirin), and coagulation disorders.

Organic causes of symptomatic epistaxes are traumas, surgery (in particular transsphenoidal surgical approaches [3]), facial tumors, vascular malformations such as hereditary hemorrhagic telangiectasias (Rendu-Osler disease), or rarely carotid-cavernous fistulae [4].

Whatever their cause may be, epistaxes can be serious and life-threatening. As soon as the patient is taken into care, it is necessary to assess the abundance and repetition of blood losses and to perform a general and biological checkup (hemostasis, CBC, blood grouping). In case of serious epistaxis, the patient must be taken into a specialized ENT care unit.

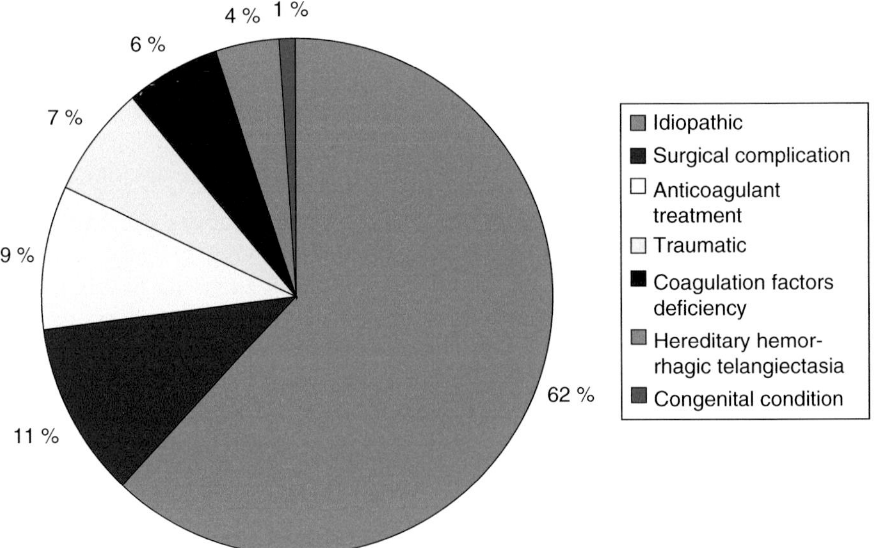

Refractory epistaxes etiologies

3.1.2 *Relevant Radiological Anatomy* (Fig. 3.1)

A perfect knowledge of the branches of the carotid artery is an essential prerequisite. They must be located on conventional angiography after a selective catheterism of the external carotid artery.

The sphenopalatine artery, a branch of the internal maxillary artery, vascularizes the nasal septum and the lateral wall of the nasal fossae. Hence, it is the artery that is the most commonly involved in idiopathic epistaxes.

Some potential anastomoses between the internal and external carotid branches are at risk for an embolization and must be systematically looked for. These are:

- Anterior ethmoidal arteries
- Posterior ethmoidal arteries
- Foramen lacerum arteries
- Pterygoid arteries
- Botallo's foramen arteries
- Foramen rotundum arteries
- Angular arteries (a branch of the facial and ophthalmic artery)
- Transclival branches of the carotid siphon

3.1.3 *Epistaxes Treatment: Techniques and Indications*

3.1.3.1 Initial Epistaxes Treatment Is Local

- Manual compression using two fingers when treating a very anterior bleeding
- Anterior gauze plugging using plugs (Merocel®)
- Endoscopic electrocoagulation using bipolar forceps under local anesthetics
- Anterior gauze plugging using inflatable balloons (e.g., Bivona®, Portex®)

Severe epistaxes are most commonly posterior epistaxis that induce oral cavity and nasal fossa bleeding. They should be treated by anterior and posterior nasal packing using a double-balloon probe. However, packing can be inefficient in a number of cases (25–52 % of cases according to series). In such cases, it is necessary to resort to surgery or to an endovascular treatment.

3.1.3.2 Surgical Treatment of Epistaxes

Surgery can be useful in case of uncontrolled bleeding. Several types of surgery are possible:

Ligation of the external carotid artery by cervicotomy: this technique is abandoned except in exceptional cases and makes any future embolization impossible.

Ligation of the internal maxillary artery: via a vestibular approach; it requires specialized skills and is not suitable for emergency treatment.

Endonasal ligation of the sphenopalatine artery: this technique consists in clipping the sphenopalatine artery at its emergence (sphenopalatine foramen) in the posterior part of the nasal fossa. It is effective in 75–85 % of cases (even more when performed by a highly experienced radiologist). Its limits are deterioration of the mucosa, which makes visualization of the artery difficult, as well as abundant bleeding linked to a hemostasis disorder. It is only used in case of unilateral and idiopathic epistaxes.

Ligation of the ethmoidal arteries: most often, it is performed when embolization fails and control angiography depicts show a revascularization of the nasal cavity via the anterior or posterior ethmoidal artery. Ligation of the anterior ethmoidal artery is more often performed through an internal canthal surgical approach rather than an endonasal approach. Ligation of the posterior ethmoidal artery is performed in the case of a hemorrhagic recurrence despite ligation of the anterior ethmoidal artery.

Generally, severe epistaxes must be treated by using anteroposterior packing. In the case of persistent or life-threatening bleeding, or in an unfavorable etiological context, they will be treated through surgical or endovascular radiologic approach.

3.1.3.3 Endovascular Treatment (Fig. 3.2)

Essential anterior epistaxes only require an embolization treatment if the local and/or surgical treatments fail.

Posterior epistaxes are a good indication of embolization if two posterior packings in 48 h are ineffective and if deglobulinization is important (hemoglobinemia under 8 g/dl).

Embolization technique: femoral approach using a valve introducer, then selective catheterism of the primitive carotid artery (if possible using a carrier catheter), internal and external homolateral to the bleeding (if necessary contralateral if the bleeding side is not identified during the ENT examination), and then microcatheterism (0.021 in.) of the target artery.

The arterial architecture and the bleeding area must be identified on frontal and lateral angiograms. Anastomoses with the arterial territories of the brain and ophthalmic arterial territories must be imperatively identified as well as anastomoses between the sphenopalatine and anterior ethmoidal arteries via turbinal and infraorbital arteries.

Catheterism of cervical arteries (subclavian artery and its branches) usually is not necessary in the case of idiopathic epistaxes. However, it is essential in other causes of ENT hemorrhages, especially postoperative in patients who have had a laryngectomy with blood on the tracheostomy tube.

Hemorrhages of the anterior ethmoidal artery require surgery and should not be treated with an endovascular approach because of the risks of ophthalmic artery microcatheterism.

Ipsilateral embolization of the sphenopalatine artery is sufficient in most cases. It can be associated with an embolization of the homolateral facial artery, which is often anastomosed with the sphenopalatine artery via the infraorbital artery. In the case of bilateral epistaxes, both sphenopalatine and both facial arteries can be embolized.

In some cases, the other branches of the external carotid artery can take over the terminal branch of the sphenopalatine and internal maxillary arteries via counter-current anastomoses. Sometimes they only appear after occlusion of the main truncus and must then be catheterized and occluded.

3.1.3.4 Occlusion Material

Occlusion material can either be microparticles or microcoils or glue.

Nonresorbable microparticles with a caliber higher than 500 μm have an excellent effectiveness. However, they must be avoided in the case of anastomoses between the sphenopalatine and anterior ethmoidal territories, particularly if these two territories take part in the epistaxis. The use of microparticles requires a free-flow injection and fluoroscopic control to avoid any backflow and to locate anastomoses that would appear around the area. These microparticles can be a source of complications during embolization of the facial artery (skin necrosis, pain).

The use of microcoils can be a good alternative with pushable coils or controlled-release coils. Their positioning must be distal within the hemorrhagic area. The main drawback of this technique lies in the fact that it permanently fills the artery and, in the event of a recurrence, occludes one of the possible targets for a re-embolization.

The use of cyanoacrylate glues (Glubran 2® or Histoacryl®) is delicate and must be performed by specifically trained radiologists [5]. This technique has an immediate efficiency and is only used when the condition is life-threatening. Onyx embolization is easier and exposes to less off-target embolizations than cyanoacrylates. It requires a good knowledge of the toxicity and delivery of the product [6].

3.1.4 Epistaxes Embolization: Practical Factsheet

Environment:

Multidisciplinary team in angiography room: ENT surgeon, anesthetist, and interventional radiologist

Indications:

- Posterior epistaxis refractory to a 48-h proper medical treatment
- Severe epistaxis with immediate life-threatening condition

Assessment of the patient's situation:

In all cases

Laboratory tests: PT, APTT, INR, CBC, platelets, and blood grouping

Controlled hemorrhage:

Etiologic investigation and technique assessment of the feasibility: angioscan of the supra-aortic trunks from the aortic arch to the circle of Willis and CT scan of the facial bones

Hemodynamic instability uncontrolled by resuscitation:

Endovascular (embolization) or surgical treatment must be discussed with ENT surgeon and anesthetist.

In the angiography suite:

Informed and reassured patient in supine position with a head rest, sedation, intravenous infusion, and monitoring
An interventional radiologist, an assistant, and a radiology technician
Anesthetist for sedation and general anesthetics if necessary, for monitoring and correction of hemodynamic parameters

On the angiography table:

6F valved introducer. Discuss 35-cm-long introducer according to the morphology of the iliofemoral arterial axis. 6F guide catheter (Envoy®, 100-cm type) on 0.035" hydrophilic guidewire (Terumo® type) and anti-backflow valve.
Microcatheter (minimum length 135 cm) suited for embolization agents (if necessary compatible with Onyx®) with straight or preformed tip (45° or 90°) with two radiopaque markers if controlled-release coils are used. 45° and 90° curved hydrophile microguides. Introducers, catheters, and microcatheters must be rinsed and infused using pressure infusion bags.

On the trolley in the angiography room:

Microcoils corresponding to the microcatheter
Calibrated microparticles (500–700-μm pre-filled Luer-Lock syringe)
Hemostatic and resorbable porcine gelatin (Gelita-Spon® type)
Cyanoacrylates (Histoacryl® or Glubran2® type)
Ethylene vinyl alcohol copolymer (Onyx®), rarely used in emergency

"Common" Procedure

Femoral arterial approach, rinsed and perfused valved introducer, and rinsed and perfused guide catheter:

- Injection in the primitive carotid artery after ipsilateral selective catheterism, with an evaluation of the jugular venous return on late acquisition phases
- Frontal and lateral selective acquisitions after injection of the internal carotid artery (study of the ophthalmic and anterior ethmoidal arteries)
- Frontal and lateral selective acquisitions including nasal fossae after injection of the external carotid artery
- Identification of hemorrhagic site and of dangerous anastomoses: foramen lacerum artery, clival artery, pterygoid artery, Botello's foramen artery, foramen rotundum artery, and ophthalmic artery

Use of a microguide and a microcatheter: the latter is positioned at the origin of the external carotid artery. Hyperselective microcatheterism of the target (by default sphenopalatine artery).

Use of arterial tracing: catheterization of external carotid branches with 0.035 guide should be avoided to prevent spastic phenomena.

In the case of a dangerous anastomosis, place the microcatheter beyond that anastomosis, but always consider the risk of backflow during embolization. If necessary, perform a proximal (truncal) embolization of the dangerous anastomosis with microcoils before using microparticles.

In the case of arterial spasm and to enable free-flow embolization, use an in situ intra-arterial infusion of nitrates (1 mg RISORDAN®), in agreement with the anesthetist.

Systematic post-procedure control angiography is obtained to detect collaterals and takeover of the target. If the facial artery takes over the sphenopalatine artery, the facial artery must be embolized by very distal microspheres or microcoils.

Final control will search for a revascularization of the nasal fossa, notably of the ethmoidal arteries.

Leave the femoral introducer in place as long as hemorrhagic and neurologic control is not clinically confirmed by the ENT team in the angiography room.

3.1.5 Embolization Results

Technical success of embolization is important: 80–88 % [7].

Complications can occur in 8–13 % of cases [7–9]. The most recent studies show better results, probably due to progress in the techniques, in the training of the radiologists, in the material, and in embolization agents (microcoils, microparticles, etc.).

Complications of endovascular treatment of an epistaxis include hemorrhagic recurrences but also reported cases of facial neuralgia, septal perforation, sinusitis, and otitis media. Systemic complications can also occur: post-inhalation hypoxia, hypovolemia, angina, and/or myocardial infarction. Cullen's meta-analysis on 539 patients has made it possible not only to make an inventory of the various complications of endovascular treatment but also to compare its rate of occurrence to that of surgical treatment [10]. Among the complications of arterial embolization, cerebrovascular accidents and occlusion of the central retinal artery [11] are the most serious. The radiologists' experience, the patient's arterial condition, and the embolization agents are likely to play a determining role in its occurrence. Few authors have made a critical analysis of the material and embolization agents used for this indication. Systematic use of microcatheterism contributes to its reduction [12].

In terms of costs of the procedure, studies data are controversial, possibly because of the uneven price of the various embolization agents that can be used. It seems the technical cost of embolization is higher than that of endoscopic ligations of the sphenopalatine artery [13]. On the other hand, the length of hospitalization is shorter with embolization [14].

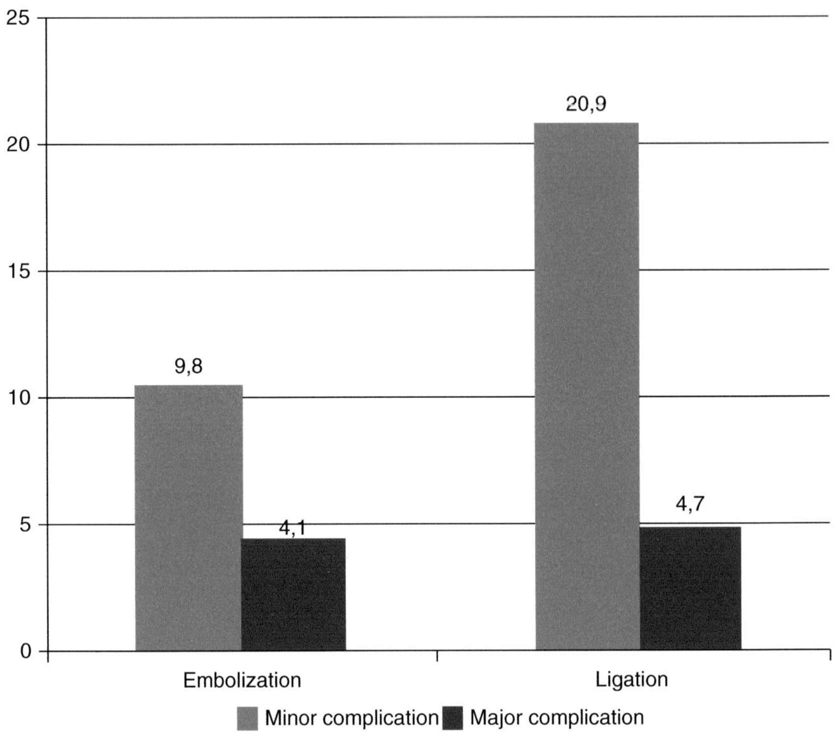

Comparison of minor and major complications of internal maxillary artery ligation versus embolization for refractory posterior epistaxis (Cullen [10])

3.1.6 Recurrence and Complications

Early rebleeding should be treated by embolization, except if ethmoidal arteries take over. Angiography will study collaterals (anterior ethmoidal, contralateral external carotid). Occlusion of both facial arteries and both sphenopalatine arteries is possible.

CVAs in relation to off-target embolization will be treated the usual way.

Post-embolization neuropathies will be treated with corticosteroids.

3.2 Other ENT Embolizations

3.2.1 Embolization of the Branches of the External Carotid Artery in Cancerology (Fig. 3.3)

Acute hemorrhage can affect all ENT neoplastic locations: face, rhinopharynx, oropharynx and oral cavity, larynx and hypopharynx, and external auditory canal. It's occurrence in head and neck surgery remains low (4.3 % [14]). External radiotherapy multiplies the risk by a 7.6 factor [15, 16].

The hemorrhage can originate from the tumor, by erosion of the invaded vascular structures, notably in case of progressive disease. It can be the result of a tumoral necrosis in patients with an excellent therapeutic response. The hemorrhage can occur in a context of full remission by radio-induced lesion. It is then favored by a local inflammatory factor (ostéoradionecrosis, tracheostomy probe, orostoma).

Rarely during the immediate post-procedure phase, the hemorrhage can be linked to vascular suture failure (reconstruction flap). Hemostatic endovascular treatment is an acknowledged therapeutic option [15].

The general principles for the embolization of the branches of the external carotid artery are the same as for epistaxes.

Selective primitive and external carotid arteries angiographic series allow the detection of the embolization target and of possible dangerous internal-external carotid or vertebro-carotid anastomoses.

The occlusion material and the microcatheter will be chosen according to topography and radiologist's habits.

Arteriography can depict tumor blush with or without extravasation of the contrast media, pseudoaneurysms, and arteriovenous fistulae [16]. On some cases, extravasation of the contrast media is only detectable with hyperselective catheterism, when the injection mobilizes the hemostatic plug.

To avoid retrograde bleeding recurrences, the hyperselective catheterism will attempt to get beyond the affected area to embolize the incriminated artery either side of the affected area, using a so-called "sandwich" technique.

If the catheterism fails to get beyond, glue embolization is discussed with an increased risk of ischemic complications. The proximal part of the affected artery branch can be occluded with controlled-release microcoils in the proximity of the internal carotid artery.

Withdrawal of the valved introducer is only considered after clinical assessment by the surgeon.

Technical feasibility and immediate clinical results are excellent (100 % immediate hemostatic control [16, 17]).

Medium-term evolution is linked to the type of the initial lesion, and hemorrhagic recurrence is the most frequent medium-term complication (20 % [16]).

3.2.2 *Carotid Blowout* (Fig. 3.4)

Common, internal, or external carotid rupture or "carotid blowout syndrome" is due to trauma or linked to oropharyngeal cancers. Radiotherapy increases its occurrence. It is characterized by a mouth and/or throat or a laterocervical bleeding, or consists in an impending threat of that type of bleeding.

Treatment for this complication has been surgical for a long time, at the cost of high-risk interventions due to the fragility of irradiated tissues and/or to the local septic context (40 % mortality and 60 % neurologic morbidity [18]).

Since 1995, series on endovascular treatment have been published, first with embolization of the affected arteries and positioning of a permanent occlusion balloon in the carotid (± carotid occlusion test), thus improving prognosis [18–20] with 15–20 % ischemic neurologic complications [18, 19, 21–23]. Since then, a more conservative approach was adopted by many teams, by covering the affected artery with a stent graft, more or less preceded by an embolization of the efferent branches of the external carotid to avoid countercurrent takeover. Immediate results for this type of procedure are excellent, close to 100 % [19, 21, 24–28] with a lower rate of neurologic complication.

3.2.3 *Rendu-Osler Disease*

Rendu-Osler disease, or hereditary hemorrhagic telangiectasia, is an autosomal dominant inheritance angiomatosis, of the phacomatoses group. Patients are managed by multidisciplinary teams in reference centers.

Epistaxes are the most frequent clinical manifestation with frequent recurrences.

ENT embolization is only discussed for patients having frequent hemorrhagic episodes, making it impossible for them to have a decent social life.

Embolization will be performed using microparticles, as distal as possible and maintaining the artery pedicles that vascularize the nasal fossae, in order to enable repeated embolizations.

3.2.4 *Preoperative Embolization of Benign Tumors* (Fig. 3.5)

Nasopharyngeal (angio-) fibromas, and rarely paragangliomas, can benefit from a preoperative embolization to reduce the risk of surgical hemorrhage [29, 30].

Angiofibromas sometimes have an important vascularization originating from the internal carotid artery. Embolization of the internal carotid territory presents neurologic risks and must be performed at hyper-specialized centers. Embolization of the sphenopalatine artery is usually insufficient, and devascularization requires embolization of the facial and ascending pharyngeal arteries, sometimes bilaterally.

Embolization of the latter artery can induce mixed nerves paralyses and should be performed cautiously with a preference in preoperative care for microcoils. Anastomoses with the vertebrobasilar territory can exist and will be searched for carefully during diagnostic arteriography.

3.3 Conclusion

Embolization is valuable option in the treatment of arterial hemorrhages of the ENT area. Its results are improved by multidisciplinary collaboration (surgeons, anesthetists), by the strict selection of its indications, by a precise knowledge of vascular anatomy, and by the mastering of the microcatheterism technique and of the various embolization agents.

Key Points

- Arterial embolization is the treatment of choice for refractory epistaxes and for some hemorrhages of the ENT area.
- Its acknowledged indications are:
  - Posterior epistaxis refractory to a 48-h proper medical treatment or with immediate life-threatening condition
  - Severe hemorrhages in ENT cancerology, pre- or postoperative
  - Preoperative devascularization of hypervascular tumors (paragangliomas or nasopharyngeal fibromas)
  - Carotid blowout due to trauma or linked to a progressive tumor or complicating radiotherapy
- Initial management of epistaxes is a local treatment.
- Hemorrhages originating in the anterior ethmoidal artery require surgery.
- Anterior essential epistaxes require surgery.
- Anterior essential epistaxes only require embolization when the symptomatic and/or surgical treatment has failed.
- A perfect knowledge of the anatomy of the external carotid artery branches is an essential prerequisite.
- Occlusion material can either be microparticles or microcoils or glues.
- The use of microparticles is only possible in the absence of dangerous anastomoses with the internal carotid or ophthalmic territories and requires a free-flow injection and fluoroscopic control.
- Using microcoils can be a good alternative. The main drawback of this technique lies in the fact that it permanently fills the artery (no possible re-embolization in case of a recurrence).
- Among the arterial embolization complications, the most serious are cerebrovascular accidents and occlusion of the central retinal artery.
- The rate of complication for a trained radiologist is not higher than that of surgery.

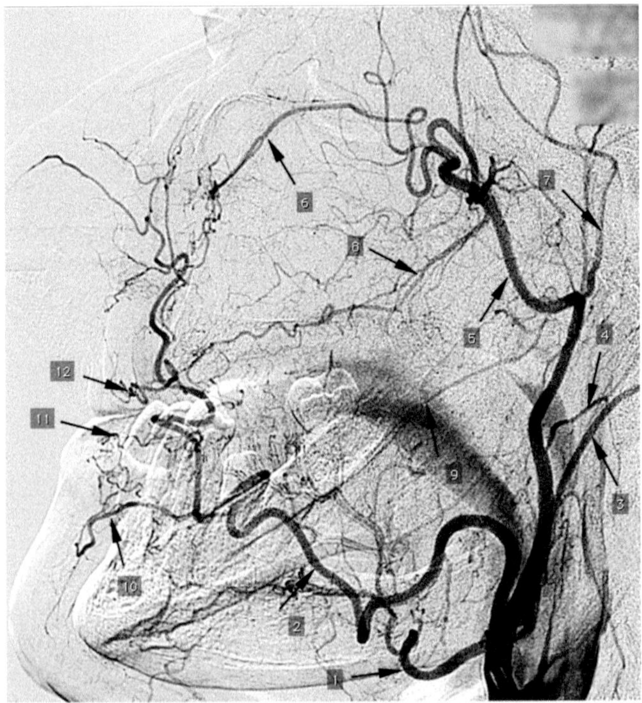

Fig. 3.1 Radio-anatomy of the external carotid branches. *1* lingual artery, *2* facial artery, *3* occipital artery, *4* posterior auricular artery, *5* internal maxillary artery, *6* sphenopalatine artery, *7* superficial temporal artery, *8* zygomatical orbital artery, *9* transverse facial artery, *10* sublingual artery, *11* inferior labial artery, *12* superior labial artery

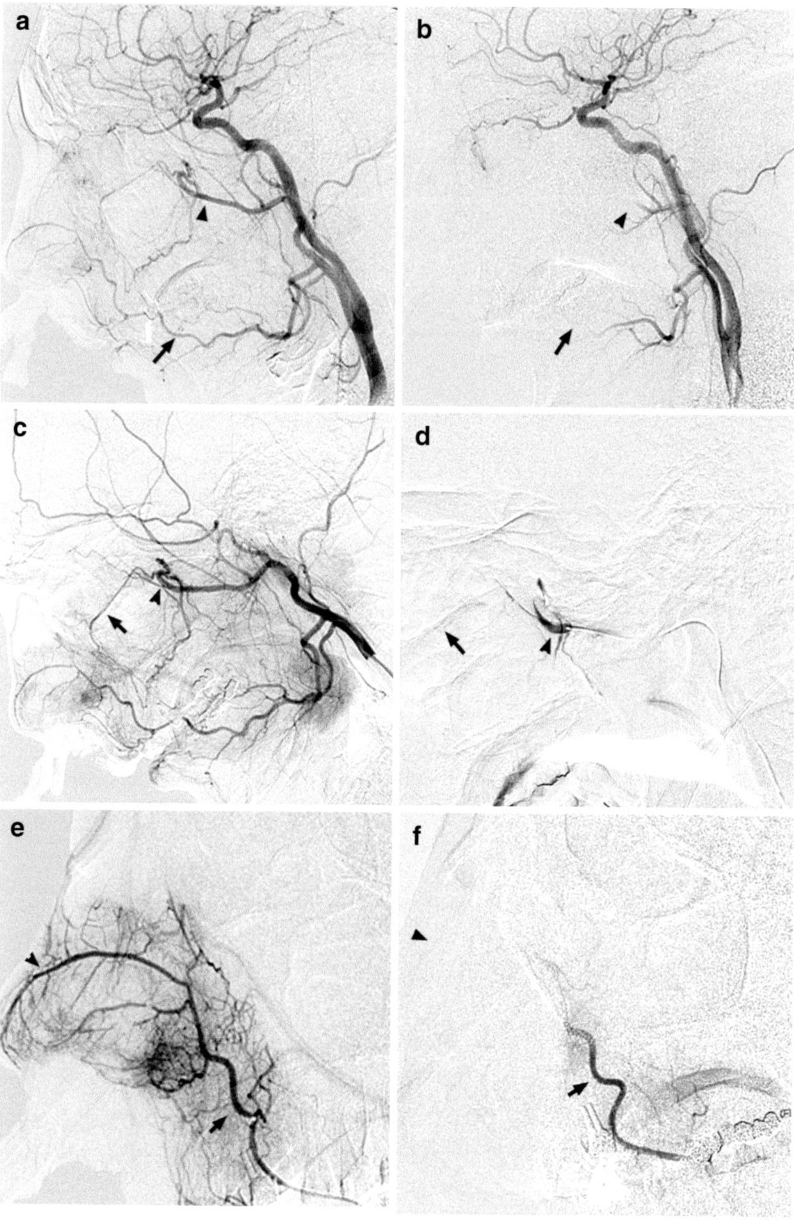

Fig. 3.2 Embolization of a refractory essential epistaxis. 34-year-old female patient presenting a left refractory essential epistaxis despite a medical treatment. Embolization performed with 500–700-μm calibrated microparticles (EmboGold®, BioSphere® medical). Left primitive carotid arteriography before (**a**) and after (**b**) embolization, showing a complete devascularization of the nasal fossa by occlusion of the maxillary artery (*black arrowheads*) and of the facial artery (*black arrows*). Arteriography before (**c**) and after (**d**) embolization by hyperselective catheterism of the left maxillary artery showing an occlusion of the internal maxillary artery (*black arrowheads*) and of the sphenopalatine artery (*black arrows*). Arteriography before (**e**) and after (**f**) embolization by hyperselective catheterism showing an occlusion of the facial artery (*black arrows*) and of the external and lateral nasal arteries (*black arrows*); note the visible microparticles at the facial artery termination (*black arrowheads*)

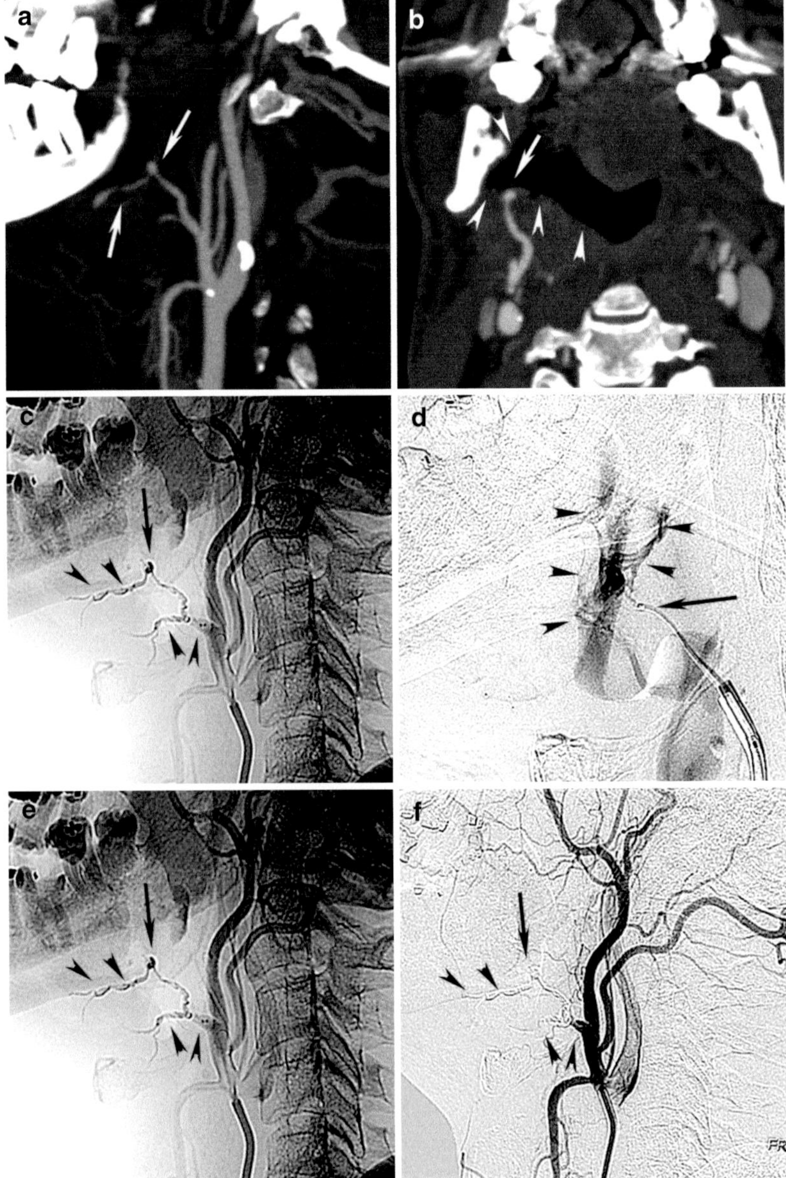

Fig. 3.3 Embolization of a hemostasis of a lingual neoplasia. Acute hemorrhage externalized by mouth in a 62-year-old male patient presenting an epidermoid carcinoma of the tonsillar glossal groove undergoing radio/chemotherapy. Angioscan (**a**, **b**) performed before embolization showing the presence of a millimetric pseudoaneurysm of the facial artery (**a**, **b**, *white arrows*) within an ulcerated lesion of the tonsillar glossal groove (**b**, *white arrowheads*). Selective diagnostic angiography (**c**) also shows the pseudoaneurysm and post-aneurysm arterial lesions (*black arrowheads*). Hyperselective diagnostic angiography using a microcatheter (**d**, Rapid Transit®, Cordis®, *arrow*) unmasks active leakage by flooding the oral cavity (**d**, *arrowheads*). Since catheterizing beyond the pseudoaneurysm is impossible, the use of a liquid embolization agent (**e**, **f**, Onyx®) enabled to occlude the pseudoaneurysm (**e**, **f**, *arrow*) and all facial and lingual arterial lesions (**e**, **f**, *arrowheads*)

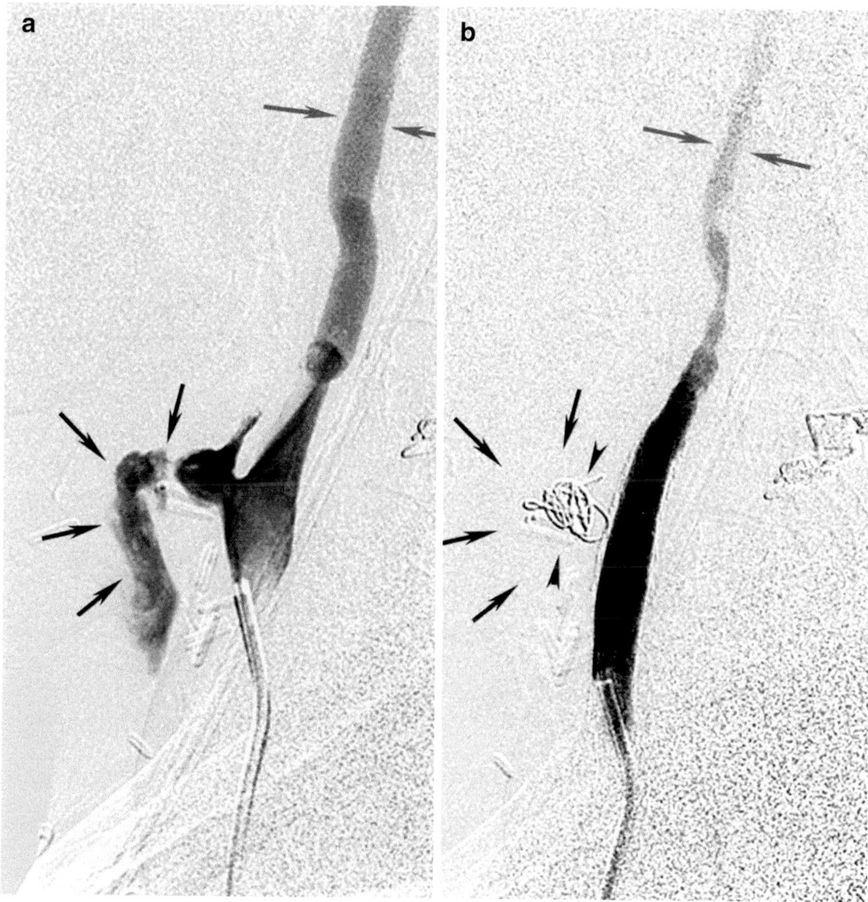

Fig. 3.4 External carotid (ExtC) rupture. Massive hemorrhage externalized by mouth in a 61-year-old male patient with a past history of external radiotherapy in 2003 (well-differentiated malpighian carcinoma of the right vocal cord) followed by a recurrence in 2008. Diagnostic angiography (**a**) postostial rupture of the ExtC (*black arrows*). Endovascular treatment (**b**) consisted in distal occlusion of the ExtC artery branches using glue (cyanoacrylate), then the pseudoaneurysm using controlled-release microcoils (IDC® 8×20 mm, *black arrowheads*), and, finally, the ostium of the ExtC using stent grafts (Advanta V12® 7×22 and 8×38). Note a spasm of the internal carotid on final control (**a**, **b**, *grey arrows*). Absence of hemorrhagic recurrence after 1 year

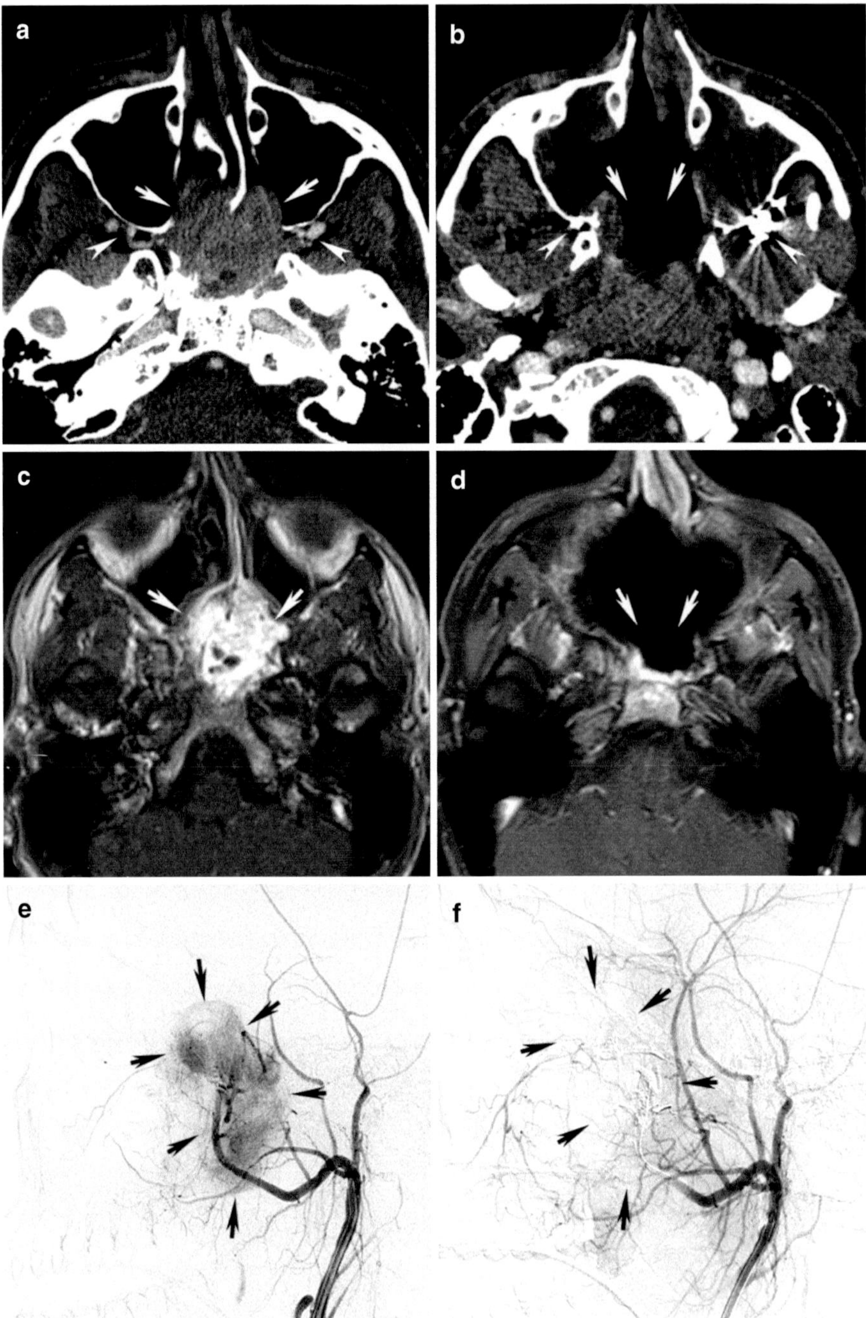

Fig. 3.5 Preoperative embolization of a nasopharyngeal fibroma. Pre-embolization (**a**, **c**, **e**), post-embolization (**f**), and postsurgical (**b**, **d**) imaging. Post-contrast CT (**a**, **b**), MRI (**d**), and subtraction digital angiography (**e**, **f**). Hypervascular nasopharyngeal tumor (**a**, **b**, **e** *arrows*). Feeding artery: distal branch of internal maxillary artery (**a**, *arrowhead*). Distal embolization of both maxillary arteries using a liquid agent (Onyx®) allows complete presurgical tumor devascularization (**e**: *arrows*)

References

1. Small M, Murray JA, Maran AG. A study of patients with epistaxis requiring admission to hospital. Health Bull (Edinb). 1982;40(1):20–9.
2. Leppänen M, et al. Microcatheter embolization of intractable idiopathic epistaxis. Cardiovasc Intervent Radiol. 1999;22(6):499–503.
3. Cockroft KM, et al. Delayed epistaxis resulting from external carotid artery injury requiring embolization: a rare complication of transsphenoidal surgery: case report. Neurosurgery. 2000;47(1):236–9.
4. Luo CB, et al. Transarterial embolization of acute external carotid blowout syndrome with profuse oronasal bleeding by N-butyl-cyanoacrylate. Am J Emerg Med. 2006;24(6):702–8.
5. Pollak JS, White Jr RI. The use of cyanoacrylate adhesives in peripheral embolization. J Vasc Interv Radiol. 2001;12(8):907–13.
6. Elhammady MS, et al. Onyx embolization of carotid-cavernous fistulas. J Neurosurg. 2010;112(3):589–94.
7. Christensen NP, et al. Arterial embolization in the management of posterior epistaxis. Otolaryngol Head Neck Surg. 2005;113(5):748–53.
8. Moreau S, et al. Supraselective embolization in intractable epistaxis: review of 45 cases. Laryngoscope. 1998;108(6):887–8.
9. Tseng EY, et al. Angiographic embolization for epistaxis: a review of 114 cases. Laryngoscope. 1998;108(4 Pt 1):615–9.
10. Cullen MM, Tami TA. Comparison of internal maxillary artery ligation versus embolization for refractory posterior epistaxis. Otolaryngol Head Neck Surg. 1998;118(5):636–42.
11. Mames RN, Snady-McCoy L, Guy J. Central retinal and posterior ciliary artery occlusion after particle embolization of the external carotid artery system. Ophthalmology. 1991;98(4):527–31.
12. Elden L, et al. Angiographic embolization for the treatment of epistaxis: a review of 108 cases. Otolaryngol Head Neck Surg. 1994;111(1):44–50.
13. Klotz DA, et al. Surgical management of posterior epistaxis: a changing paradigm. Laryngoscope. 2002;112(9):1577–82.
14. Strong EB, et al. Intractable epistaxis: transantral ligation vs. embolization: efficacy review and cost analysis. Otolaryngol Head Neck Surg. 1995;113(6):674–8.
15. Bates MC, Shamsham FM. Endovascular management of impending carotid rupture in a patient with advanced head and neck cancer. J Endovasc Ther. 2003;10:54–7.
16. Chen YF, et al. Transarterial embolization for control of bleeding in patients with head and neck cancer. Otolaryngol Head Neck Surg. 2010;142(1):90–4.
17. Bhansali S, Wilner H, Jacobs JR. Arterial embolization for control of bleeding in advanced head and neck carcinoma. J Laryngol Otol. 1986;100(11):1289–93.
18. Citardi MJ, et al. Management of carotid artery rupture by monitored endovascular therapeutic occlusion (1988–1994). Laryngoscope. 1995;105(10):1086–92.
19. Chaloupka JC, et al. Endovascular therapy for the carotid blowout syndrome in head and neck surgical patients: diagnostic and managerial considerations. AJNR Am J Neuroradiol. 1996; 17(5):843–52.
20. Chaloupka JC, et al. Recurrent carotid blowout syndrome: diagnostic and therapeutic challenges in a newly recognized subgroup of patients. AJNR Am J Neuroradiol. 1999;20(6):1069–77.
21. Lesley WS, et al. Preliminary experience with endovascular reconstruction for the management of carotid blowout syndrome. AJNR Am J Neuroradiol. 2003;24(5):975–81.
22. Chazono H, et al. Carotid artery resection: preoperative temporary occlusion is not always an accurate predictor of collateral blood flow. Acta Otolaryngol. 2005;125(2):196–200.
23. Macdonald S, et al. Endovascular treatment of acute carotid blow-out syndrome. J Vasc Interv Radiol. 2000;11(9):1184–8.
24. Warren FM, et al. Management of carotid 'blowout' with endovascular stent grafts. Laryngoscope. 2002;112(3):428–33.

25. Pyun HW, et al. Placement of covered stents for carotid blowout in patients with head and neck cancer: follow-up results after rescue treatments. AJNR Am J Neuroradiol. 2007;28(8):1594–8.
26. Chang FC, et al. Patients with head and neck cancers and associated postirradiated carotid blowout syndrome: endovascular therapeutic methods and outcomes. J Vasc Surg. 2008;47(5):936–45.
27. Chang FC, et al. Brain abscess formation: a delayed complication of carotid blowout syndrome treated by self-expandable stent-graft. AJNR Am J Neuroradiol. 2006;27(7):1543–5.
28. Desuter G, et al. Carotid stenting for impending carotid blowout: suitable supportive care for head and neck cancer patients? Palliat Med. 2005;19:427–9.
29. Nicolai P, et al. Endoscopic surgery for juvenile angiofibroma: a critical review of indications after 46 cases. Am J Rhinol Allergy. 2010;24(2):e67–72.
30. Santaolalla F, et al. Efficacy of selective percutaneous embolization for the treatment of intractable posterior epistaxis and juvenile nasopharyngeal angiofibroma (JNA). Acta Otolaryngol. 2009;129(12):1456–62.

Suggested Reading

Kaufman JA, Lee MJ, 1. Vascular and interventional radiology: the requisites. St. Louis: Mosby; 2003. p. 510.

Klurfan P, Lee SK. Vascular embolotherapy: a comprehensive approach. 1st ed. Berlin/New York: Springer; 2006.

Part III
Situations and Strategies: Thorax

Chapter 4
Massive Hemoptysis: Radiological Management

Louis Boyer, Lucie Cassagnes, Hélène Vernhet, Jean-Marc Garcier, and Pascal Chabrot

4.1 Background

The expectoration of blood from the lower respiratory tract defines hemoptysis (H). One must distinguish "H as a symptom" (small or moderate blood loss, sometimes over several days) and "H as a disease", which can be life-threatening: small but recurring H or massive H (more than 100 or more than 400 cc per day, depending on the authors). The risk of death is due to asphyxiation secondary to intra-alveolar hemorrhage rather than exsanguination.

In 90 % of cases, the source of H is the bronchial circulation, in an area of chronic or active inflammation, with reduced or occluded pulmonary circulation, causing proliferation and enlargement of bronchial artery (BA). Rupture of enlarged BA may be due to arterial wall erosion by bacterial agents or elevated regional blood pressure (BP). In 5 %, bleeding is due to aorta (aortobronchial fistula, ruptured thoracic aorta aneurysm) or non-bronchial systemic arteries (NBSA). The usual course of these NBSA is transpleural, through a thickened and adherent pleura due to a chronic disease. Each parieto-thoracic systemic artery can be involved in this hypervascularization. At last pulmonary arteries (PA) are the source of bleeding in 5 % of the cases.

The prevalence of causes of massive H depends from the continent: in the Western countries, tuberculosis (TB) (active, intracavitary aspergillomas, fibrous

L. Boyer, MD, PhD (✉) • L. Cassagnes, MD • P. Chabrot, MD, PhD
Department of Radiology, University Hospital of Clermont-Ferrand, Clermont-Ferrand, France
e-mail: lboyer@chu-clermontferrand.fr; pchabrot@chu-clermontferrand.fr

H. Vernhet, MD, PhD
Department of Radiology, University Hospital of Montpellier, Montpellier, France

J.-M. Garcier, MD, PhD
Department of Anatomy and Radiology, University Hospital of Clermont-Ferrand, Clermont-Ferrand, France

P. Chabrot, L. Boyer (eds.), *Embolization*,
DOI 10.1007/978-1-4471-5182-1_4, © Springer-Verlag London 2014

sequels, etc.) is the most frequent etiology, followed by primary bronchiectasis, bronchogenic carcinoma, pneumoconiosis, intrabronchial ruptured vessels, etc.

Massive H requires an immediate hospitalization and an active multidisciplinary approach, with intensive pulmonary and cardiovascular care.

Percutaneous endovascular embolization is the first-line treatment of refractory massive arterial bleeding or less severe H despite medical treatment (local or systemic administration of vasoconstrictive drugs, reversal of antiplatelet and anticoagulant drugs). To determine which vessel to occlude, pretherapeutic investigations must answer to two questions: where is the site of bleeding?, and what is its cause?

Multidetector CT (MDCT) shows the site of bleeding as localized ground glass opacity, with or without alveolar consolidation. The visualization of the causes or the consequences of bleeding are of less localizing value. The size of the intra-alveolar hemorrhage is correlated with severity of H.

CT also depicts physiopathological features such as enlarged BA, with or without aneurysm, ectopic and aberrant BA, tortuous hypertrophic NBSA within extrapleural fat and through pleural thickening, as well as abnormal PA (hilar neoplasm, Rasmussen aneurysm, TB, necrotizing pneumopathy, Behcet disease, traumatisms, PAVM, etc.)

CT allows the identification of all bleeding BA that can be catheterized; however, BA depicted only by angiography but not on CT are never involved in the bleeding: thus CT should nowadays be the first-line modality. The visibility of a BA up to the pulmonary hilum pleads in the favor of its responsibility with respect to the bleeding. Fiberoptic bronchoscopy (FOB) is not always mandatory but has to be performed if CT is not informative. According to the results of chest plain film and CT (and if necessary FOB), bronchial arteriography and/or pulmonary angiography is then performed.

4.2 Relevant Radiological Anatomy

Most commonly, BA originate from descending aorta between the levels of the fifth and sixth thoracic vertebrae (T5 and T6), in an area between the lower end of the trachea, the aortic knob, and the middle part of the left main bronchus.

Typically two to four BA are present; Cauldwell described four classical branching patterns (2 left BA + 1 intercostobronchial trunk (ICBT), 1 left BA + 1 ICBT, 1 right BA and 1 ICBT + 2 left BA, 1 right BA and 1 ICBT + 1 left BA). A right ICBT is seen on angiography in 80 % of cases. A right-left common trunk is quite often seen, as well as interbronchial right-left anastomosis (10–30 %). On CT scans, a BA diameter larger than 2 mm is abnormal. Variant BA anatomy is not infrequent (8.3–35 %). Ectopic BA originates from the aortic arch (75 %) or from descending aorta below the level of T6. Aberrant BA should be looked for in cases of discordances between large BA on CT and small orthotopic BA on arteriography, when a significant BA supply to areas of abnormal pulmonary parenchyma is not demonstrated, when the source of bleeding has not been detected, and in case of recurrent

H despite of successful embolization. It can originate from SCA, ITA, thyrocervical trunks, primitive carotids, BCA, pericardic and phrenic A, and coronary A (right +++); they enter in the pulmonary parenchyma via the hilum; they extend along the course of the major bronchi. They have to be distinguished from NBSA and from anastomosis between NBSA and BA, whose diameter is smaller than BA.

NBSA originate from various parieto-thoracic trunks, most often ICA, SCA, ITA, arteries of the pulmonary ligament, and diaphragmatic A. Their course is not parallel to that of the bronchi. They are most often contiguous to chronic pleural or pulmonary diseases with a pleural thickening, and they enter the pulmonary parenchyma through the adherent pleura or via the pulmonary ligament.

From T3 to T8, the spinal cord is supplied by one or two anterior radiculomedullary arteries, among which the most constant originates at the level of T5 or T6, usually on the left side, with angiographically a characteristic "hair spin" configuration (rarely seen). It may also arise from the right ICBT, classically in 5–10 % of the patients, but the true prevalence is probably lower. The visualization of a spinal artery is not a contraindication to embolization.

At-risk anterior spinal A arising from right ICBT may be unmasked during embolization procedure, and reflux may become possible in spinal cord branches not detected initially. So during embolization, step-by-step angio controls are mandatory.

On CT scans, the visualization of SA is unusual, even with the thinner collimations.

4.3 Systemic Arterial Bleeding: Bronchial Arteries and NBSA

4.3.1 Angio and Embolization Techniques

- Informed consent is required.
- The examination is carried out under local anesthesia; intensive pulmonary and cardiovascular care may be necessary. The quality of the angiographic system is essential (digital subtraction technique, spatial resolution, high frame rate, etc.).
- Femoral arterial access.
- A careful arterial evaluation is then based upon CT and thoracic aortogram, with injections in the descending aorta and in the aortic arch, and selective search of BA (arising from aorta or from abnormal origin, to begin with SCA). Selective catheterization must be performed even if the caliber of BA is normal: they can be responsible for the bleeding even in these cases. Catheterization of subclavian arteries and eventually of intercostal arteries and other possible origins of aberrant BA and NBSA is performed when no abnormal BA is observed. If there is a slight doubt, these selective opacifications must be done by manual injections.

- Hypertrophic BA can be depicted: with or without aneurysms (but BA with a normal diameter can be responsible of a massive H); PA or PV shunts, hypervascularity, neovascularization, and extravasation of contrast media (CM) which is specific but inconstant. Systematic detection of spinal A or dangerous anastomoses with supra-aortic or coronary arteries must also be undertaken.
- To embolize, the catheterization must be stable and safe. It should be superselective, using a microcath, if: (a) there is unstable catheterization and/or in case of ostial stenosis; (b) an arterial rupture occurs during CM injection; (c) at risk A: BA collaterals (spinal cord branch, or esophageal A), or NBSA at risk, originating from supra-aortic trunks or coronary arteries.
- Embolization should not be too distal to avoid necrosis nor too proximal to preserve future arterial access; it should be peripheral enough to avoid recruitment and development of NBSA.
- A nonionic contrast agent must be used in order to limit risks of medullar ischemia.
- In embolic agents, the goal is to reduce the perfusion pressure in pathological pulmonary areas where there are fragile vessels, carrying out occlusion as close as possible to the pathological bronchopulmonary anastomoses, in order to prevent recurrences originating from collateral NBSA.

  – Liquid embolic agents, as glue or absolute alcohol, are not currently used because of high risk of necrosis and definitive occlusion.
  – Thrombin has been used in some cases
  – Absorbable gelatine sponge (Gelfoam) is easy to use, even with a microcatheter, but it is resolvable after 10–15 days, so recurrences are possible.
  – Coils must be deployed distally because hilar anastomoses make proximal occlusions ineffective.
    We choose microcoils when BA arises from ICBT to occlude aneurysms and to prevent embolization of normal territories, i.e., in case of ITA embo. Coils are immediately safe, but may be ineffective if used proximally, and may preclude repeated embolizations. BA aneurysms are usually located near the ostium and are at risk of rupture. Their exclusion if possible must be preceded by the exclusion of outcoming branches, to avoid recanalization.
  – To avoid distal occlusion as well as embolization of bronchopulmonary shunts, most authors choose particles of 350 μm or more. We use particles of 500 μm in diameter. Even if these agents are considered as nonabsorbable, the concept of a definitive occlusion with microparticles remains very controversial.
  – Particles and then microcoils can also be used.

4.3.2 Results

- 70–90 % rate of immediate success; most of the failures correspond to unstable catheterism or identification of a spinal cord branch.

- Complications: transient pain is rather frequent; sometimes a transitory dysphagia is observed. The main complication is the spinal cord ischemia: from 1.4 to 6.5 %.
- The other complications are rare: bronchial necrosis, bronchoesophageal fistulas, pulmonary infarctions, myocardial necrosis (especially in case of coronaro-bronchial arterial anastomosis in Takayasu's disease), nontargeted embolization, or aortic subintimal dissection or hematoma.
- Initial nonrecurrence rates of 73–98 % during the first month have been reported
- Early recurrences must call into questions the origin of H: PA, an unknown aberrant BA or NBSA, or a proximal interbronchial anastomosis.
- The long-term (1–46-month follow-up) recurrence rates vary from 10 to 52 %, depending on recanalization and/or incomplete initial occlusion (notably with gelatine sponge), revascularization by collaterals and/or NBSA supply, inadequate medical treatment, or progression of underlying disease. But should H recur, repeated embolization can be safely performed.

4.3.3 Indications

The high mortality and morbidity rates of systemic hemorrhages (B and NBSA) make necessary a multidisciplinary approach, in which embolization is the first-line treatment.

In case of focal lesion, embolization is a *symptomatic* treatment preceding medical and/or surgical management of the underlying disease.

When H complicates diffuse chronic lesions or occurs in at surgical risk patients, embolization is a *palliative* treatment, to be conceived in a long-term view, with or without associated medical treatment, in order to preserve a vascular access and to avoid recruitment of pedicles difficult to catheterize. This strategy makes possible re-embolization in the future.

4.4 Pulmonary Arterial Bleedings

The erosion of PA may be caused by various evolutive lesions: infections (TB, aspergillosis, necrotizing pneumopathy, septic emboli); traumatisms, especially iatrogenic lesions with Swan–Ganz catheter; inflammation (especially during Behcet disease); tumors (necrosis of hilar masses); and PAVM for which H is one of the spontaneous complications. All these erosions can be nowadays diagnosed directly on angio CT, which can depict an aneurysm or a necrosis, pointing toward the PA responsible for the bleeding. A vaso-occlusion of this PA can then be proposed.

4.4.1 Technique

The technique of PA vaso-occlusion is the classical technique used to treat PAV aneurysm (see Chap. 5).

At first, the exact location must be determined on CT and then on pulmonary angiography if indication of PA vaso-occlusion has been validated. A selective catheterization is the first step of embolization procedure.

Coils are normally used. We prefer to use AVP plugs. Embolization should be released as close to the sac as possible, to preserve normal parenchyma.

4.4.2 Results

Among varied etiologies, only results of the PAVM vaso-occlusion are codified: they will be detailed in Chap. 5. Let us recall that:

- Technical success is observed in 98 % of the cases.
- Complications : less than 10 % : emboli (critical in case of arteriovenous communication); pulmonary infarction, eventually with an associated pleural effusion.
- 84–96 % of good results are maintained in the long term.

But recanalizations are possible, such as systemic hypervascularization reperfusing the vaso-occluded zone, justifying a control CT scan 1 year after.

4.4.3 Indications

Vaso-occlusion is the first-line treatment to treat PAVM.

In the case of erosion of the pulmonary artery, in order to treat or prevent an H, percutaneous vaso-occlusion will be discussed taking into account the prognosis on one hand and other therapeutic options on the other hand (abstention, medical or surgical treatments, which must then be carried out without delay). This vaso-occlusion may concern the feeding artery, a false aneurysm, the neck of an aneurysm, etc.

In case of iatrogenic rupture of a pulmonary arterial branch, reinflating the Swan–Ganz catheter (to occlude of the arterial breach) can be life saving, allowing the transfer to the angio suite.

4.5 Double Systemic Arterial and Pulmonary Embolization

The intertwining of a pulmonary arterial origin and of a systematic hypervascularization is well displayed by CT. A multidisciplinary approach is mandatory. The following may be responsible:

- Behcet disease, in which a vaso-occlusion of the arterial pulmonary aneurysm will firstly be realized, and then followed by embolization of the BA and NBSA.
- Tuberculosis.
- Takayasu's disease in which H is the consequence of a pulmonary infarction, which is the complication of PA stenosis and/or their compensation by systemic hypervascularization. One therefore has to attentively search for coronary anastomoses. The treatment may associate an angioplasty of the PA and a BA embolization.

Key Points

- Multidisciplinary management.
- Pretherapeutic assessment must answer two questions: what is the site of the bleeding?, and what is the cause of the bleeding?
- Workup must include the following: a chest plain film, a CT scan, and possibly a FOB (when the CT is noncontributory) so as to determine which vessel must be occluded.
- In case of bronchial arterial bleeding, an embolization is the first-line treatment.
- If hemoptysis is of systemic arterial origin and is caused by a focal lesion, embolization is a symptomatic treatment, preceding medical and/or surgical management of underlying disease.
- In the case of systemic arterial H caused by diffuse and chronic lesions, palliative embolization is associated with a medical treatment, in a long-term strategy, preserving a vascular access and thus avoiding the recruitment of pedicles that can be difficult to catheterize.
- In the case of H of PA origin (5 %), percutaneous vaso-occlusion is to be discussed taking into account the prognosis and other therapeutic options (emergency surgery or abstention)
- The PA vaso-occlusion requires a CT follow-up.

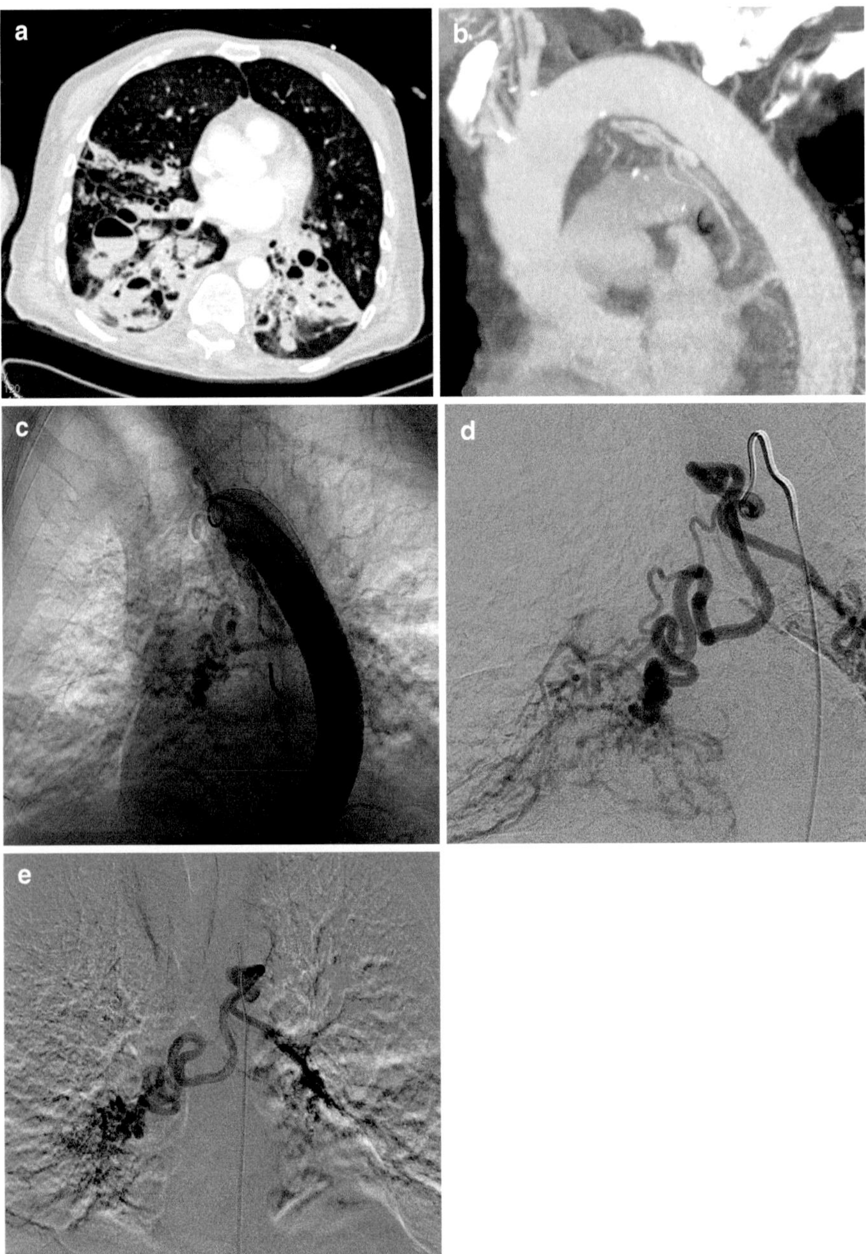

Fig. 4.1 Abundant repeated hemoptysis, complications of an old bronchiectasis. (**a**) CT, parenchymal windows: bilateral basal severe bronchiectasis. (**b**) Mediastinal window, sagittal oblique reconstructions: voluminous BA arising from the aorta at T5 level; bilateral alveolar condensation. (**c**) Descending aorta angiography showing this BA. (**d**) Selective angiography (Mikaelsson catheter); frontal view: right–left common BA, hypervascularization of the left inferior lobe and of the right base. The CT/angio confrontation leads to decide a bilateral embolization. (**e**) Selective microcatheterization: bilateral distal particular embolization, authorizing the preservation of the arterial access, in order to later re-embolize if necessary

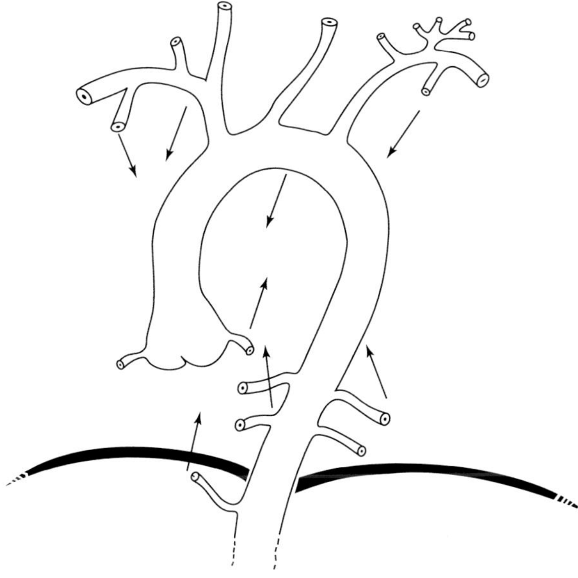

Fig. 4.2 Possible origins of ectopic BA (from aortic arch or descending aorta below T6) and possible origins of aberrant BA (from subclavian, internal thoracic A, thyro bicervical trunk, coronary A, etc.)

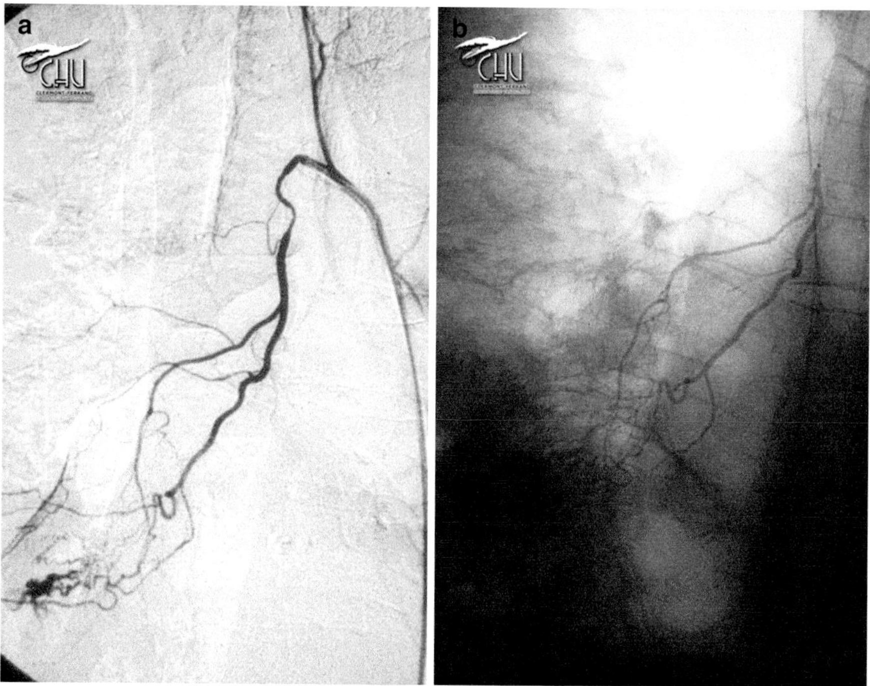

Fig. 4.3 Common right intercostobronchial trunk. (**a**) Semi-selective catheterization: hilar hypervascularization. (**b**) Hyperselective catheterization, downstream intercostal arteries, which warrant embolization without out-of-target occlusion (anterior radiculo-medullary artery arising from an intercostal artery)

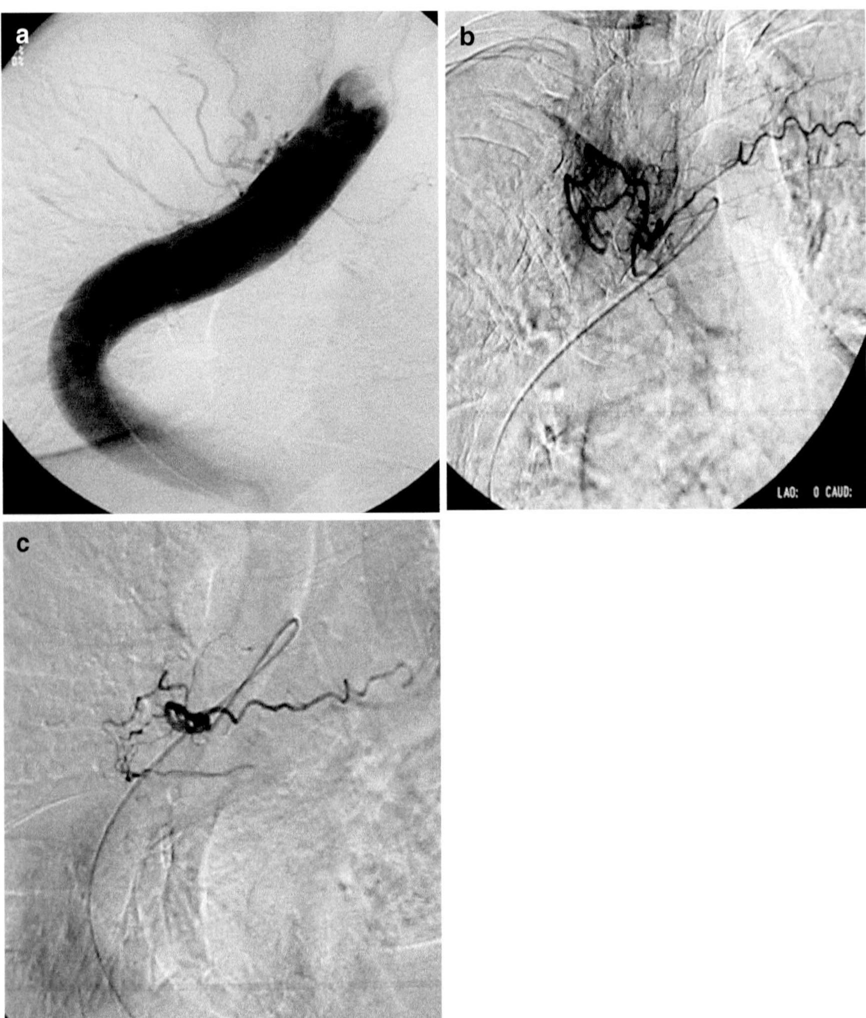

Fig. 4.4 Abundant and repeated hemoptysis in a severely scoliotic old woman: CT has localized the bleeding coming from right superior lobe. (**a**) Aortogram: extremely sinuous thoracoabdominal aorta; large right BA. (**b**) Selective catheterization: common right+left BA trunk, with a right intercostobronchial trunk. This unstable catheterization led us to use absorbable gelatine sponge (Gelfoam) as occlusion agent. (**c**) Post-embo angiogram

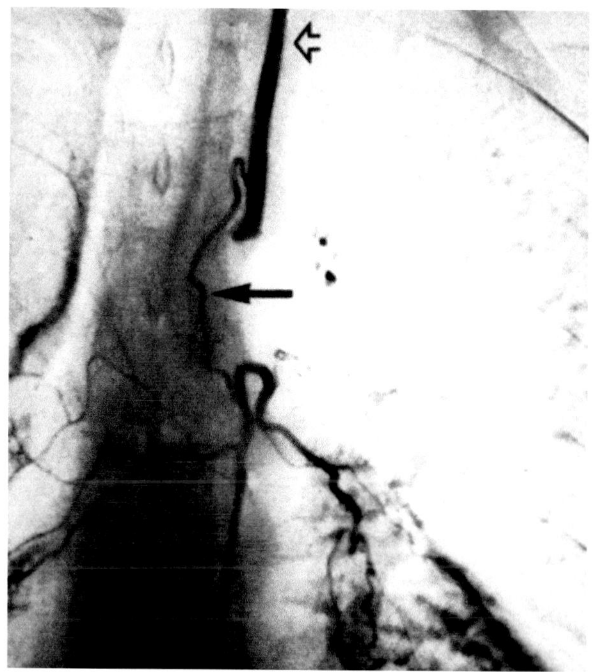

Fig. 4.5 Anastomosis between left BA and left vertebral A (*arrow*)

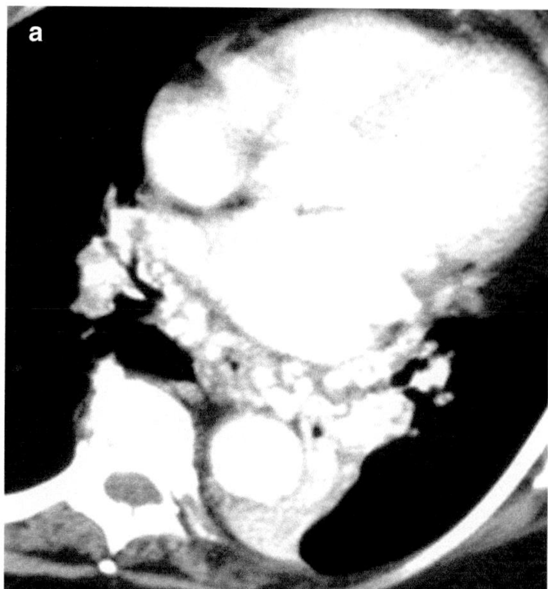

Fig. 4.6 Repeated abundant hemoptysis, complication of an old tuberculosis in an old patient. (**a**) Important systemic right bronchial hypervascularization; a right BA origin is suspected on lung CT analysis. (**b**) Right BA selective catheterization: voluminous proximal BA aneurysm. (**c**) Post-embo (coils + Gelfoam) angio control

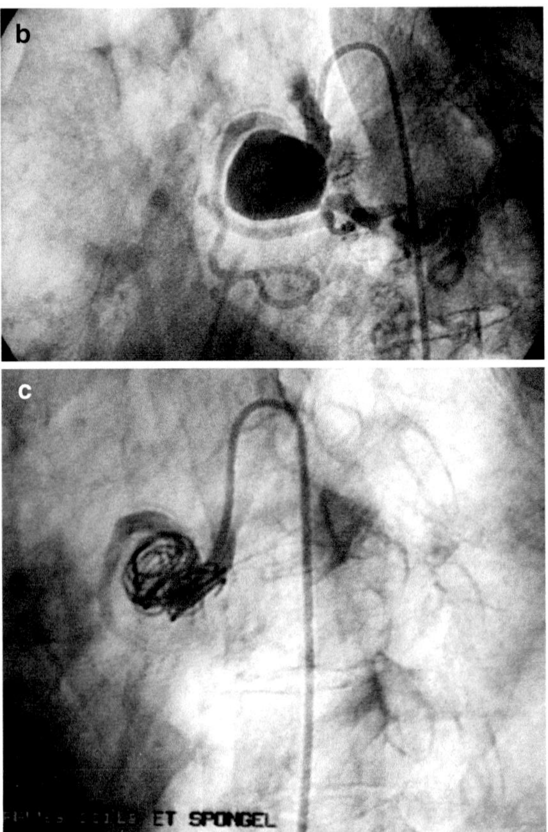

Fig. 4.6 (continued)

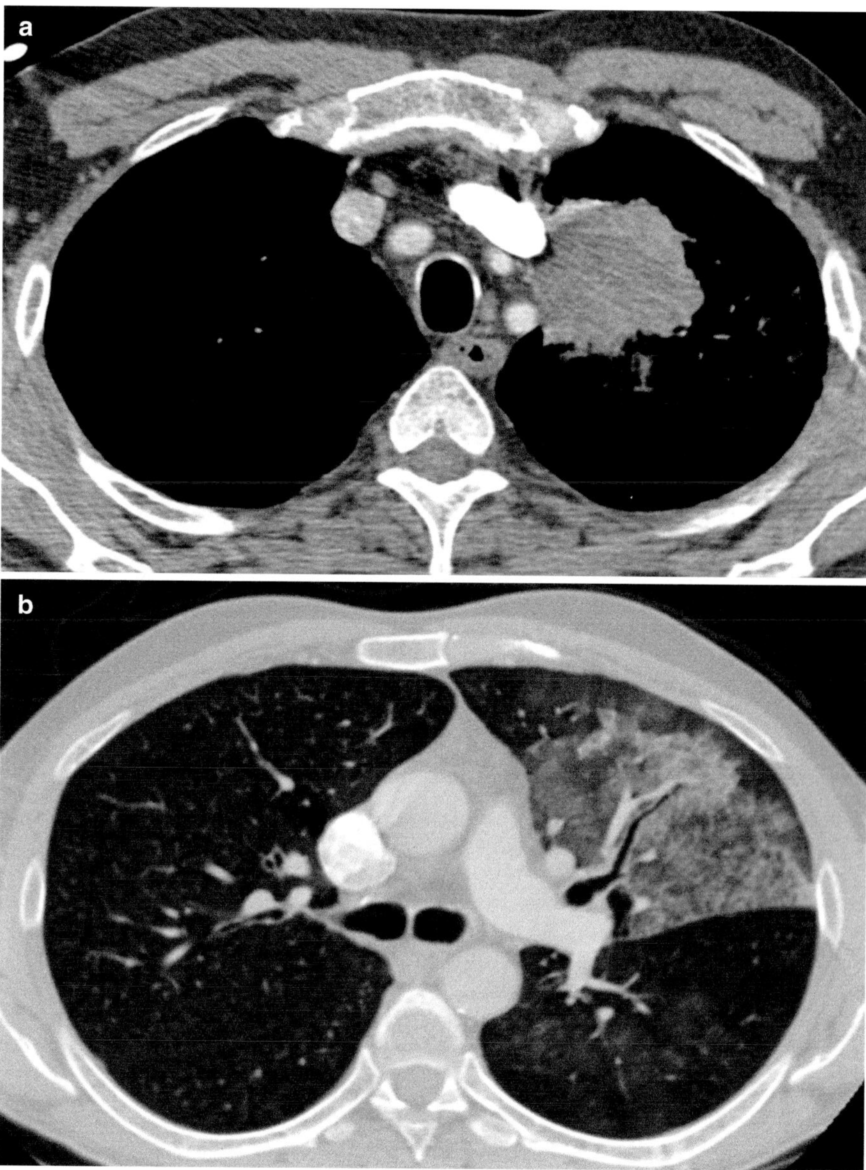

Fig. 4.7 Severe hemoptysis, complication of an extended bronchial adenocarcinoma. (**a**) CT (mediastinal window) showing the tumor. (**b**) Left superior lobar alveolar condensation. (**c**) Selective catheterization: common right–left BA trunk, right superior lobar hypervascularization, which has been excluded using microparticles and then coils. (**d**) Angio control: patent right intercostobronchial artery

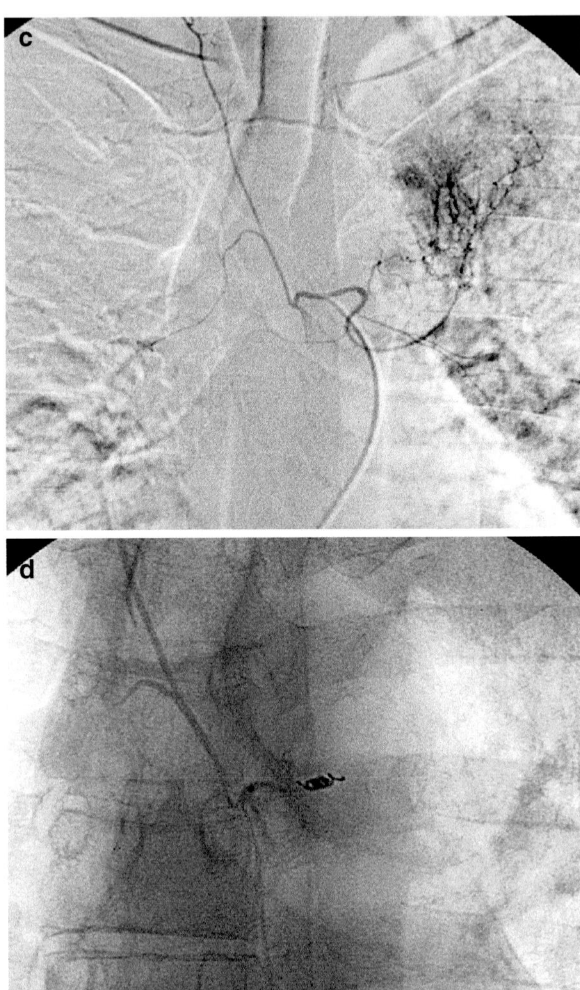

Fig. 4.7 (continued)

Suggested Reading

Haponik EF, Fein A, Chin R. Managing life threatening hemoptysis: has anything changes? Chest. 2000;118:1431–5.

Hartmann IJC, Remy-Jardin M, Menchini L, Teissiere A, et al. Ectopic origin of bronchial arteries: assessment with multidetector helical CT angiography. Eur Radiol. 2007;17:1943–53.

Hsu A, et al. Thoracic embolotherapy for life threatening hemoptysis: a pneumologist's perspective. Respirology. 2005;10:138–43.

Khalil A, Fartoukh M, Parot A, et al. Impact of MDCT angiography on the management of patients with hemoptysis. AJR Am J Roentgenol. 2010;195:772–8.

Lacombe P, EL Hajjam M, Lagrange C, et al. Dualité vasculaire pulmonaire: substratum anatomo pathologique et implications thérapeutiques. In: sous la dir. de JM Bigot, editors. Formation Médicale Continue 2003, Paris: Société Française de Radiologie; 2003. p. 475–84.

Remy Jardin M, Bouaziz N, Dumont P, et al. Bronchial and non bronchial systemic arteries at multidetector row CT angiography: comparison with conventional angiography. Radiology. 2004;233:741.

Remy J, Remy Jardin M, Wattines L, et al. Pulmonary arterio venous malformations: evaluation with CT of the chest before and after treatment. Radiology. 1992;182:809–16.

Remy J, Remy Jardin M, Giraud F, et al. Angioarchitecture of PAVM: clinical utility of 3D helical CT. Radiology. 1994;191:657–64.

Revel MP, Fournier LS, Hennebicque AS, et al. Can CT replace bronchoscopy in the detection of the site and cause of bleeding in patients with large or massive hemoptysis ? AJR Am J Roentgenol. 2002;179:1217–24.

Thony F, Gaubert JY, et Varoquaux A. Embolisations des urgences médicales-hémoptysies. In: sous la direction d'H. Vernhet-Kovacsick, SFICV, editor. Recommandations de bonne pratique de la SFICV en radiologie vasculaire interventionnelle. Paris: SFICV; 2007.

Vernhet H, Dogas G, Bousquet C, et al. Hémoptysies sévères: apport de la TDM thoracique. J Radiol. 2003a;84:685.

Vernhet H, Dogas G, Serre-Cousine O, et al. Prise en charge d'une hémoptysie chez l'adulte: imagerie et radiologie thérapeutique Feuillets de. Radiologie. 2003b;43(2):119–27.

Yoon W, Kim JK, Kim HY, et al. Bronchial and non bronchial systemic artery embolization for life threatening hemoptysis: a comprehensive review. Radiographics. 2002;22:1395–409.

Chapter 5
Embolization of the Pulmonary Artery

Louis Boyer, Lucie Cassagnes, Hélène Vernhet, Jean-Marc Garcier, and Pascal Chabrot

5.1 Pulmonary Arteriovenous Malformations (PAVMs)

Pulmonary arteriovenous malformation is the main indication of pulmonary artery embolization.

5.1.1 Background

These direct arteriovenous communications create a left-to-right shunt. In 60–90 % of the cases, PAVMs are congenital and related to a Rendu-Osler-Weber syndrome: hereditary hemorrhagic telangiectasia (HHT). Diagnosis is confirmed when at least three of the following criteria are present: family history (autosomal dominant transmission), mucocutaneous telangiectasia, recurrent epistaxis, and visceral lesions (liver, GI tract, neurological, or lung). In these cases, PAVMs are commonly multiple and bilateral. Isolated PAV fistulas are in general associated with the Fanconi syndrome, following a thoracic traumatism or surgery; more rarely it is secondary to cirrhosis or pulmonary arterial hypertension. Neurological complications (ischemic strokes and abscesses by paradoxical embolism) are observed in 30–40 % of the patients presenting at least one PAV communication

L. Boyer, MD, PhD (✉) • L. Cassagnes, MD • P. Chabrot, MD, PhD
Department of Radiology, University Hospital of Clermont-Ferrand, Clermont-Ferrand, France
e-mail: lboyer@chu-clermontferrand.fr; pchabrot@chu-clermontferrand.fr

H. Vernhet, MD, PhD
Department of Radiology, University Hospital of Montpellier, Montpellier, France

J.-M. Garcier, MD, PhD
Department of Anatomy and Radiology, University Hospital of Clermont-Ferrand, Clermont-Ferrand, France

P. Chabrot, L. Boyer (eds.), *Embolization*,
DOI 10.1007/978-1-4471-5182-1_5, © Springer-Verlag London 2014

with a feeding artery diameter equal or superior to 3 mm. Systemic oxygen desaturation can lead to intolerance to effort (more frequent with diffuse PAVM, where nearly all the segmentary arteries of at least a pulmonary lobe are affected by small PAVM fed by subsegmentary branches). Hemoptysis and hemothorax, due to the rupture of the aneurysmal sac, especially during pregnancy, are the other potential complications.

Two thirds of the PAVMs are localized in the lower lobes, which means the interest of an orthoxymetry for these patients. Schematically, simple PAVMs (80 % of the cases, with a segmental feeding artery and a draining vein) are distinguished from complex ones (20 %, which present several afferent arteries and one or several draining veins). But an apparently unique feeding artery can be associated with other afferent ones which can go undiagnosed even on a selective angiography, because of a preferential backflow phenomenon.

CT plays an essential role in the detection, the diagnosis, and the pre-therapeutic work-up. The diagnosis can be incidental, on the work-up of a complication, or at the time of a medical work-up for Rendu-Osler-Weber syndrome, which commonly includes a screening of the PAVM, either by echocardiography with contrast agent or directly on a chest plain film or MRI or CT which has a higher sensibility.

5.1.2 Relevant Radiological Anatomy

The pulmonary artery (PA) divides into its left and right branches immediately below the level of the tracheal bifurcation. The right PA courses horizontally and ventrally to the primary bronchus in the mediastinum and the pulmonary hilum; the left PA courses superiorly and posteriorly to the primary bronchus.

The division of the pulmonary arteries follows that of the bronchi:

On the right side, the mediastinal artery of the upper lobe is constant.

On the left side, the culminal arteries run ventrally and medially to the bronchus; lingular arteries are more dorsal and lateral. A common trunk of the segmental arteries of the lower lobe is frequent.

The scissural arteries, originating from the corresponding lobar branch, are frequent, complements or substitutes of the corresponding "modal" segmental branch.

5.1.3 Technique

- Simple sedation.
- Systematic antibiotic prophylaxis if the context may cause infectious complications (dental care, ENT infections).
- Femoral venous access, alternating puncture sides when several sessions are necessary, to avoid peripheral venous complication.

- A selective bilateral pulmonary angiography, using a Grollman catheter in comparison to angio CT scan in order to define more precisely the size and the angio-architecture of the PAVM. The aneurysmal sac should not be directly embolized: an upstream occlusion of the feeding artery is to be attempted. So as to protect the healthy arterial branches originating from the efferent artery (and to avoid a large amputation of the pulmonary arterial bed), the vaso-occlusion must be as distal as possible but has also to take into account all the feeding arteries, even those of small size, to avoid a residual shunt.
  Larguable balloons have been used for a long time. Today a great majority of the authors prefer using steel coils, which must be carefully deployed to avoid gas embolism during release.
  An occlusion balloon can also be used to control the flow during coils' release in large feeding arteries with high flow rate.
  We willingly use Amplatzer Vascular Plug (AVP) occluders. The diameter of the plug must be oversized: at least 150 % of the feeding artery diameter. Angiographic controls via the introducer sheath, before the deployment, allow an optimal positioning. The length and diameter of the coils are determined by the pre-angiographic work-up. The occlusion must be complete, in order to avoid a recanalization in the center of the coils. These plugs have several advantages: precise and fast setup and good quality of the occlusion.
- Several sessions are necessary for 20–40 % of the patients, in order to obtain the exclusion of multiple PAVMs.

5.1.4 Results

The PAVM exclusion is obtained in almost all of the cases, rapidly followed by a correction of the hypoxemia.

Complications occur in less than 10 % of the patients such as per procedure embolic accidents (gas embolism, paradoxical embolism by occlusion material), thrombophlebitis at the puncture site, bacterial contamination of the thrombus, pleural effusion, post-procedure lung infarction in the days following, and secondary migration of spontaneously deflated larguable balloons (the reason why they are today abandoned).

The rapidity and the quality of the occlusion obtained using Amplatzer VP occluders contribute to limit the morbidity and obtain sustainable results.

The risk of an embolic relapse after embolization is low (5 %), in direct relation with the quality of the embolization techniques.

A CT scan control after 6–9 months is necessary: it depicts a diminishing aneurysmal sac; if it remains unchanged, one must look for a recanalization of the embolized branch, a persistent feeding by undiagnosed branches, or by a systemic artery.

The possibility of these reperfusions and/or growth in the size of untreated PAVMs requires to remain precautious with respect to the sustainability of a good technical result in patients suffering from HHT.

5.1.5 *Indications*

The vaso-occlusion, sparing the pulmonary parenchyma, is today considered to be the reference treatment for PAVM, indicated in three situations:

- Effort intolerance
- Prevention of neurological complications in patients having PAVMs with afferent artery's diameter superior or equal to 3 mm
- Prevention of hemorrhagic complications

Reports of emergency embolization due to the rupture of PAVM are exceptional.

Surgery may be required in isolated PAVM with a large, short, and proximal afferent pedicle, and in case of vaso-occlusive failure.

5.2 Other Indications of PA Embolization

They are rare. The risk of a rupture can lead to occlusion in the following situations:

- A posttraumatic false aneurysm, in particular iatrogenic trauma caused by the balloon of a Swan–Ganz catheter: embolization is required in emergency to treat a hemoptysis that can sometimes be of sudden onset. Inflation of the Swan–Ganz catheter (obstructing the arterial breach) can then be lifesaving, allowing the transfer of the patient to the angio suite. PA false aneurysms have also been reported after a radio-frequency tumor ablation.
- A Rasmussen's aneurysm, which is a rare but severe complication of tuberculosis.
- PA false aneurysms found in patients presenting Behcet's disease, for which embolization has been advocated in case of bilateral lesions.
- Neoplastic PA erosions.
- Infectious PA pseudoaneurysms (secondary to a septicemia/endocarditis or to a necrotizing pneumopathy such as tuberculosis or invasive aspergillosis).

Key Points

- PAVMs are at risk of systemic embolic neurological complications, of right-to-left shunt (especially for diffuse PAVM), and of hemorrhages.
- 60–90 % of them are congenital and are to be found in patients with the Rendu-Osler-Weber syndrome (HHT).
- Embolization must be carried out for fistulas with afferent artery diameter of more than 3 mm.

- As it is effective and safe in experienced hands and spares the pulmonary function, the complete vaso-occlusion by coils today is the standard of care for PAVMs and for PA aneurysms or false aneurysms.
- A CT is essential for the screening, the pre-therapeutic evaluation, and the follow-up that takes place 6–12 months after the embolization, in order to search for a reperfusion which can lead to a risk of recurrence.

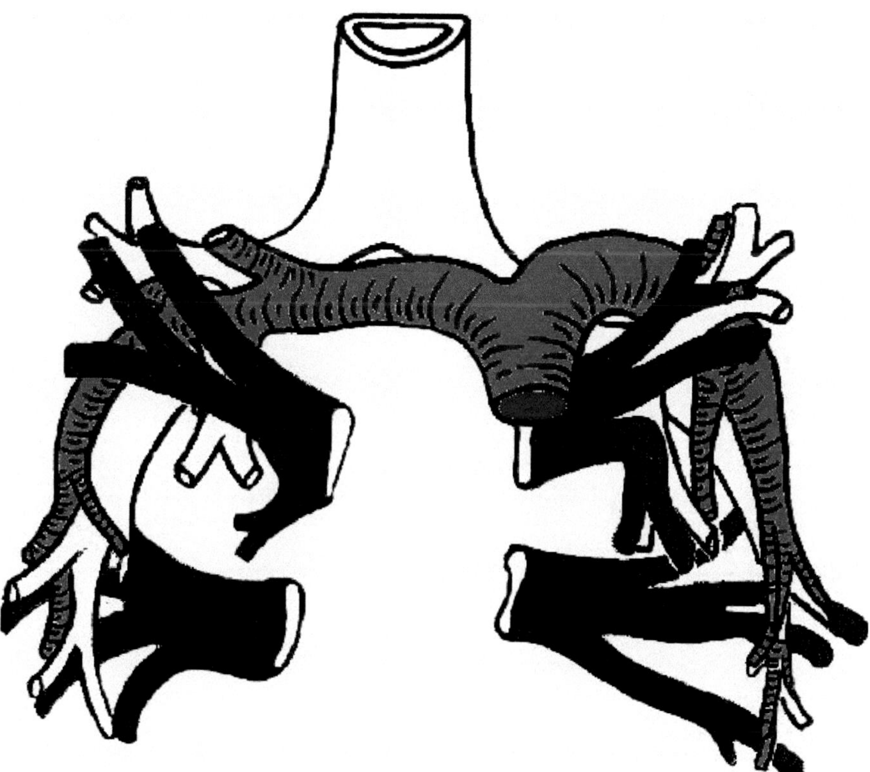

Fig. 5.1 Pulmonary pedicle (pulmonary arteries)

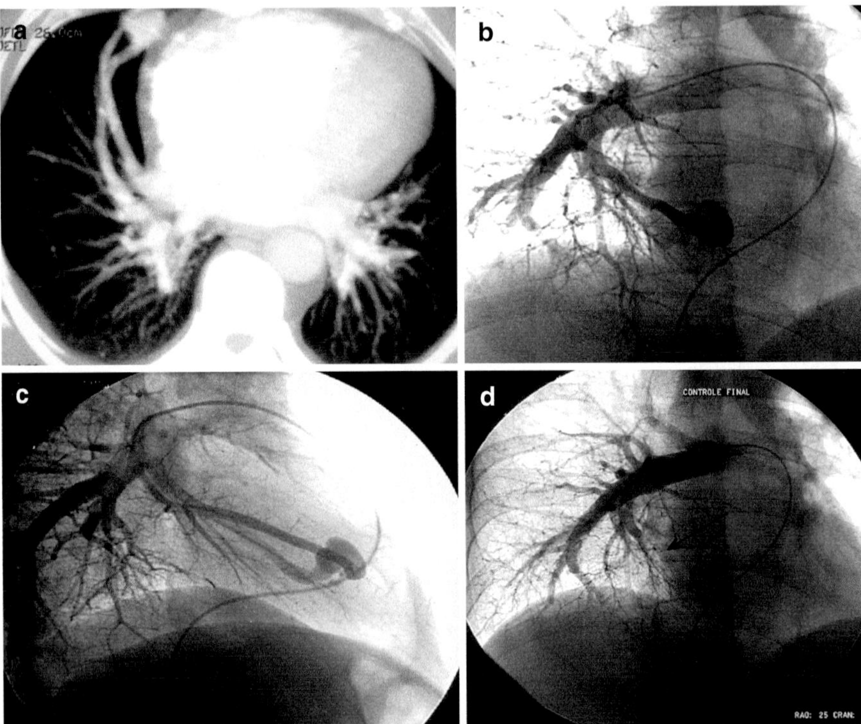

Fig. 5.2 Repeated hemoptysis, consequence of a bleeding single right basal PAVM. (**a**) Axial MIP thick CT scan: voluminous PAVM, with indentified afferent artery and efferent vein. (**b**, **c**) Pulmonary angiography (frontal (1–2) and lateral (1–3) views), well correlated with CT data: voluminous mediobasal feeding artery, large saccular aneurysm, and early venous flow. (**d**) Control angio after endovascular exclusion using AVP occluder, delivered just upstream the sac

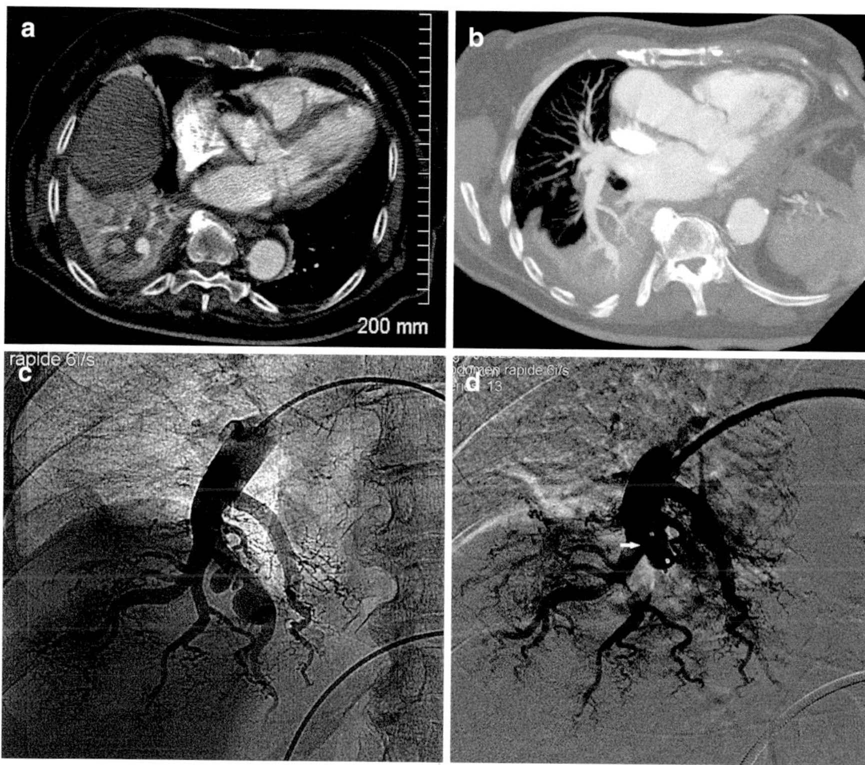

Fig. 5.3 Right basal bronchial cancer: massive hemoptysis. (**a**, **b**) CT: bleeding pulmonary, a false aneurysm. (**c**) Selective right pulmonary angiography: false aneurysm caused by tumoral erosion. (**d**) Exclusion with AVP (*arrow*)

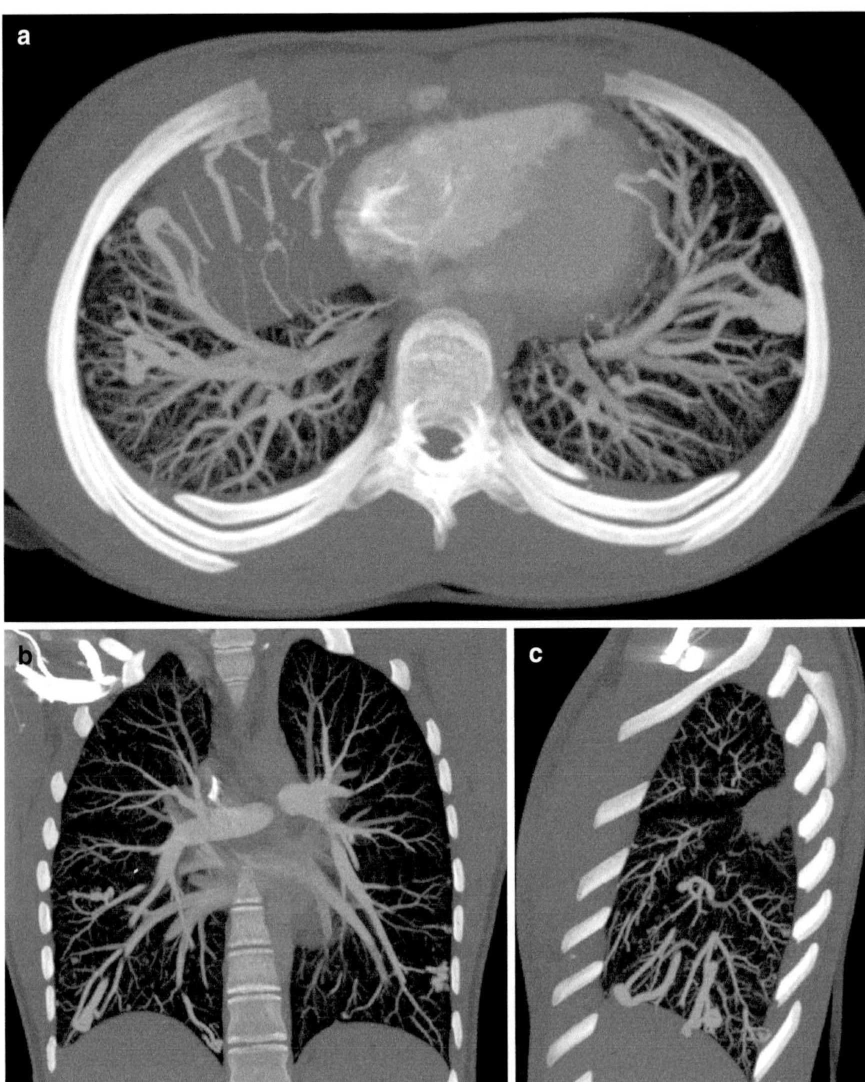

Fig. 5.4 16-year-old, family history of Rendu-Osler-Weber syndrome: hypoxia, severe left–right shunt, and pulmonary hypertension. (**a–c**) MIP: multiple PAVMs, of which the most voluminous in the right inferior lobe. (**d, e**) Right selective pulmonary angio: large middle lobe PAVM. Arterial phase (**d**) and then massive early venous flow (**e**). (**f**) Selective right inferior lobar injection: at least 2 other PAVMs. (**g**) First session: middle lobe PAVM AVP exclusion. Left shunts have been secondarily treated (delay between the 2 procedures: 2 months). (**h–j**) Angio CT 6 months after the last embolization session

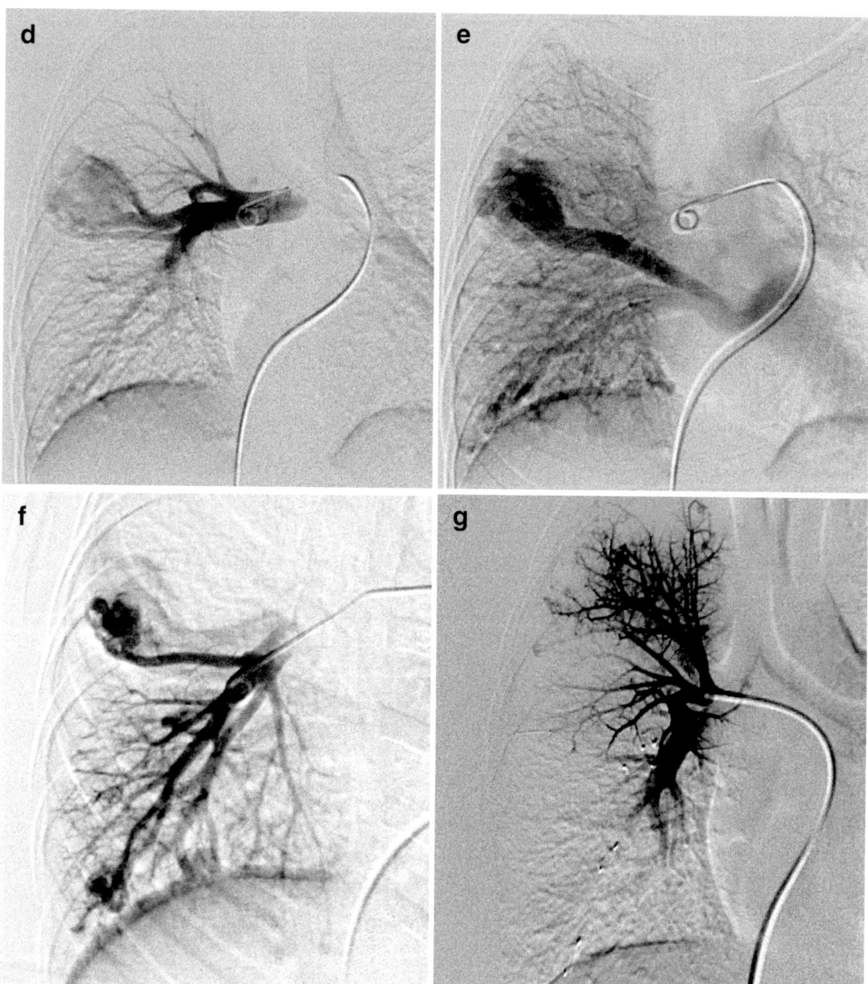

Fig. 5.4 (continued)

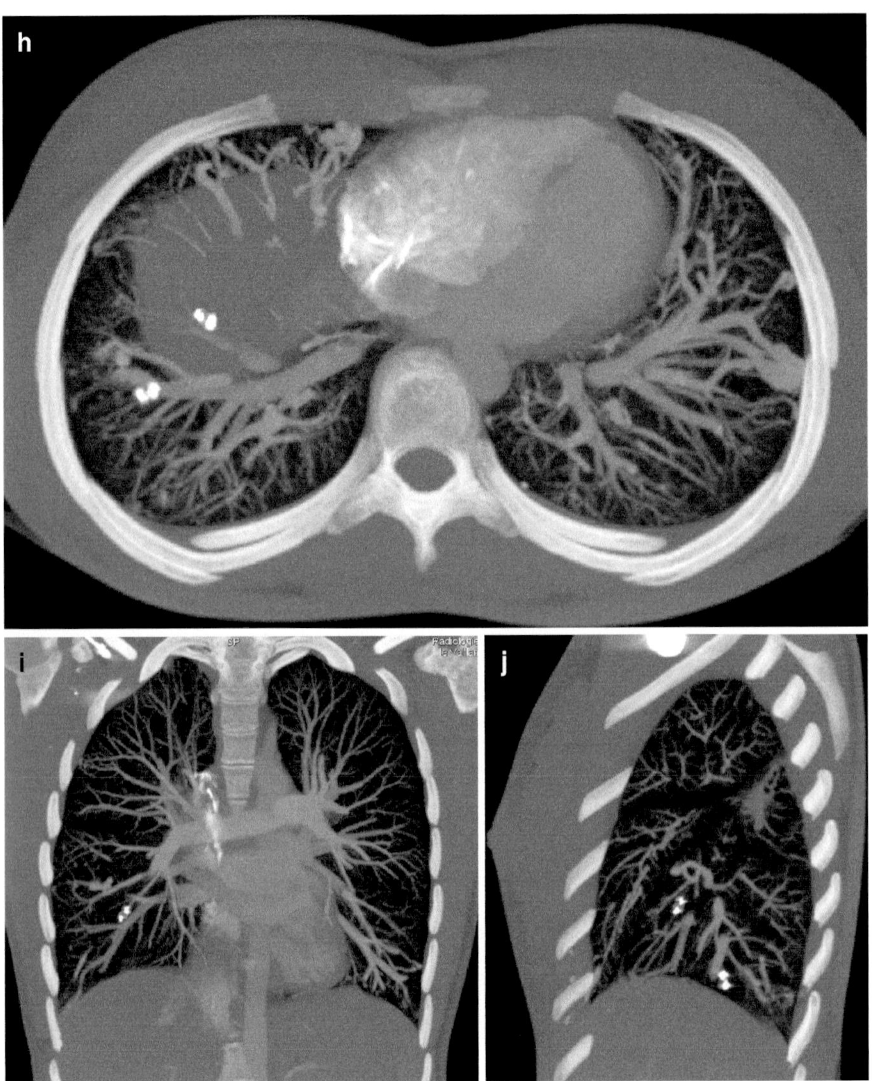

Fig. 5.4 (continued)

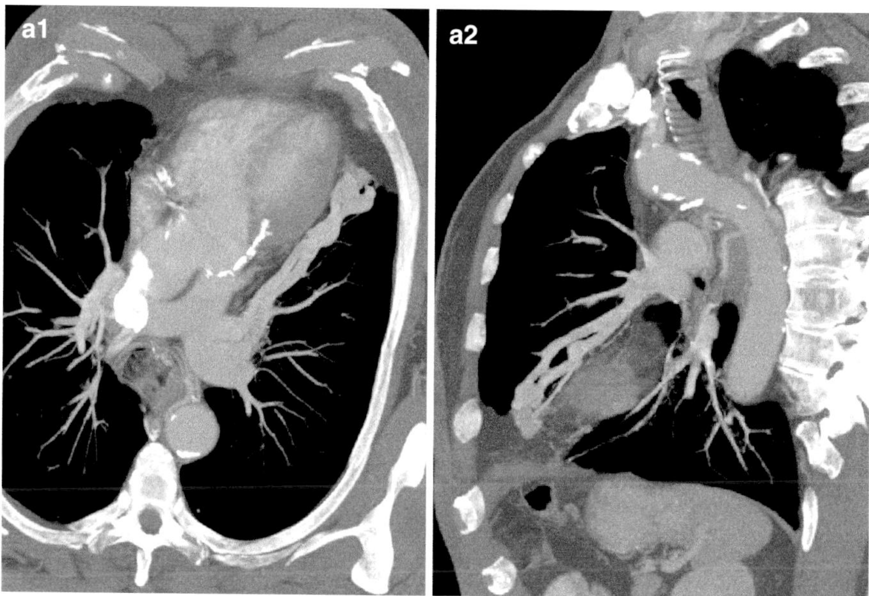

Fig. 5.5 72-year-old respiratory insufficient W, recurrent right base lung abscesses. On CT: voluminous lingular large AV shunt. The size of the shunt and the severity of hypoxia make an exclusion necessary. (**a**) CT MIP reconstruction. (**b**) Left PA injection (left anterior view): voluminous PA feeding a large PAVM sac. (**c**) Hyperselective lingular PA injection and calibration. (**d**) Control angio via the guiding catheter before AVP release. (**e**) Final pulmonary angiogram control

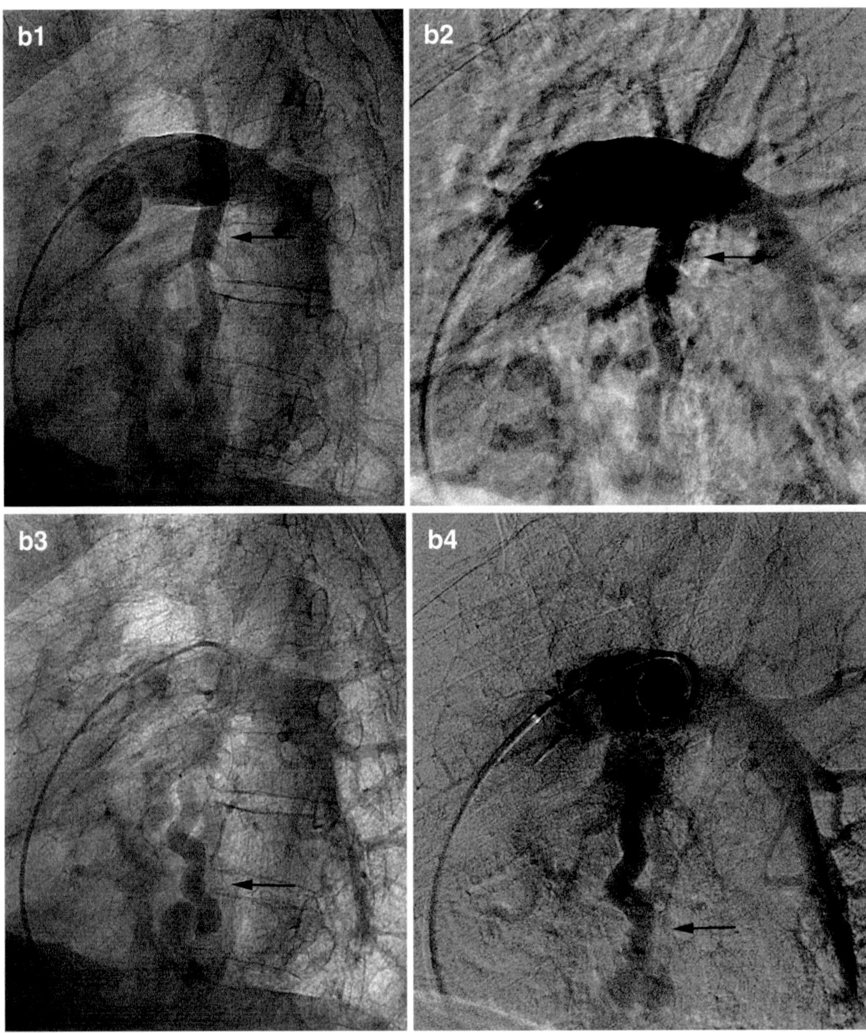

Fig. 5.5 (continued)

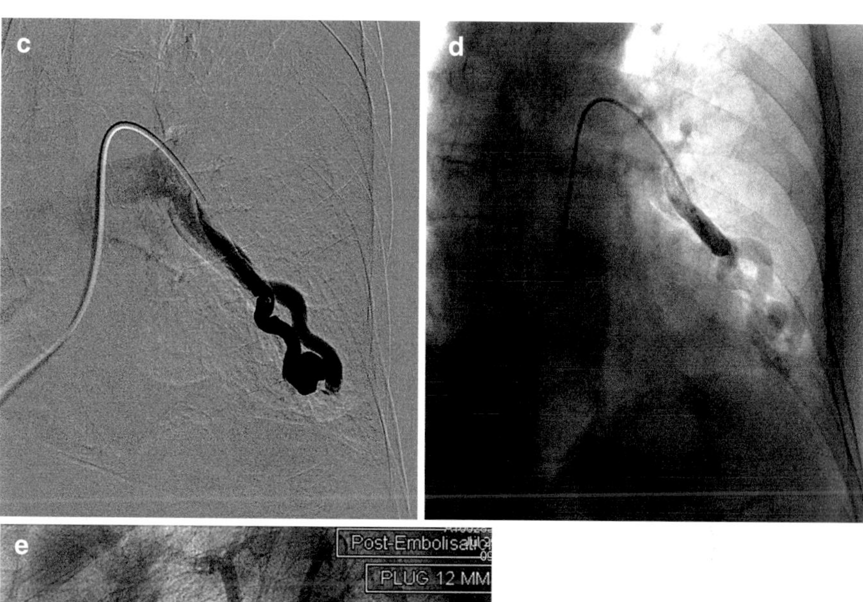

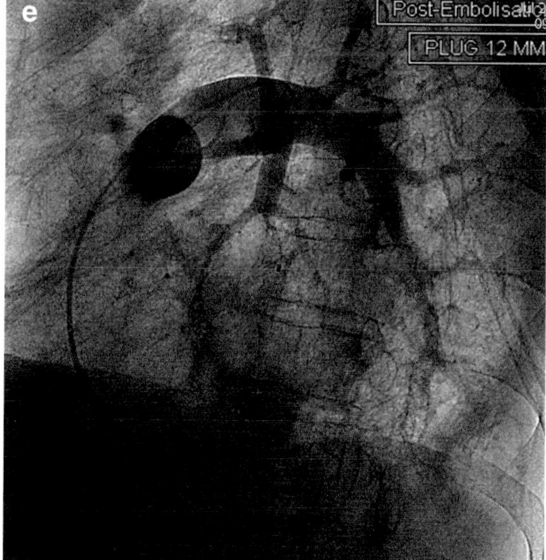

Fig. 5.5 (continued)

Suggested Reading

Chan RF, Faughnan M, White R. Pulmonary AV malformation treated with embolotherapy. Radiology. 2007;244(3):932.

Hart JL, Aldin Z, Braude P, et al. Embolization of pulmonary arteriovenous malformations using the Amplatzer vascular plug: successful treatment of 69 consecutive patients. Eur Radiol. 2010;20:2663–70.

Letourneau-Guillon L, Faughnan ME, Soulez G, et al. Embolization of pulmonary arteriovenous malformations with Amplatzer vascular plugs: safety and midterm effectiveness. J Vasc Interv Radiol. 2010;21:649–56.

Pelage JP, Lagrange C. Chinet T Embolisation des malformations artério veineuses pulmonaires localisées de l'adulte. J Radiol. 2007;88:367–76.

Remy J, Remy-Jardin M, Giraud F, et al. Angioarchitecture of pulmonary arteriovenous malformations: clinical utility of three-dimensional helical CT. Radiology. 1994;191:657–64.

Shovlin CL, Guttmacher AE, Buscarini E, et al. Diagnostic criteria for hereditary hemorrhagic telangiectasia (Rendu-Osler-Weber syndrome). Am J Med Genet. 2000;91:65–7.

Part IV
Situations and Strategies: Liver

Chapter 6
Hepatic Artery Embolizations

Louis Boyer, Emmanuel Buc, Denis Pezet, Tan Duc Vo, and Pascal Chabrot

6.1 Background

Embolization techniques are largely used to treat vascular and traumatic disease of hepatic arteries as well as hepatic tumors.

The specific rationale of each one of these situations will be developed in the paragraph (see Sec. 6.4)"indications and results." However, one must constantly keep in mind: — that the liver has a double afferent vascular supply, arterial and portal; — terminal arterial vascular bed; — and that the exclusion of the arterial flow even for large zones only rarely has functional hepatic consequences, as the liver is endowed with an important regeneration potential.

6.2 Relevant Radiological Anatomy

Hepatic artery usually originates from the celiac trunk, immediately below the medial arcuate ligament of the diaphragm, at the level of T12. The common hepatic artery, which is its right ending branch, then divides into the gastroduodenal and the proper hepatic arteries, the latter assuming the perfusion of the hepatic lobes through its left and right branches.

L. Boyer, MD, PhD (✉) • P. Chabrot, MD, PhD
Department of Radiology, University Hospital of Clermont-Ferrand, Clermont-Ferrand, France
e-mail: lboyer@chu-clermontferrand.fr; pchabrot@chu-clermontferrand.fr

E. Buc, MD, PhD • D. Pezet, MD, PhD
Department of Abdominal Surgery, University Hospital of Clermont-Ferrand, Clermont-Ferrand, France

T.D. Vo, MD
Department of Radiology, Medical Sciences University, Ho Chi Minh Ville, Viet Nam

P. Chabrot, L. Boyer (eds.), *Embolization*,
DOI 10.1007/978-1-4471-5182-1_6,

Arterial variations are frequent:

- Common hepatic artery originating directly from the aorta.
- Right hepatic branch originating from the superior mesenteric artery, in place of or in association with the normal right hepatic artery.
- Left hepatic artery originating from the left gastric artery.
- Proximal division of the proper hepatic artery with the left hepatic artery branching off before the gastroduodenal artery.

6.3 Technique

- The procedures are carried out in collaboration with an anesthesiologist.

Hepatic arterial embolization, no matter what the target, can rapidly be painful, and for the long interventions, abrupt movements linked to the pain can interfere with the continuation of the intervention.

The sedation starts in the angiographic room, at the time of the occlusion. It continues accordingly to patient's needs, ideally with a PCA pump (patient-controlled analgesia).

- An antibiotic prophylaxis targeted against cutaneous pathogens is recommended each time that the patient is at risk of an infarction which can lead to a significant volume of necrotic tissue.
- A preprocedure analysis of multislice imaging is very important in order to evaluate the vascular anatomy of arteries, portal and hepatic veins (with many of anatomic variants), and the status of the hepatic parenchyma and to define the arterial and portal vascularization of the embolization target. CT and/or MRI shows with precision and reliability the abnormal vascular supplies of the liver (tumor perfused by phrenic artery, internal thoracic artery, etc.) and eventually the development of collateral vessels.

The preprocedure localization of the ostia of the celiac trunk and of the superior mesenteric artery on multislice imaging can allow a rapid selective catheterization. In case of difficulty or in case of stenosis, lateral view aortogram can guide selective catheterization.

We systematically begin the procedure by a selective injection in the superior mesenteric artery, which allows us to detect or to confirm the branching off of a right hepatic artery branch, to ensure the patency of the portal vein and the direction of its flow.

A selective injection into the celiac trunk then allows us to confirm the layout of its terminal branches. The common hepatic artery is then selectively catheterized: an injection allows the localization of the gastroduodenal artery, the confirmation of the direction of its circulation, and eventually the detection of the cystic artery.

We routinely use the Michaëlson catheter or a Cobra catheter for the selective catheterizations of the celiac trunk and the superior mesenteric artery; a hydrophilic guide wire is introduced into the right or left hepatic arterial branches, on which can be pushed a straight or Cobra hydrophilic catheter, which allows the release of embolic agents, or the access to a microcatheter.

- The embolization agents used (which can be associated with other agents: drugs, Lipiodol, etc.) and the site of their release depend on the indication. In this chapter, we limit ourselves to simple bland embolizations; intra-arterial chemoembolizations and chemotherapy will be treated in Chap. 7.

Each embolization must be preceded by a selective injection to ensure the coverage of the entire target, to define the angioarchitecture, to study the pathologic vessels, and to detect eventual arterio-portal or hepatic artery-vein fistulas.

When embolizing tumors, it may be necessary to occlude first the branches which may be at the origin of bypass (and above all the gastroduodenal artery), so as to avoid any reflux, notably in the area of the gastroduodenal artery.

- In our group, the patient is then left fasting for 12 h. The hydration is adapted to the kidney function. The antibiotic prophylaxis is indicated in patients at risk (biliary-intestinal anastomosis, sphincterotomy, etc.).
  Fever is a common phenomenon after a tumor embolization, usually lasting for 48 h. It may be if necessary treated with antipyretics (paracetamol which must be used in respect to liver disease, or NSAID). The criteria allowing patient discharge in our center are pain control by oral medication (Visual Analog Pain Scale: EVA <3), if the temperature is inferior to 38 °C, and absence of discomfort when patient is re-fed.
- After each hepatic embolization, a morphological CT or MRI control is carried out; the delay depends on the indications (early and regular follow-up after traumatisms, 1-month follow-up for tumors). The subsequent strategy then depends on the results of these follow-up imagings.

6.4 Indications and Results

6.4.1 Liver Traumatisms

6.4.1.1 Indication

Hemorrhage spontaneously amends in at least 50 % of liver traumatisms.

Unstable patients (uncompensated hemorrhagic shocks) require surgery by laparotomy with hepatic packing. Surgery can also be required for associated visceral or peritoneal lesions.

One must therefore identify stable patients at risk of re-bleeding, in order to treat them by embolization.

- Embolization is indicated in case of active arterial bleeding on CT scan and in patients who are hemodynamically stable or who have had a compensated hemodynamic shock, no matter what the AAST injury grade is (see Appendix 6.1). In some reports, arteriography is recommended for patients with AAST grades 4 and 5 lesions.

Gelatin, coils, particles, or glue can be used.

Semi-proximal embolization using microcoils and/or gelatin sponge, sparing the anastomotic arterial network, reduces the risk of ischemic complication of the bile ducts. However, a proximal embolization can be insufficient in case of centro-hepatic arterial impairments, due to the hepatic arterial collaterality.

- A combined interventional radiology + surgery treatment can also be carried out: laparotomy allows homeostasis by packing and if necessary an appropriate complementary treatment for associated injuries; after suture closure, an arterial embolization can be performed.
- Embolization is not suitable for caval or portal venous bleedings, which are indications for surgery.

6.4.1.2 Results

- The success rate for hepatic arterial embolization varies from 80 to 100 %. A second embolization is rarely needed.
- Mortality for isolated liver lesions does not exceed 10 %, but liver injuries can occur in a polytraumatic context with higher mortality rates.
- The main complication is ischemic cholecystitis due to embolization of the cystic artery, a condition which is in fact frequently asymptomatic.
- In the specific case of hepatic arterial embolization for postsurgical hemorrhage (pancreatic or liver surgery), the absence of collateral pathways favors a hepatic failure during the follow-up [1].

6.4.2 Aneurysms of Hepatic Artery (See also Chap. 9)

Eighty percent of the aneurysms of the hepatic artery concern its extrahepatic proximal segment and therefore revealed by a hemoperitoneum. Other circumstances leading to such a diagnosis are GI hemorrhage, hemobilia (cf. Chap. 8), or incidental finding.

6.4.2.1 Technique (See also Chaps. 8 and 9)

Depending on the angioarchitecture, several options are available: parent vessel occlusion, packing, thrombin injection, exclusion of the aneurysmal segment by a covered stent or a multilayer stent (flow diverter), or the combination of a surgical bypass prior to an endovascular occlusion.

6.4.2.2 Results

Only small series have been published.

Successful results are obtained in 60–90 % of the cases, with few complications; however, technical failures are possible, as well as accidental migration of embolization agent and preprocedure rupture (notably in case of false aneurysm).

Exclusions of hepatic arterial aneurysms are generally well tolerated, except in the case of an associated occlusion of the portal flow, which is possible after severe hepatic traumatisms. Ischemic tolerance problems can also be observed when there is a history of hepatobiliary surgery, notably of bile duct dissections and even more so of biliary-intestinal anastomosis, and in the postoperative period after hepatectomy.

Imaging follow-up is recommended, notably in cases of false aneurysms, so as to eliminate reperfusions, which are not exceptional. In our team, a cross-sectional imaging (CT or MRI) is carried out at 1 month and at 1 year after the procedure.

6.4.2.3 Indications

- In case of ruptured aneurysm, the mortality rate for the surgical series remains high (at least 25 %); therefore, endovascular treatment can be an alternative after taking into account the configuration of the lesions, the experience, and the availability of operator. By carrying out an upstream occlusion with a temporary balloon first, one can limit the amount of blood loss during the exclusion of the ruptured aneurysm.
- Excluding Emergency Situations
  Arteriography is essential to decide the therapeutic indications, but it only gives information on luminography and thus must always be preceded by CT (which is our preference) or MRI.
  - False aneurysms must always be treated, without delay, no matter what their size. Endovascular treatment is the first-line treatment.
  - Aneurysms: According to the 2006 recommendations of AHA, prophylactic treatment of aneurysms rupture is indicated when their diameter is of 2 cm or more, in women of childbearing age (to be performed outside of any pregnancy) (class I, level of evidence B).

The treatment of visceral aneurysms of more than 2 cm, according to the same recommendations, is "probably indicated" in older women and in men (class IIa, level of evidence B). When it is possible, endovascular techniques are often the first-line treatment. Their low morbidity has led to proposals of lowering this threshold of 2 cm and taking into account the diameter of the parent artery. A critical threshold should therefore be considered over twice the diameter of the parent artery. With this threshold, one would be able to treat aneurysms of 20 mm or less: — especially in young patients and in women of childbearing age who have a desire of pregnancy;

— when these aneurysms are symptomatic; — in the case of dissecting aneurysms or *with distal embolizations*; — if there is an obvious increase in size shown during imaging follow up: — and for hepatic aneurysms in the cases of periarthritis nodosa or of fibromuscular dysplasia. Hence the therapeutic indications are not totally clear: therefore, all of the alternatives must be discussed.

- In the case of therapeutic abstention, imaging follow-up is mandatory; we carry out a yearly multislice imaging control.

6.4.3 Spontaneous Hemoperitoneum of Hepatic Origin

In the absence of aneurysm, traumatism, or anticoagulation treatment, a spontaneous hepatic bleeding is rare. It is in general a complication of a hypervascular liver tumor.

- *HCC:* Large subcapsular tumors are the most susceptible to bleed.

Clinically, a hemodynamic shock is common, associated with hepatalgia when the bleeding is contained in the capsule.

Ultrasound and above all CT can show intrahepatic and/or subcapsular hematoma, eventually intraperitoneal hematoma; it can localize a blush and sometimes reveals an underlying hepatopathy. Visualization of the primitive tumor is not systematic.

In this unfavorable context for surgery, embolization is a first choice treatment.

- *Adenomas:* The context is different: women of childbearing age, often having a prolonged history of estroprogestative contraception.

With respect to imaging, the framework is quite similar than previously described with HCC, but without the underlying hepatopathy.

A selective embolization, when it is possible, is an interesting therapeutic option rather than emergency surgery.

- The spontaneous rupture of the *focal nodular hyperplasia* is rare, and it is difficult to diagnose given the presence of necrotic changes.
- *Angiomas:* Situations with major risks of rupture are pregnancy, preeclampsia, or the use of cocaine.

  The typical angioma radiological semiology is modified by the hematoma. Selective embolization is an interesting therapeutic option.

- *Liver Metastases:*
  Hemoperitoneum is rare, observed with the following primary tumors: bronchial, renal colonic, pancreatic, vesicular, testicular, and melanomas.

Subcapsular localization, large tumor or necrosis, hemostasis disorders, and intra-abdominal hyperpression (cough, defecation) are all risk factors for rupture.

Embolization allows a rapid palliative hemostasis.

- *HELLP Syndrome:*
  Hemolysis, elevated liver enzymes, and low platelet count, found in a context of preeclampsia or eclampsia, characterize this syndrome which comes about before or immediately after delivery and can be complicated by DIC, hepatic necrosis, and hemorrhagic infarction.

Clinically, pain in the right hypochondrium usually leads to the discovery of a subcapsular and/or intrahepatic hematoma, with an eventual hepatic rupture and intraperitoneal hemorrhage. Peripheral hepatic infarctions can also be observed.

6.4.4 Bland Embolization of Liver Tumors Excluding Hemorrhaging Situations

6.4.4.1 Indications

In some cases, liver tumors cannot be surgically resected in respect to intrahepatic growth, patient's clinical status, or the risk of liver decompensation. Intra-arterial chemotherapy or chemoembolization techniques (which will be developed in Chap. 7) can however be sometimes indicated. In the same context, bland embolizations can also be realized to treat hypervascular benign or malignant (primary or secondary) tumors which are fed by an afferent artery and characterized by an intense contrast enhancement at the arterial phase, on a CT angiography or a dynamic angio-MRI but with variable patterns on the portal and late phases: persistent enhancement, early washout, etc.

- Unresectable HCC occurring on Child A and B7 cirrhosis can be embolized (Child C stage is not an indication). Selection criteria are similar to those used for the chemoembolization (see Chap. 7). The superiority of chemoembolization with respect to bland embolization remains controversial for some authors. Simple bland embolization has as the advantage to spare hepatic artery patency. The meta-analysis (1978–2002) of Llovet and Bruix [2] comparing chemoembolization versus conservative treatment found a significant 2-year improvement survival with chemoembolization but not with bland embolization. Recent findings [3] however suggest that the hypoxia induced by the arterial embolization can activate growth factors such as the vascular endothelial growth factor (VEGF), leading to a tumor growth. Occlusion has to be performed as distally as possible, inducing necrosis of the tumor. There is no formal consensus concerning the optimal embolization agent, but if gelatin and PVA have been used for a long time, particles of a reduced diameter (100–300 μ) are nowadays preferred.

- *Hypervascular liver metastases* of endocrine, gastrointestinal stromal tumors, as well as sarcoma, ocular melanoma, and breast/kidney/prostate tumors can also be embolized.

Embolization can be chosen to treat a unique metastasis.

It may also be a palliative treatment for symptomatic or secreting metastases: with some metastatic endocrine tumors, the symptoms can be linked to hepatic secreting metastases, even though the original tumor is very small.

These embolizations of endocrine liver metastases or of other origins in noncirrhotic patients are certainly not indicated if more than 75 % of the hepatic parenchyma is concerned by the tumor; however, should these patients be treated, notably to ameliorate the endocrine syndrome, the embolization must be carried out in 2 or more sessions.

- One must not expect favorable outcomes concerning arterial ischemia when embolizing hypovascular tumors such as secondary hepatic localizations of most GI tract tumors.
- As indicated in Chap. 7, randomized trials comparing embolization and chemoembolizations of malignant liver tumors other than HCC are necessary to prove the interest of associated use of chemotherapy (with its own toxic potential) with embolization.
- *FNH* [4]
  There are reports of embolization of non-resectable FNHs responsible for pain symptoms.
- *Adenomas* [5–8]
  Besides hemostatic embolization to treat a hemorrhagic complication, adenomas must be treated as they can degenerate. Surgical resection is the first-line treatment. Embolization has however been reported for tumoral volume reduction, in inoperable and/or symptomatic patients as a first-line treatment or after hemostatic embolization, to treat isolated adenomas or multiple hepatic adenomatosis.

6.4.4.2 Results

- A post-embolization syndrome is very frequent (80 %), associating pain, fever, nausea, and vomiting: this must be considered as a collateral effect and not as a complication and treated for 2–3 days by analgesics, antipyretics, and antiemetics.

- The embolization of the cystic artery can cause an extended post-embolization syndrome. A vesicular transhepatic percutaneous drainage can be discussed as an alternative to a cholecystectomy when confronted with these ischemic cholecystitises.
- *A liver abscess* is a rare complication, occurring between 7 and 10 days after embolization. It appears most frequently in patients with bilio-intestinal anastomoses or when the sphincter of Oddi is not intact (in particular after a sphincterotomy). A change in patients' general status, a fever, or a hyperleukocytosis are indications for an imaging exploration (keeping in mind that the hypodense layers with little bubbles constitute a normal pattern immediately after embolization).

In patients at risk (bilio-intestinal anastomosis, sphincterotomy), a prophylactic antibiotic therapy is mandatory.

Key Points

- Before embolization: arterial and portal cartography, angioarchitecture of the lesions, detection of arterio-portal fistulas, or hepatic arteriovenous fistulas.
- Liver traumas: arterial embolization is efficient on arterial bleeding; it is indicated in hemodynamically stable patients who have an active bleeding on the CT scan; bleeding caused by portal, hepatic, or caval veins is an indication for surgical treatment.
- Hepatic aneurysms: endovascular methods are today the first-line treatment; AHA recommendations: threshold = 2 cm, but smaller aneurysms can in some cases be treated.
- Spontaneous hemoperitoneum evokes a hypervascular tumor; excellent indication of embolization in case of hemorrhagic HCCs, metastases, and angiomas.
- Bland embolization can also concern non-resectable HCC, hypervascular metastases (if they take up less than 75 % of the parenchyma), painful non-resectable FNHs, adenomas in inoperable patients, or in case of multiple adenomatosis.
- Post-embolization syndrome is very frequent: if extended, it must lead one to think of an ischemic cholecystitis by occlusion of the cystic artery.
- A liver abscess appearing 7–10 days after the embolization can be seen, most notably in cases of bilio-intestinal anastomoses or after a sphincterotomy: these particular cases justify an antibiotic prophylaxis.

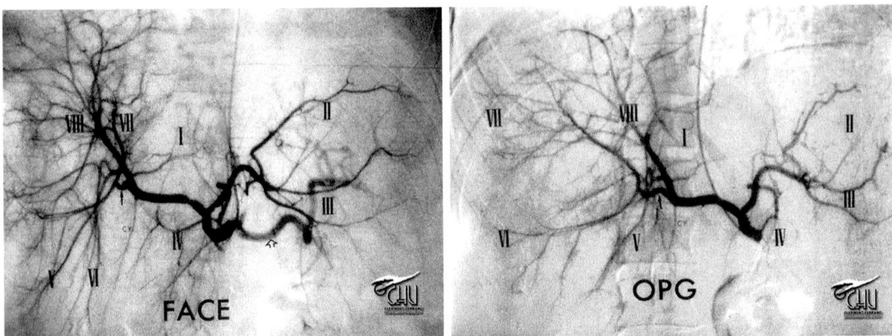

Fig. 6.1 Arterial segmentation of the liver (selective injection of the CT via a humeral access, front and left oblique posterior view) (Courtesy Pr JL Lamarque)

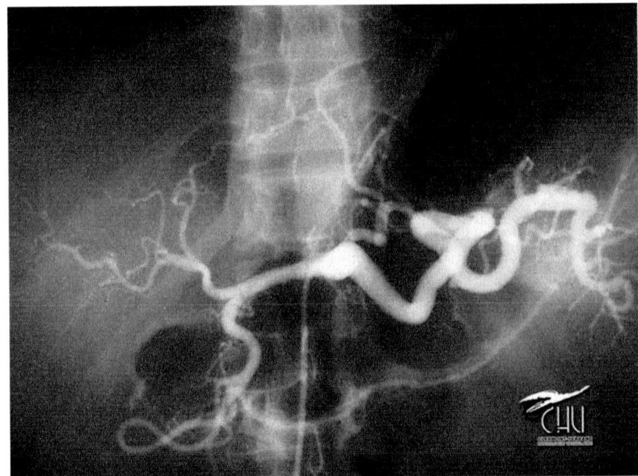

Fig. 6.2 Selective injection of the CT via a femoral access (Courtesy Pr JF Viallet)

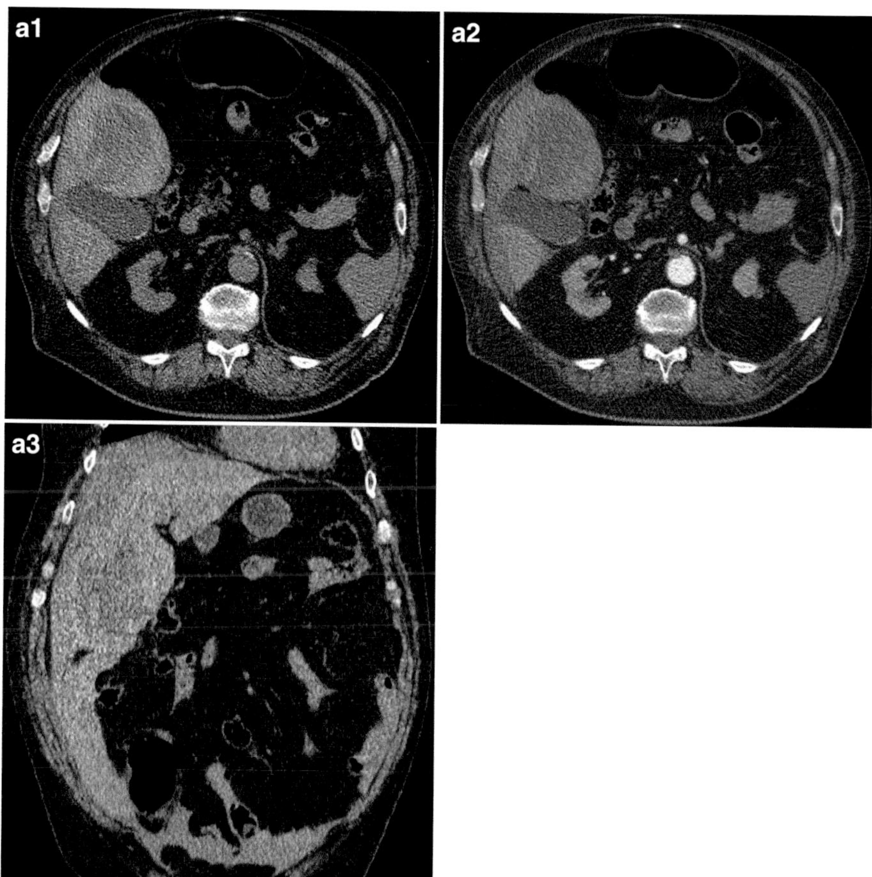

Fig. 6.3 68-year-old male, violent right hypochondrium pain: CT. (**a**) Subcapsular hematoma of the liver, heterogeneous segment V mass spontaneously hyperdense: these data and a clinical hypovolemic collapsus led to perform in emergency an angio. (**b**) Proper hepatic A selective injection: the liver is far from the abdominal wall; old costal fracture callus; heterogen hepatography. (**c**) Hyperselective segment VIII branch (arterial branch injection): massive extravasation, consequence of a hemorrhagic tumoral rupture; embolization using microparticles completed with Gelfoam. (**d**) Clinical aftereffects were simple; CT control 1 m later: residual hyperdensity inside a hypodense tumor. (**e**) Same CT: not any other tumor focus

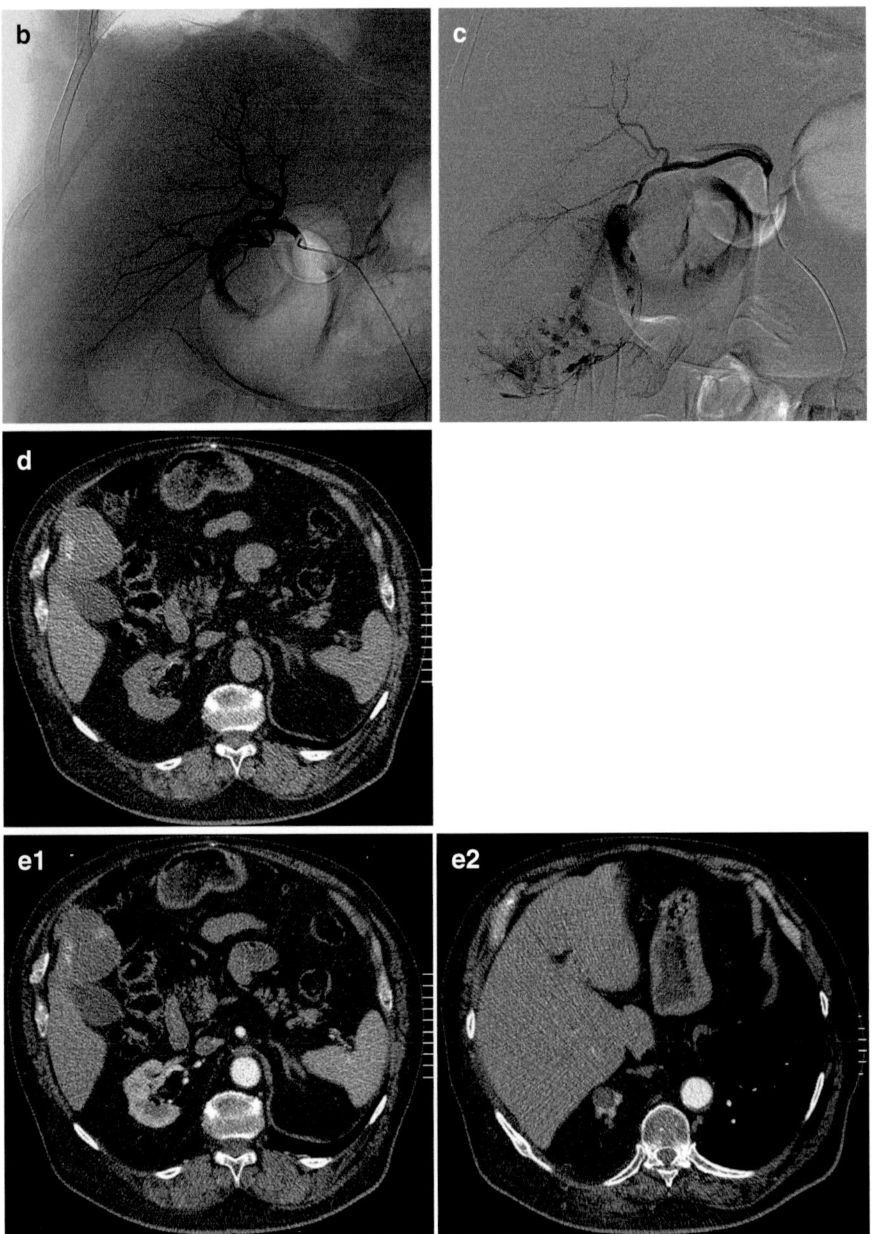

Fig. 6.3 (continued)

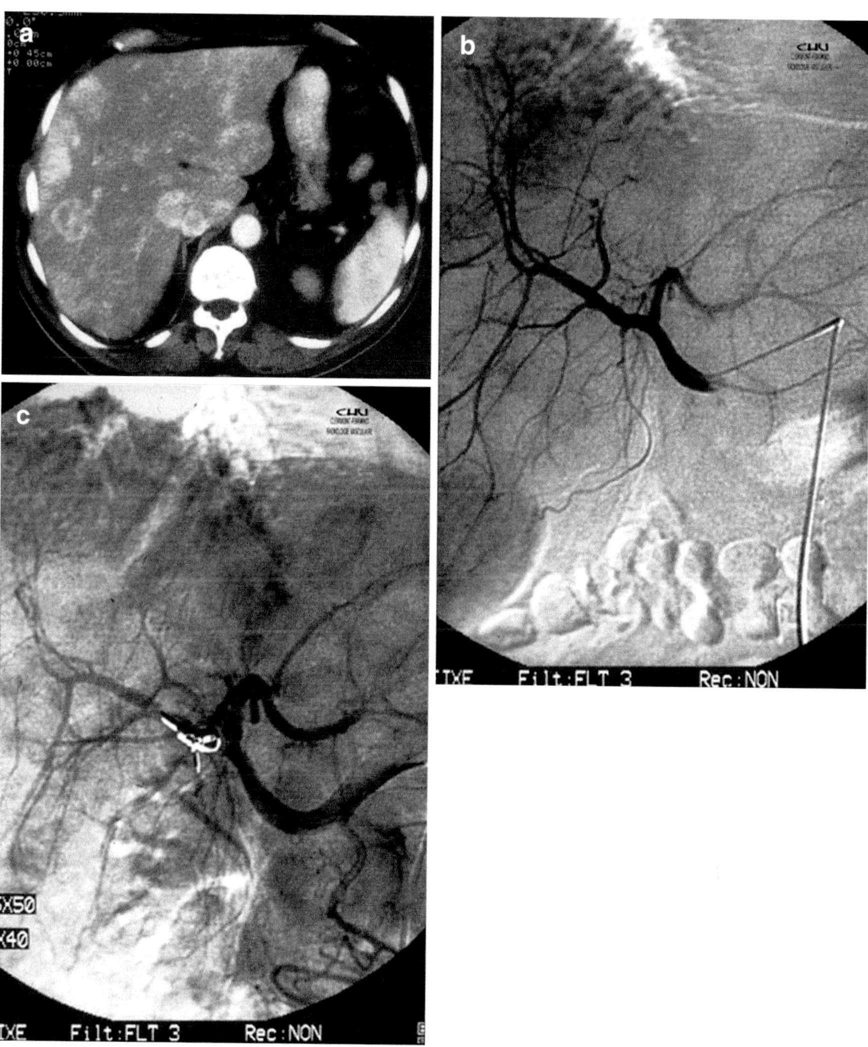

Fig. 6.4 Carcinoid secreting liver metastasis (primitive tumor unknown). Severe flushes led to decide an embolization to treat these symptoms. (**a**) Multiple hypervascular metastases. (**b**) Selective hepatic A injection. (**c**) CT scan after arterial tumoral-feeding microparticles embolization

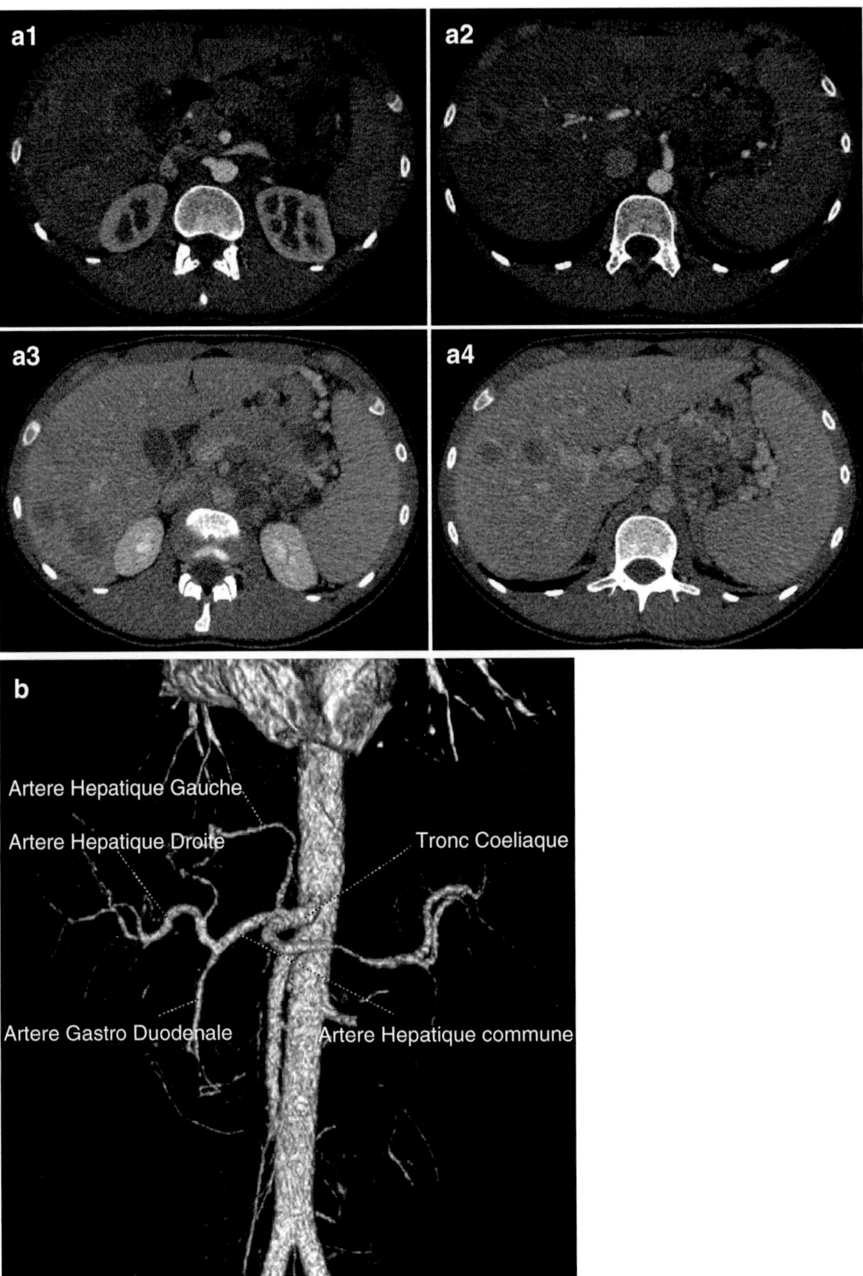

Fig. 6.5 21 years old, malignant pancreatic insulinoma surgically treated, multiple liver metastases. A complementary embolization has been decided to try to normalize the glycemia. (**a**) Multiple liver hypervascular metastases, among which some are heterogeneous. (**b**) CT angio: origin of the left hepatic A from the CT. (**c**) Selective catheterization of the right hepatic A, arterial and late phases: heterogeneous hepatography. Lateral and medial right liver sector particles embolization. (**d**) CT 5 weeks later: relative devascularization of the right masses; persistent segment IV hypervascularization and enhanced left liver metastasis. (**e**) Recurrence of hypoglycemias led to a re-embolization. Semi-selective injection of the CT: relative devascularization of the right liver, patent segment IV, and left hepatic A

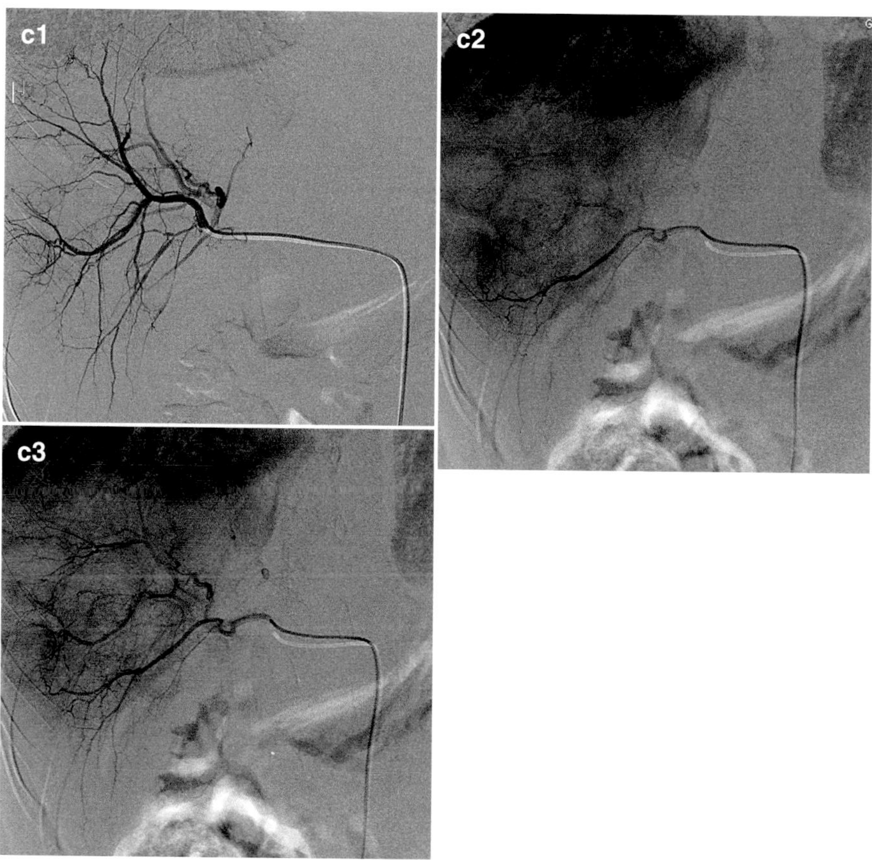

Fig. 6.5 (continued)

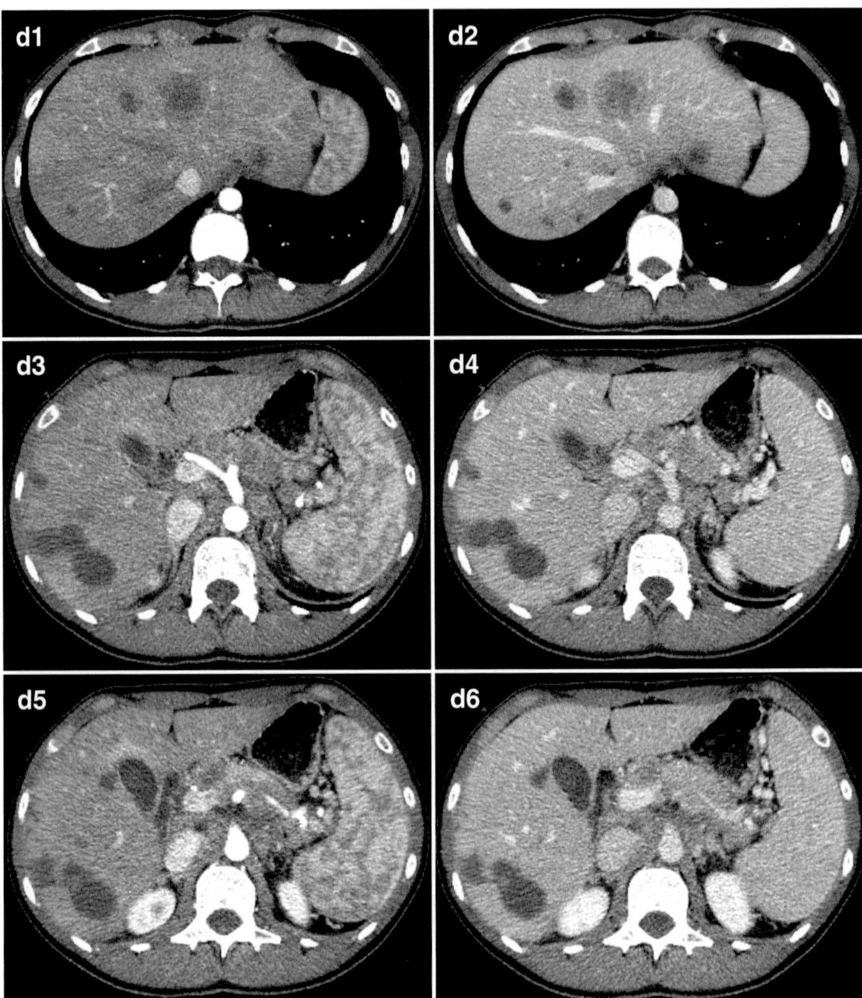

Fig. 6.5 (continued)

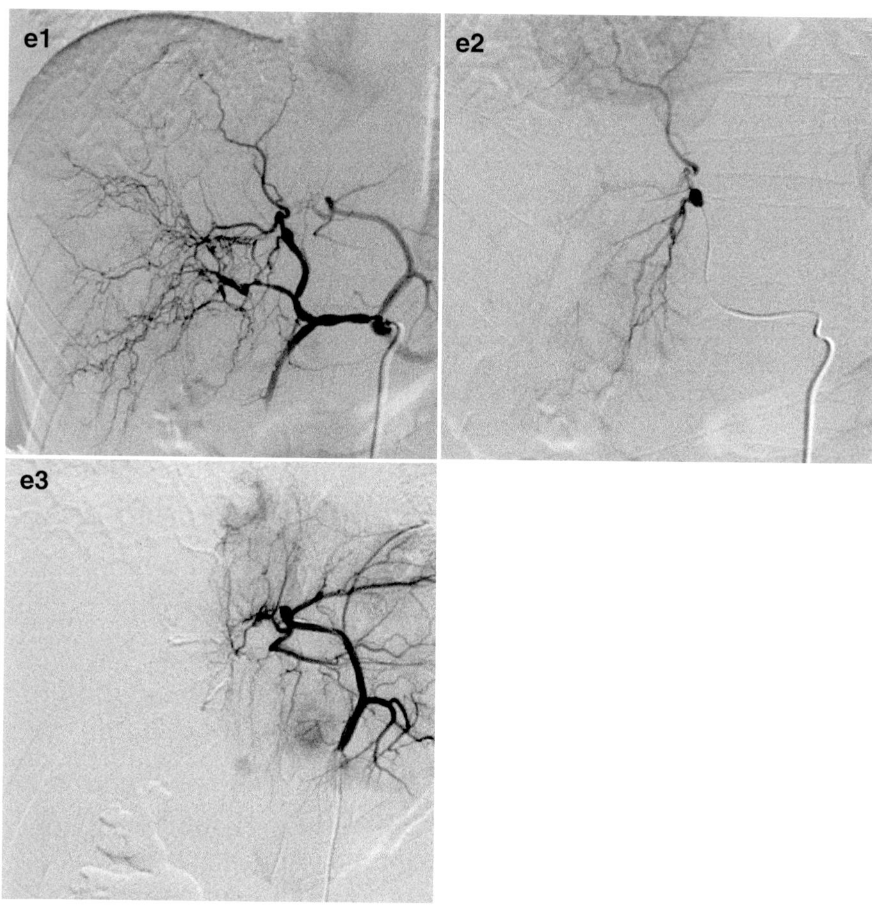

Fig. 6.5 (continued)

Appendix: Liver Trauma: AAST Classification [9]

Grade[a]	Type of injury	Description of injuries	AIS
I	Hematoma	Subcapsular, <10 % of surface area	2
	Laceration	Capsular tear, <1 cm of parenchymal depth	2
II	Hematoma	Subcapsular, 10–50 % surface area: intraparenchymal <10 cm in diameter	2
	Laceration	Capsular tear: 1–3 cm parenchymal depth, <10 cm length	2
III	Hematoma	Subcapsular, >50 % surface area of ruptured subcapsular, or parenchymal hematoma	3
	Laceration	Intraparenchymal hematoma >10 cm or expanding >3 cm of parenchymal depth	3
IV	Laceration	Parenchymal disruption involving 25–75 % hepatic lobe or 1–3 Couinaud's segments	4
V	Laceration	Parenchymal disruption involving >75 % of hepatic lobe or >3 Couinaud's segments within a single lobe	5
	Vascular	Juxtahepatic venous injuries, i.e., retrohepatic vena cava/ central major hepatic veins	5
VI	Vascular	Hepatic avulsion	6

AIS: Abbreviated Injury Scale
[a]Advance one grade for bilateral injuries up to grade III

References

1. Sato A, Yamada T, Takase K, et al. The fatal risk in hepatic artery embolization for hemostasis after pancreatic and hepatic surgery: importance of collateral arterial pathways. J Vasc Interv Radiol. 2011;22:287–93.
2. Llovet JM, Bruix J. A systematic review of randomized trials for unresectable hepatocellular carcinoma chemoembolization improves survival. Hepatology. 2003;37:429–42.
3. Liapi E, Geschwind JFH. Intra-arterial therapies for hepatocellular carcinoma: where do we stand? Ann Surg Oncol. 2010;17:1234–46.
4. Amesur N, Hammond JS, Zajko AB, et al. Management of unresectable symptomatic focal nodular hyperplasia with arterial embolization. J Vasc Interv Radiol. 2009;20:543–7.
5. Kim IY, Chung JW, Park JH. Feasibility of transcatheter arterial chemoembolization for hepatic adenoma. J Vasc Interv Radiol. 2007;18:862–7.
6. Lee SH, Hahn ST. Treatment of multiple hepatic adenomatosis using transarterial chemoembolization. Cardiovasc Intervent Radiol. 2004;27:563–5.
7. Erdogan D, Van Delden OM, Busch ORC, Gouma DJ, van Gulik TM. Selective transcatheter arterial embolization for treatment of bleeding complications or reduction of tumor mass of hepatocellular adenomas. Cardiovasc Intervent Radiol. 2007;30:1252–8.
8. Deodhar A, Brody LA, Covey AM, Brown KT, Getrajdman GI. Bland embolization in the treatment of hepatic adenomas: preliminary experience. J Vasc Interv Radiol. 2011;22:795–9.
9. Tinkoff G, Esposito TJ, Reed J, et al. American Association for the Surgery of Trauma organ injury scale 1: spleen, liver and kidney, validation based on the national data bank. J Am Coll Surg. 2008;207:646–55.

Suggested Reading

Liapi E, Geschwind JFH. Intra-arterial therapies for hepatocellular carcinoma: where do we stand? Ann Surg Oncol. 2010;17:1234–46.

Llovet JM, Bruix J. A systematic review of randomized trials for unresectable hepatocellular carcinoma chemoembolization improves survival. Hepatology. 2003;37:429–42.

Monnin V, Sengel C, Thony F, et al. Place of arterial embolization in severe blunt hepatic trauma: a multidisciplinary approach. Cardiovasc Intervent Radiol. 2008;31:875–82.

Otal P, Auriol J, Chabbert V, et al. Urgences vasculaires: prise en charge des états de choc hémorragiques. In: Taourel P, Schouman-Claeys E, editors. Imagerie des urgences. SFR éd; Paris, 2008.

Tinkoff G, Esposito TJ, Reed J, et al. American Association for the Surgery of Trauma organ injury scale 1: spleen, liver and kidney, validation based on the national data bank. J Am Coll Surg. 2008;207:646–55.

Chapter 7
Chemoembolizations and Hepatic Intra-arterial Chemotherapies

Pascal Chabrot, Agaïcha Alfidja Lankoande, Eric Dumousset, Armand Abergel, Denis Pezet, and Louis Boyer

Intra-arterial chemoembolization allows the administration of embolic agents and/or drugs to treat arterialized liver tumors, thus reducing the systemic side effects and sparing the disease-free liver parenchyma. Various techniques can be performed: transarterial embolization (TAE), transcatheter arterial chemo-infusion (TACI) with a high concentration of chemotherapy agents and minimal embolization, transarterial chemoembolization (TACE), and chemoembolization with drug-eluting beads (DEB TACE). Irradiation techniques are also therapeutic alternatives such as radioembolization with yttrium 90 and injection of radioactive Lipiodol (I 131): these highly specialized techniques are at the crossroads of interventional radiology, nuclear medicine, and radiotherapy, thus will not be developed in this chapter.

7.1 Hepatocellular Carcinoma (HCC)

7.1.1 Background

The incidence of HCC is high in sub-Saharan Africa and in Southeast Asia but is also increasing in the Western countries due to the high number of viral cirrhosis.

L. Boyer, MD, PhD (✉) • P. Chabrot, MD, PhD • E. Dumousset, MD • A.A. Lankoande, MD
Department of Radiology, University Hospital of Clermont-Ferrand, Clermont-Ferrand, France
e-mail: lboyer@chu-clermontferrand.fr; pchabrot@chu-clermontferrand.fr

A. Abergel, MD, PhD
Department of Hepatogastroenterology, University Hospital of Clermont-Ferrand, Clermont-Ferrand, France

D. Pezet, MD, PhD
Department of Abdominal Surgery, University Hospital of Clermont-Ferrand, Clermont-Ferrand, France

P. Chabrot, L. Boyer (eds.), *Embolization*,
DOI 10.1007/978-1-4471-5182-1_7, © Springer-Verlag London 2014

Nowadays, the diagnosis of HCC is based on biopsy for lesions occurring in non-cirrhotic liver, and by the updated Barcelona criteria otherwise (AASLD 2010 recommendations) [1, 2], a supra-centimetric nodule with arterial wash-in and portal washout on a contrast-enhanced imaging (CT or MRI) is considered as an HCC. In case of atypical findings on one imaging modality (MRI or CT), confirmation must be obtained with the other technique. If both imaging techniques are inconsistent with HCC, then the lesion must be biopsied. For nodules of less than 1 cm, a follow-up imaging is recommended after 3 months. A cirrhotic liver is characterized by morphological modifications (lobulated contours, dysmorphy due to modifications of the volume ratios of hepatic segments), more or less associated with cirrhotic nodules, modifications of liver signal (steatosis, iron overload), and complications (ascites, portal hypertension, etc.).

The staging of the disease is essential in defining therapeutic indications: number, size, localization of the lesions, portal and/or hepatic vein invasion, and status of tumor-free liver. According to the Barcelona Clinic Liver Classification (BCLC) treatment algorithm [3–5], surgery (resection and transplantation) and percutaneous tumor ablation techniques constitute the curative treatments for HCC. Only about one third of the patients are eligible for a curative treatment. Surgery is indicated for patients with a preserved liver function and a limited number of lesions. Transplantation is also recommended in patients with liver failure, as long as the Milan criteria are respected: a unique tumor of less than 5 cm and 1–3 lesions of less than 3 cm [6]. Percutaneous ablation is indicated in patients with few tumors (less than 3) of less than 3 cm.

Palliative treatments such as intra-arterial therapies are indicated in patients with a preserved liver function for which percutaneous ablations (radiofrequency, alcohol injection) are not possible due to the excessive number, the size, and/or the localization of the lesions.

7.1.2 Relevant Radiological Anatomy: *See Chap. 6*

7.1.3 Techniques

- *Hepatic intra-arterial chemotherapy*: Its aim is to increase the concentration of the electively administrated drugs in the targeted lesions, thus diminishing the general systemic effects of chemotherapy. It can be carried out after surgical or percutaneous placement of catheters linked to subcutaneous chambers, or by iterative percutaneous catheterizations.
- Transarterial *embolization* (*TAE*) of HCC (simple bland embolization), excluding hemorrhagic complications, has been developed in Chap. 6.
- *Hepatic infusions of chemotherapy* can be carried out with infusion pumps or subcutaneous implantable devices connected to a hepatic arterial catheter, implanted surgically or via a percutaneous femoral or left brachial arterial access, under local anesthesia. The percutaneous method can be carried out in an

ambulatory setting but has higher complication rates. They can also be carried out by iterative catheterizations (*TACI*: *transcatheter arterial chemo-infusion*), which correspond to a very selective injection of highly concentrated drugs, followed by a minimal embolization so as to limit ischemic and cytotoxic complications. It allows optimal delivery of drugs to the tumor but requires repeated catheterizations.

- *Lipiodol chemoembolization*: It is the most frequently used technique: cytotoxics are emulsified with Lipiodol (chemo-lipiodol), before intra-arterial administration. Complementary embolization agents can secondarily be administered.

Administration of cytotoxic with a high level of hepatic extraction and high extrahepatic clearances allows the increase of drug concentration (by a factor of up to ×100). The emulsion with Lipiodol constitutes a "vectorization"; a temporary embolization increases the contact time of drugs with the endothelium. The internal micelles are delivered into the distal arteries.

Anthracyclines are used, among which is Adriamycin (doxorubicin): it is the most often used in our center (1–2 mg/kg, in our center: 50 mg/m^2). Monotherapy is most often carried out, with doxorubicin in most cases. If a double therapy is carried out, the most commonly associated drugs are doxorubicin (or epirubicin) + mitomycin C or doxorubicin + cisplatin. In the USA, the association of CAM (cisplatin + Adriamycin + mitomycin) is used. The superiority of cisplatin (50 mg/m^2) with respect to Adriamycin has been suggested. But no drug has proven its superiority [7].

Chemotherapy must be prepared in a centralized reconstitution unit, transferred, and manipulated in the angiographic unit according to specific recommendations.

Usually, 10 ml of Lipiodol is used. For some authors, the volume of Lipiodol must take into account tumor size as well as its vascularization: 2–3 ml/cm in highly vascularized tumors and 1 ml/cm for lesions with poor arterial supply [8]. Beyond 20 ml, one must fear the risk of pulmonary embolism, as well as higher toxicity on disease-free liver.

Complementary embolization with various embolization agents allows the increase of tumor ischemia volume, of contact time, as well as of intracellular drug retention by the inhibition of the transmembrane pumps of tumor cells. To obtain a stagnation of the contrast agent, absorbable gelatin sponges are often used but also particles (Ivalon; Embosphère from 300 to 700 μm, 1 to 3 cm^3), which have not however proven their superiority.

- *Chemoembolization with loaded microspheres*: DEB TACE (drug-eluting beads) are injected into the arteries feeding the tumor, allowing simultaneous embolization and progressive chemotherapy release. Two types of beads are available [7]: the DC Bead microspheres (Biocompatibles, UK) and more recently the HepaSphere microspheres (superabsorbent polymers (SAP) QuadraSphere in USA) (Biosphere Medical).

Most reports are related to the DC Bead microspheres, loaded with doxorubicine, which have the "CE" marking for treatment of malignant hypervascular tumors. They are nonbiodegradable calibrated PVA microspheres, impregnated with doxorubicin or sometimes with irinotecan used for palliative treatment of metastatic colorectal cancers. The Precision Bead (Biocompatibles, UK) were the first preloaded microspheres (with doxorubicine) available; their diameter varies from 100 to 900 μm.

The HepaSphere microparticles are biocompatible, hydrophilic, nonabsorbable, and capable to absorb up to 64 times their dry volume state. The rate of expansion depends on the surrounding ionic concentration. The expansion sizes vary from 200 to 800 μm. They can be impregnated with doxorubicin or cisplatin. With doxorubicin, they have the "CE" marking for chemoembolization of HCC. The dose of doxorubicin is calculated on the basis of body surface (75 mg/m^2), or at fixed dose ≤150 mg [8].

The procedure must be performed on an overhydrated patient, under pre- and post-procedure sedation, and requires administration of analgesics and antiemetic drugs. The administration of antibiotics for gram-negative enteric organisms is performed by some authors, even though this practice is not universal and has not been proven by prospective studies to be beneficial for all patients. The risk of post embolization infection seems to decrease when a bowel preparation is performed prior to embolization.

The protocols in our center are in common cases: preventive antibiotics (amoxicillin and clavulanic acid or 3rd-generation cephalosporin during 48 h); in case of bilio-intestinal anastomosis, the treatments are prolonged because of an important risk of abscess.

Using femoral Seldinger's technique, procedures must begin with an abdominal aortography followed by selective injections in the celiac trunk and the superior mesenteric artery, allowing the evaluation of portal system patency and of a precise splanchnic arterial anatomy workup so as to avoid undesired injections of drugs in the digestive tract or the cystic artery. The presence of aberrant feeding arteries (phrenic, mammary, parietal, visceral arteries), which is sometimes suspected on initial CT or MR, must be precised.

Schematically, a selective catheterization of the arterial branches feeding one or more tumors is to be attempted if there are few localized tumors and/or in case of massive hypervascular zones, thus increasing tumor response and limiting hepatic toxicity. Otherwise, the embolization is performed downstream of the gastroduodenal artery. A French study including 184 patients in two centers [9] compared nonselective chemo-lipiodol + nonselective embolization using gelatin sponge and nonselective chemo-lipiodol + selective embolization: tumor response was best with the two selective techniques, and patient tolerance was best with selective chemo-lipiodol.

To avoid untimely diffusions of chemotherapy, occlusion of gastroduodenal and/or gastric arterial branches with coils can be useful and necessary.

A 4F hydrophilic catheter is often sufficient for the selective catheterization; in case of catheterization difficulties and/or small arterial caliber, large lumen microcatheters can be used. Chemoembolization agents must in all cases be injected until blood flow stagnation is obtained in the lobar arteries. Blood flow interruption must be avoided, as it can preclude future embolization sessions. The choice of catheters and microcatheters depends on their compatibility with the drugs used, keeping in mind the frequent fragility of the catheter's base to some chemotherapies, inducing leaks or catheter ruptures around the connection with the syringe.

Recently, the role of cone beam CT during superselective TACE of HCC undepicted on angiography (or for hypovascular metastases) has been emphasized.

A post-embolization syndrome (abdominal pain, fever, and cytolysis) is nearly always present; it requires analgesics and bacteriological samples and blood tests, searching for an infection. If fever is associated with a leukoneutropenia, a systematic antibiotic therapy adapted to febrile neutropenia should be discussed. A transitory impairment of liver function is frequently observed. Patient hydration aims to limit the problem of renal insufficiency, which is linked to the tumor necrosis and to injections of iodinated contrast agent.

In our practice, patients are usually hospitalized for 72 h and have post-procedure clinical and biological monitoring. Elevation of ALATs and ASATs is normal. Early imaging controls are carried out only in case of complication; in this context, the presence of gas in the liver is not synonymous with an infection.

The number of sessions and the inter-cure interval vary considerably from one team to another. Some carry out systematically two or three sessions; others adapt the number of sessions to the tumor response. Two to 3 weeks' interval between embolization sessions is the ideal delay so as to avoid tumor growth, but it also implies the risk of ischemic liver failure. Embolization sessions should be programmed according to tumor response rather than systematically, thus allowing the reduction of complication rates and the increasing survival rates.

The inter-cure follow-up is carried out by monitoring $\propto$-fetoprotein and by control imaging performed 4–6 weeks after procedure: an abdominal CT scan is usually performed, but MRI can also be used. One takes into account the Lipiodol fixation on the lesion(s), which is predictive of tumor response and survival, and the enhancement of treated lesions, which allows the detection of active tumor zone(s) or new tumor(s). According to the EASL [10] criteria, full response is obtained when all the lesions have disappeared and a partial response when a reduction of 50 % of the viable surface of the lesions is observed at the arterial phase; the disease is progressive in case of a 25 % growth of a lesion or if new lesions appear; otherwise, the disease is stable.

In the absence of active site at the end of the program, an imaging control will be performed every 3–4 months.

7.1.4 Indications

Nonindications:

- More than 50 % of the liver concerned with the tumor process
- Metastasis and/or extrahepatic extension of the HCC

Contraindications:

- To angiography: endovascular navigation and iodine contrast media
- To chemotherapy: leukopenia, and renal and/or heart insufficiency
- To chemoembolization: cirrhosis Child C, Okuda 3, bilirubin >2 mg/dl, ASAT superior to 100 IU/l, and hepatic encephalopathy, which leads to an excess of death and morbidity rates.
  - In our team, Child B9 cirrhoses are also contraindications.
  - An obstruction in the bile duct necessitates prior drainage.
  - Portal thrombosis is a relative contraindication: classically, at least 4 noninversed patent portal branches must be depicted for a nonselective chemoembolization; otherwise, selective chemoembolization must be carried out, and additional embolization should be avoided. The related risk of parenchymal infarction depends on several characteristics, in particular the extent of thrombosis (contralateral or ipsilateral to the disease, distal or proximal). So TACE using less aggressive embolization can be performed safely. The use of radioembolization has also been advocated in these patients.

In the case of an arterioportal shunt, a downstream injection should be realized beyond the shunt. An occlusion of the shunt or of the drainage vein when it is possible can also be carried out.

The management of a hepatofugal flow remains controversial. We consider it as a relative contraindication, once an arterioportal fistula has been excluded. In these cases, we take into consideration the hepatic function and perform chemoembolization in patients with Child A or low B scores.

Indications: Chemoembolization can only be considered if the HCC is proven.

- *As curative treatment*: the results of chemoembolization are not as good as those of surgical resection or percutaneous ablation techniques, which are the first-line treatments.
- *As palliative indication*: chemoembolization is indicated for localized or multifocal tumors that are not accessible to surgery or percutaneous ablation techniques; the optimum benefit is observed for lesions of 3–4 to 8–10 cm in diameter, without vascular spread or extrahepatic extension, in asymptomatic patients, with a conserved liver function. In our group, we treat Child A cirrhoses and some Child B7 and B8 cirrhoses that are discussed on a case-to-case basis.
  This palliative treatment can be carried out after postsurgical recurrences.
- *As neoadjuvant treatment*: a review pooling 18 studies (15 observational and 3 random) [11] suggests that chemoembolization before resection is effective and sure, with high levels of response, but does not increase recurrence-free survival. Several prospective trials [12] plead in the favor of chemoembolization, but 2 randomized trials [13, 14] found no difference, notably in terms of surgical complications and recurrences.
  The neoadjuvant chemoembolization before transplantation is a widespread indication, but its impact in terms of long-term survival is not proven (an old randomized trial [15] has shown favorable effects for tumors of more than 5 cm).

- *As adjuvant treatment*: after resection, hepatic embolization prolongs survival and diminishes the number of recurrences [16]; these results were also found in a randomized trial using radioactive iodine after resection [17].
- Chemoembolization is used *both before and after radiofrequency treatment.*

In summary, the indications must be approved by a multidisciplinary team and in accordance with the BCLC treatment algorithm [2–4]:

- Chemoembolization is the first-line palliative treatment for intermediate forms (BCLC-B).
- It should not be used for advanced stages (BCLC-C) when there is a portal vein thrombosis.
- Two groups of BCLC-A patients can also be included: those with single tumors who are waiting for a transplantation so as to avoid the tumor progression and those managed by an ablative therapy (RFA).

7.1.5 Results

The analysis of the results must take into account the heterogeneity of the practices, with a large variability in indications and protocols.

The mortality after 30 days is about 1 %.

The morbidity rate is 4 % [18]. The major complications include tumor ruptures, hepatic infarction or liver failure, biliary necrosis, cholecystitis, and nontarget embolizations.

Infectious complications are much more frequent in case of bilio-intestinal anastomosis; therefore, they must systematically be prevented with prophylactic antibiotic therapy. Ischemic cholecystitis caused by injection upstream the cystic artery does not always require surgical treatment. GI tract necrosis caused by injection in the splanchnic arteries can be avoided by careful analysis of arterial cartography. Toxic arteritis is noticeably observed in the case of injection of Adriamycin.

Hepatic failure could result from the incidental damage caused by cytotoxic agent on tumor-free liver. Superselective embolization has thus been advocated to decrease this risk.

Survival: Many series are favorable to chemoembolization, but a pessimistic randomized study has for a long time been the reference [19], in which the survival rate after chemoembolization versus a control group was not significant after 1 year.

A 2002 meta-analysis of eight randomized controlled trials [20] shows a significantly decreased global mortality at 2 years with chemoembolization, and a global mortality significantly lower when using arterial embolization rather than intra-arterial chemotherapy, but there was no difference in terms of efficacy between arterial embolization and Lipiodol hepatic chemoembolization. Another meta-analysis [21] found a significant benefit in terms of 2-year survival rate with chemoembolization versus conservative treatment, but not with bland embolization.

Two randomized trials found the following results:

- Lo et al. [22] (cisplatin, Asiatic patients, 80 HCC unresectable Okuda 1 (47 %) or 2 (53 %), 80 % HVB, with an average 4.5 sessions [1–15] every 2–3 months) reports for chemoembolization 57, 31, and 26 %, for 1, 2, and 3 years' survival rates and for symptomatic treatments 32, 11, and 3 %.
- Llovet et al. [23] (112 patients generally affected by viral C infections, HCC Child A or B, Okuda 1 or 2, with an average of 2.8 sessions at M0, M2, and M6, then eventually every 6 months) observed for the chemoembolization 82 and 63 %, survival at 1 and 2 years; for the bland embolization (gelatin) 75 and 50 %; and with a symptomatic treatment 63 and 27 %.

To summarize, one must keep in mind the efficacy of the technique, with the best results when considering survival rates are obtained in selected patients and can exceed 50 % for 3-year survival rate [24].

The preliminary results of *DEB TACE* (chemoembolization with drug-eluting bead) for nonoperable HCC show a better pharmacokinetic profile, less side effects, and a better tumor response on control imaging, with respect to the conventional chemoembolization. The PRECISION V trial [25] was the first randomized prospective controlled trial evaluating microparticles loaded with doxorubicin; intermediary results showed higher rates of complete responses, objective responses, and disease controls in respect to those with conventional chemoembolization, with a marked decrease in hepatic toxicity. Further results concerning survival rates are still expected.

The preliminary results using HepaSpheres are yet to be published.

7.1.6 Technical Variations and Evolutions

7.1.6.1 Radioembolization

Conventional external radiotherapy as a palliative treatment for nonresectable liver tumors has its limits, above all the fact that the liver has a very low tolerance to irradiation, in spite of the technological advances. Also an intra-arterial injection of radioembolic materials has been advocated, in order to deliver high doses to the tumors while protecting the remainder of the liver. These radioembolization techniques associate an internal radiation of the tumor and the embolization of the feeding arteries. This means additional constraints specific to the use of radioactive agents.

- *Yttrium 90*: microspheres marked by yttrium 90 are used to treat nonresectable HCC, colorectal metastases, and metastases of endocrine tumors.

Two products are available (glass-based, TheraSphere; resin-based, SIR-Spheres), for which the vectors are different, but both are yttrium carriers and beta-emitters. The technique is interesting as it allows the downstaging of some HCCs. It is an alternative to chemoembolization for BCLC-B patients. It can be used in patients with a more advanced BCLC-C and portal vein thrombosis. Lastly, it has been indicated in BCLC-A patients (radiation segmentectomy), for patients who are not eligible for curative therapies.

- *Intra-arterial injection of Lipiodol marked with radioactive iodine* (*Lipiocis*): this technique is based on the tumor tropism of Lipiodol injected in the hepatic artery and its retention by HCC during several weeks, and up to 1 year, where it is normally eliminated by a healthy or cirrhotic liver in 4 weeks. After its administration in the hepatic artery, the Lipiodol crosses the peribiliary plexus up to the portal vein, resulting in a double embolization.

The adjunction of a radionuclide beta-emitter to Lipiodol has been used as palliative, adjuvant, or neoadjuvant treatment of HCCs.

This technique does not include embolization with microparticles at the end of the procedure: a thrombosis of the portal vein is therefore not a contraindication.

Most of the studies have not shown any benefits in terms of survival, but Lipiodol marked with iodine 131 is better tolerated (less secondary effects) than chemoembolization.

7.1.6.2 New Drugs

The ideal chemotherapy agent for the percutaneous endovascular treatment of HCC remains to be determined: it must combine antitumor effects and reduced toxicity for normal or cirrhotic liver.

The drugs that are actually used are evaluated more systematically, prospectively, and research on new drugs is conducted keeping in mind these criteria.

A better knowledge of the tumor genesis of HCCs has led to evaluate new cytostatic agents so as to overcome resistances to drugs, to inhibit angiogenesis, and to limit dose-related toxicity. Phase I, II, and III studies are currently underway, using antiangiogenic agents, growth factors/enzymes inhibitors, nonspecific inhibitors for growth, specific antagonists of HCC tumor markers, and anti-inflammatory agents.

7.1.6.3 Combined Therapeutics

Percutaneous endovascular treatments must be evaluated in combination with the other therapies: ablative treatments (e.g., RFA is combined with TACE for HCC recurrences after hepatectomy) or systemic treatments, in particular when faced with a metastatic disease (bevacizumab, Avastin; sorafenib, Nexavar).

Radiosensitization agents can also be used with radioembolization techniques.

7.2 Other Malignant Liver Tumors

Randomized trials comparing embolization and chemoembolization are necessary in order to determine benefits of chemotherapy (with its own potential toxicity) in association with embolization.

TACE has been proposed to treat other primary neoplasms such as cholangiocarcinomas but with a lack of published data.

7.2.1 Metastases of Endocrine Tumors (ET)

Chemoembolization has also been realized in hepatic metastases of ET (before all, anthracyclines as selective as possible, in two sessions in the case of important intrahepatic extension). Additional sessions are carried out at the request, based on symptomatic results.

The patients should receive premedication with somatostatin analogous to prevent severe metabolic reaction induced by arterial embolization.

The technique is interesting in case of differentiated ET with nonresectable hepatic metastases, in symptomatic patient, in order to control the secretion syndrome when the somatostatin is not efficient or if the metastases are rapidly evolving.

A clinical response is obtained in more than 86 % of the cases, among which 49 % are complete responses, for an average duration of at least 16 months, given that chemoembolization is the first-line treatment and that the primary tumor is not pancreatic.

In terms of survival, there are no randomized trials. Chu et al. [26] has shown in the follow-up of 50 pancreatic ET, among which 39 had liver metastases, that resection of the primary tumor, metachronous metastases, absence of hepatic metastases and/or the aggressive surgical treatment of hepatic metastases, and intra-arterial chemotherapy or chemoembolization were the predictive factors influencing survival.

7.2.2 Other Metastases

There are fewer reports of chemoembolization in the treatment of other hepatic metastases. The results are generally poorer to those of HCC, in part, surely because of the prognosis of the primary tumor.

Concerning metastases of colorectal carcinomas, which are usually hypovascular, the long-term benefit is considered to be limited. A randomized trial has compared chemoembolization and hepatic embolization, without showing any advantage for one technique with respect to another [27].

Intra-arterial chemotherapies have not formally shown their superiority with respect to IV administrations; however, they can be used in case of unique nonresectable hepatic metastases when systemic protocols have failed.

Drug-eluting bead and yttrium 90 microspheres have yet to be evaluated in these indications.

Key Points

- Prevalence of HCC increases in Western countries.
- Management of HCC requires a multidisciplinary team.
- Chemoembolization is a palliative treatment for HCC in patients who cannot undergo surgery or a radiofrequency treatment (BCLC-B). It must not be used in advanced stages (BCLC-C).
- In selected patients, an increase in the survival, exceeding 50 % at 3 years, is observed after chemoembolization.
- Chemoembolization is a neoadjuvant treatment in patients awaiting hepatic transplantation; it can also be used in association with RF.
- Interpretation of the results of clinical trials and meta-analyses is difficult, notably because of the great heterogeneity of the indications, practices, and results; so far, it does not allow any definitive conclusion.
- Questions remain unanswered: What is the best drug? What is the best embolization agent? And among the microparticles, what diameter should be chosen? What is the best technique protocol (global, lobar, or selective chemoembolization)? What is the "end point" of the procedure? What is the best chronology for the therapeutic sequences? What is the most efficient association of therapies? To answer to all these questions, new randomized trials are necessary.
- Radioembolization techniques are interesting in case of portal thrombosis.

  Yttrium-based treatments must be compared with the classic chemoembolization.

  These techniques implicate constraints due to the handling of radioactive elements.
- Chemoembolization is interesting to treat nonresectable hepatic metastases of rapidly evolving or symptomatic endocrine tumors.

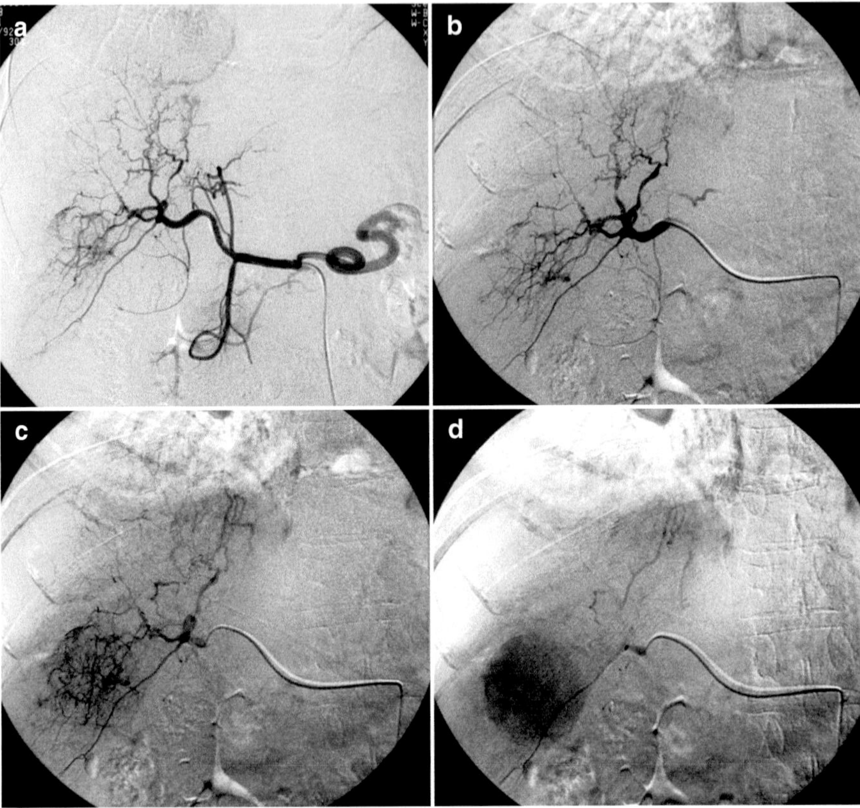

Fig. 7.1 Selective injection of the CT: *thin* helicine arteries (typical pattern of cirrhosis), heterogeneous hepatography, and segment VI tumoral hypervascularization

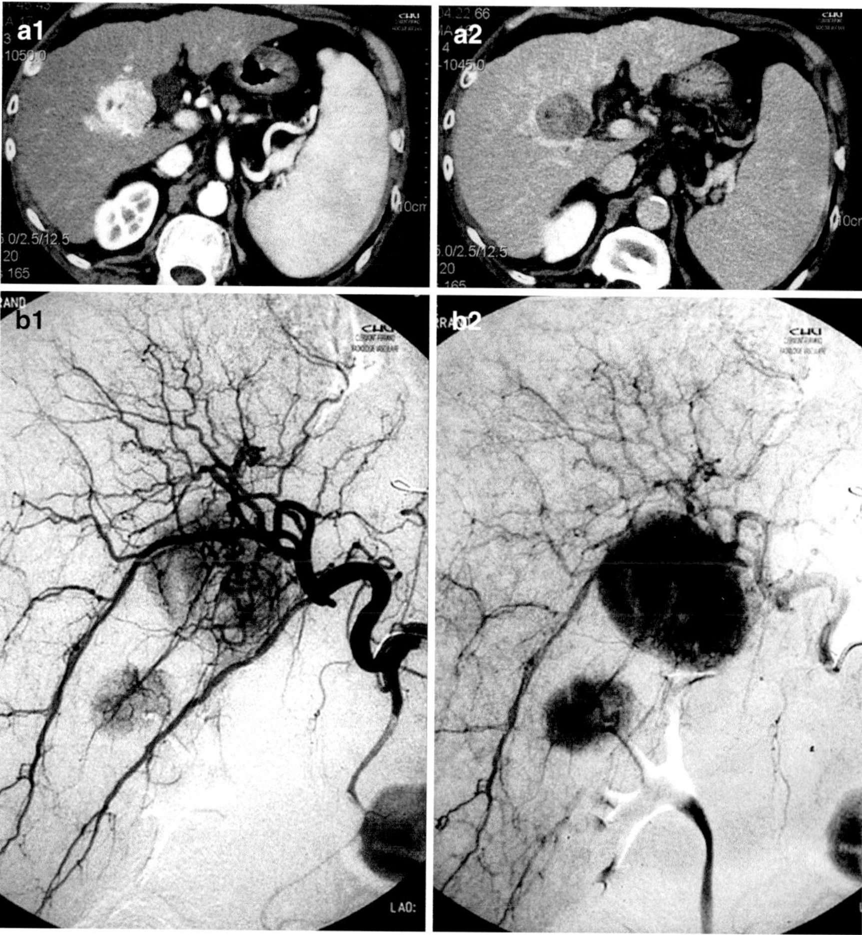

Fig. 7.2 HCC complication of HVC hepatitis. (**a**) CT, juxta-gallbladder tumor; arterial phase, massive enhancement (wash-in) and then washout on the portal phase scan. (**b**) Same patient, 2D angio correlation: 2 tumors foci

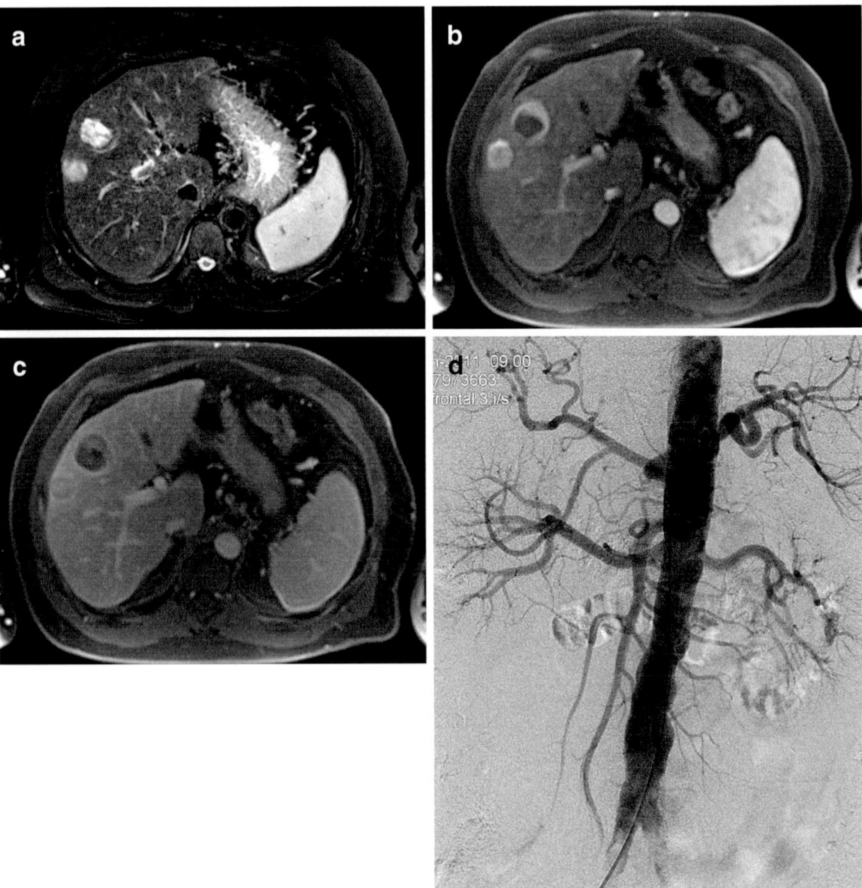

Fig. 7.3 Double HCC; the multidisciplinary concertation and a complete workup led to decide a hepatic transplantation. But a long waiting delay (months) is expected, so an adjuvant TACE has been decided. (**a**) MRI T2-weighted scan: 25 and 30 mm heterogeneous hypersignal tumors. (**b**) Dynamic MR, arterial phase: global enhancement of one of this lesion (wash-in) and peripheral enhancement of the other. (**c**) Late portal phase: washout. (**d**) Aortography (right femoral access): modal angiographic anatomy of the splanchnic collaterals of the aorta. (**e**) Selective SMA injections, arterial and venous phase: patent portal vein and hepatoportal flow direction. (**f**) Selective injection of the CT. (**g**) Common hepatic A selective injection, just upstream the gastroduodenal A (*arrow*): unusual distribution of the terminal branches of the proper hepatic A, with an accessory left hepatic artery, and then a right/left bifurcation. (**h**) Accessory left hepatic artery selective injection, early arterial and late phases: double tumorography. (**i**) Injection of this accessory hepatic A. TACE: we injected epirubicin 50 mg (25 ml) + Lipiodol (10 ml), 20 % in the accessory branch and 40 % in each of the right and left hepatic branches. 2×5 cm^3 gelatin sponge syringes were then injected, in order to observe a very slow flow. (**j**) CT 1 m later: dense Lipiodol fixation in the lesion which was previously massively enhanced and peripheral fixation in the other. No arterial enhancement

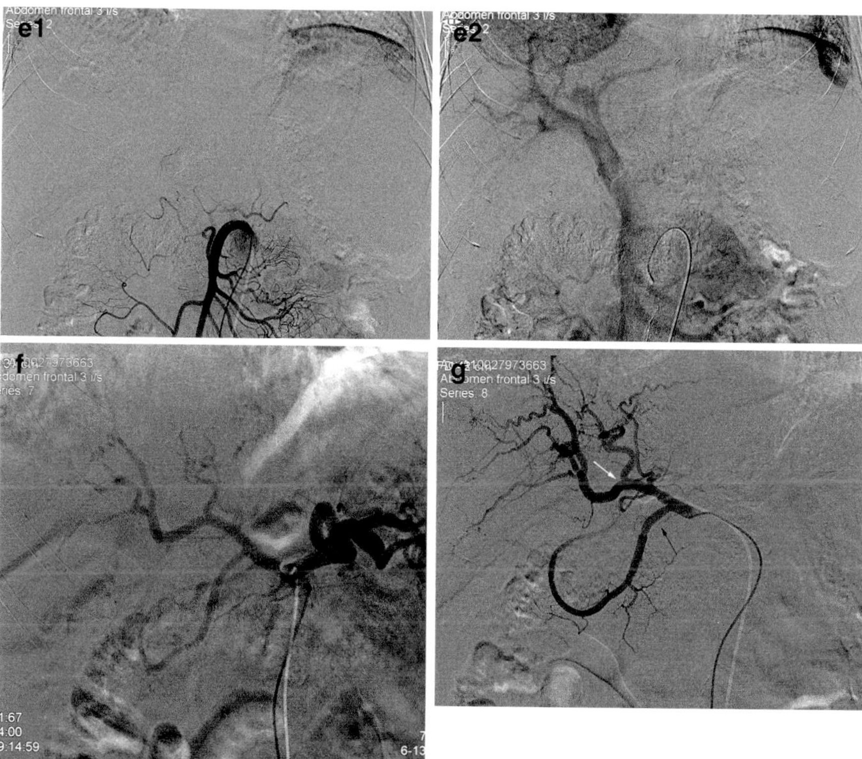

Fig. 7.3 (continued)

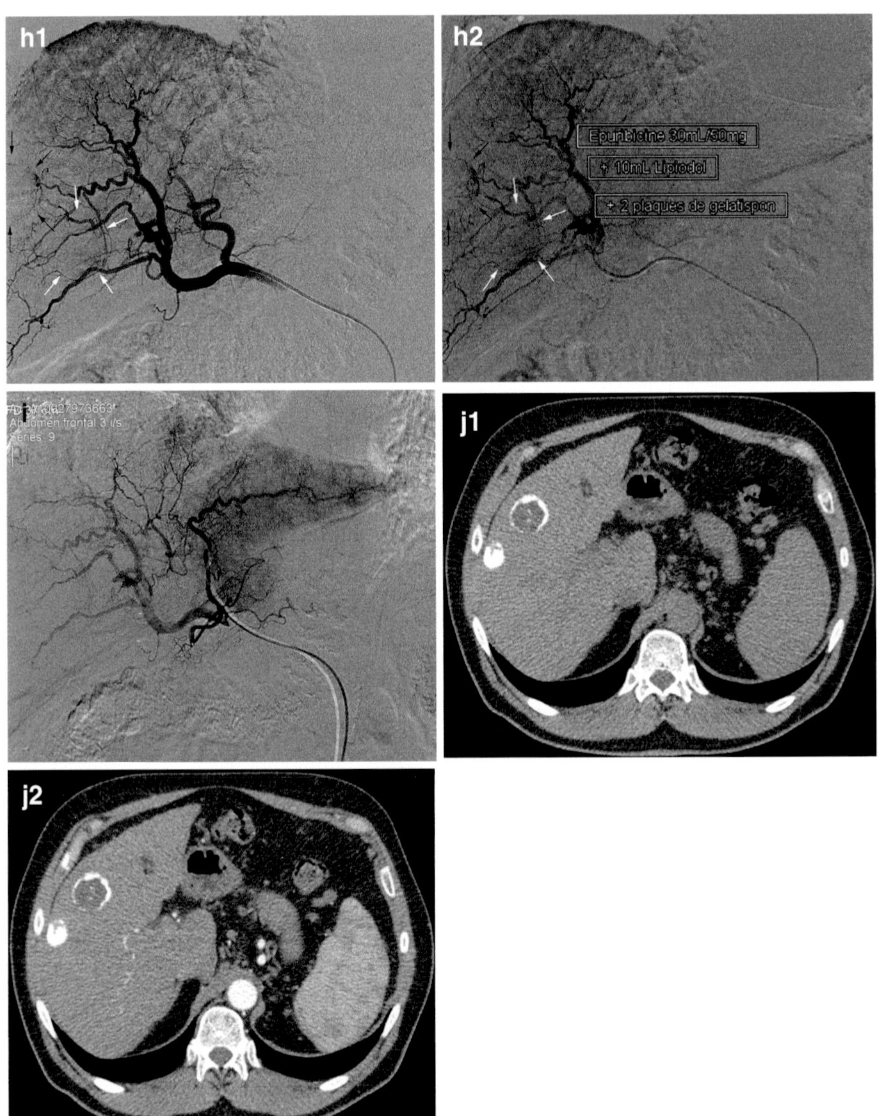

Fig. 7.3 (continued)

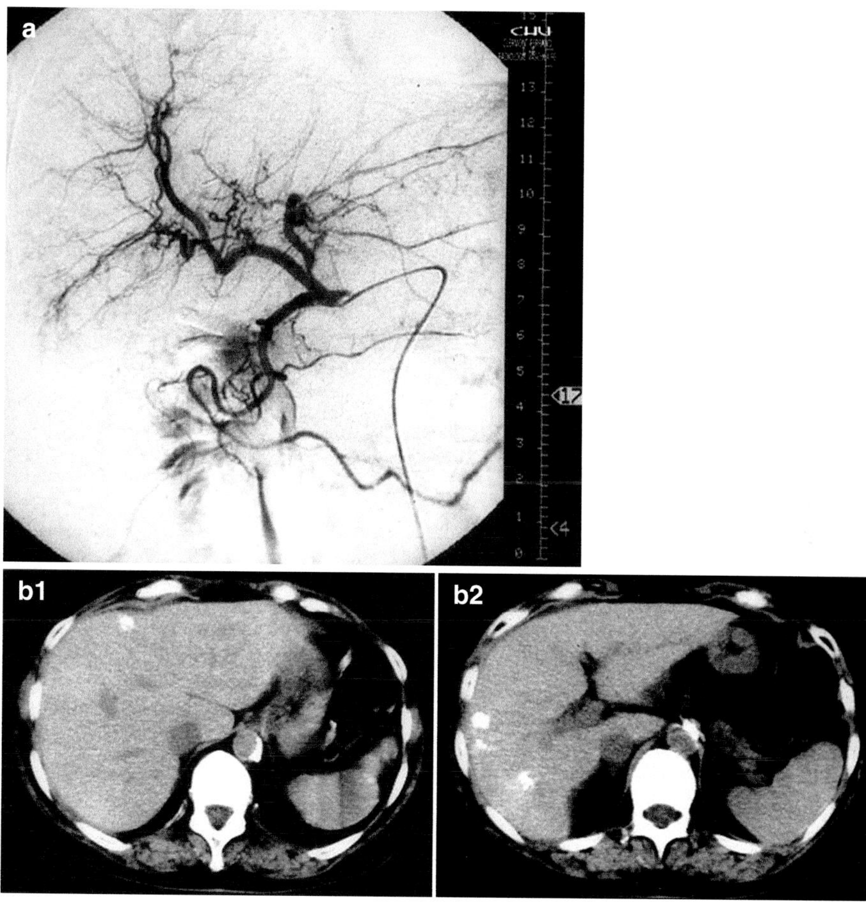

Fig. 7.4 HCC treated by TACE. (**a**) Selective common hep A injections: nonselective TACE (2/3 in the right hepatic A, 1/3 in the left). (**b**) 1 m later CT: tumoral Lipiodol fixation

References

1. Bruix J, Sherman M. Practice guidelines committee, American Association for the Study of Liver Diseases Management of hepatocellular carcinoma. Hepatology. 2005;42:1208–36.
2. Bruix J, Sherman M. Management of hepato cellular carcinoma: an update AASLD practice guidelines. Hepatology. 2010;53:1–34.
3. Grieco A, Pompili M, Caminit G, et al. Prognostic factors for survival in patients with early-intermediate hepatocellular carcinoma under-going non-surgical therapy: comparison of Okuda, CLIP, and BCLC straging systems in a single Italian centre. Gut. 2005;54:411–8.
4. Llovet JM, Bru C, Bruix J. Prognosis of hepatocellular carcinoma the BCLC staging classification. Semin Liver Dis. 1999;19:329–38.
5. Llovet JM. Updated treatment approach to hepatocellular carcinoma. J Gastroenterol. 2005;40(3):225–35.
6. Mazzafero V, Regalia E, Doci R, et al. Liver transplantation for the treatment of small hepato cellular carcinomas in patients with cirrhosis. N Engl J Med. 1996;334:693–9.

7. Liapi E, Geschwind JF. Intra-arterial therapies for hepatocellular carcinoma: where do we stand? Ann Surg Oncol. 2010;17:1234–46.
8. Basile A, Carrafiello G, Ierardi AM, Tsetis D, Brountzos E. Quality-improvement guidelines for hepatic transarterial chemoembolization. Cardiovasc Intervent Radiol. 2012;35:765–74.
9. Bouvier A, Ozenne V, Aubé C, et al. Transarterial chemoembolisation: effect of selectivity on tolerance, tumour response and survival. Eur Radiol. 2011;21:1719–26.
10. Bruix J, Sherman M, Llovet JM, Beaugrand M, Lencioni R, Burroughs AK, Christensen E, Pagliaro L, Colombo M, Rodés J, EASL Panel of Experts on HCC. Clinical management of hepatocellular carcinoma. Conclusions of the Barcelona-2000 EASL conference. European Association for the Study of the Liver. J Hepatol. 2001;35:421–30.
11. Chua CT, Liauw W, Saxena A. Systematic review of neoadjuvant transarterial chemoembolization for resectable hepatocellular carcinoma. Liver Int. 2010;30:166–74.
12. Gerunda GE, Neri D, Merenda R, et al. Role of transarterial chemoembolization before liver resection for hepatocarcinoma. Liver Transpl. 2000;6:619–26.
13. Wu CC, Ho YZ, Ho WL, et al. Preoperative transcatheter arterial chemoembolization for resectable large hepatocellular carcinoma: a reappraisal. Br J Surg. 1995;82:122–6.
14. Yamasaki S, Hasegawa H, Kinoshita H, et al. A prospective randomized trial of the preventive effect of pre-operative transcatheter arterial embolization against recurrence of hepatocellular carcinoma. Jpn J Cancer Res. 1996;87:206–11.
15. Cherqui D, Piedbois P, Pierga JY, et al. Multimodal adjuvant treatment and liver transplantation for advanced hepatocellular carcinoma. A pilot study. Cancer. 1994;73:2721–6.
16. Shimoda M, Bando T, Nagata T, et al. Prophylactic chemolipiodolization for postoperative hepatoma patients. Hepatogastroenterology. 2001;48:493–7.
17. Lau WY, Leung TW, Ho SK, et al. Adjuvant intra-arterial iodine-131-labelled lipiodol for resectable hepatocellular carcinoma: a prospective randomised trial. Lancet. 1999;353:797–801.
18. Llovet JM, Burroughs A, Bruix J. Hepatocellular carcinoma. Lancet. 2003;362:1907–17.
19. Groupe d'Etude et de Traitement du Carcinome Hepatocellulaire. A comparison of lipiodol chemoembolization and conservative treatment for unresectable hepatocellular carcinoma. N Engl J Med. 1995;332:1256–61.
20. Camma C, Schepis F, Orlando A, et al. Transarterial chemoembolization for unresectable hepatocellular carcinoma: meta-analysis of randomized controlled trials. Radiology. 2002;224:47–54.
21. Llovet JM, Bruix J. A systematic review of randomized trials for unresectable hepatocellular carcinoma chemoembolization improves survival. Hepatology. 2003;37:429–42.
22. Lo CM, Ngan H, Tso WK, et al. Randomized controlled trial of transarterial lipiodol chemoembolization for unresectable hepatocellular carcinoma. Hepatology. 2002;35:1164–71.
23. Llovet JM, Real MI, Montana X, et al. Arterial embolisation or chemoembolisation versus symptomatic treatment in patients with unresectable hepatocellular carcinoma: a randomised controlled trial. Lancet. 2002;359:1734–9.
24. Llovet JM, Fuster J, Bruix J. The Barcelona approach: diagnosis, staging, and treatment of hepatocellular carcinoma. Liver Transpl. 2004;10:115–20.
25. Lammer J, Malagari K, Vogl T, et al. Prospective randomized study of doxorubicin-eluting-bead embolization in the treatment of hepatocellular carcinoma: results of the PRECISION V study. Cardiovasc Intervent Radiol. 2010;33:41–52.
26. Chu QD, Hill HC, Douglass HO, et al. Predictive factors associated with long-term survival in patients with neuroendocrine tumors of the pancreas. Ann Surg Oncol. 2002;9:855–62.
27. Salman HS, Cynamon J, Jagust M, et al. Randomized phase II trial of embolization therapy versus chemoembolization therapy in previously treated patients with colorectal carcinoma metastatic to the liver. Clin Colorectal Cancer. 2002;2:173–9.

Suggested Reading

Basile A, Carrafiello G, Ierardi AM, Tsetis D, Brountzos E. Quality-improvement guidelines for hepatic transarterial chemoembolization. Cardiovasc Intervent Radiol. 2012;35:765–74.

Bruix J, Sherman M. Management of hepatocellular carcinoma: an update – AASLD practice guidelines. Hepatology. 2010;53:1–34.

Cleveland TJ, Kelekis AD, Kopp C, et al. CIRSE take force on clinical pratice: Hepato Cellular Carinoma. In: Clinical practice in interventional radiology CIRSE, Vienna 2007. p. 74–9.

Liapi E, Geschwind JF. Intra-arterial therapies for hepatocellular carcinoma: where do we stand? Ann Surg Oncol. 2010;17:1234–46.

Liapi E, Geschwind JF. Transcatheter arterial chemo embolization for liver cancer: is it time to distinguish conventional from drug eluting chemoembolization? Cardiovasc Intervent Radiol. 2011;34:37–49.

Llovet JM. Updated treatment approach to hepatocellular carcinoma. J Gastroenterol. 2005;40(3): 225–35.

Chapter 8
Portal Vein Embolization

Pascal Chabrot, Vincent Vidal, Laurent Poincloux, Le Thanh Dung, Gérald Gahide, Louis Boyer, and Pierre Perreault

8.1 Background

Preoperative portal embolization allows a reorientation of the portal vein flow from the segments to be resected towards the future liver remnant (FLR). This results in hypertrophy of the preserved segments and increase in the hepatic reserve. Thus, the number of patients eligible for an extended hepatic resection has increased, and the rate of postoperative complications has diminished.

In order to obtain a sufficient hypertrophy, the embolization has to be as complete as possible and must target all the segmental branches that are going to be resected: embolization of anteromedian sector (segments 5 and 8) and posterolateral sector (segments 6 and 7) in right hepatectomies and additional embolization of segment 4 in extended right hepatectomies. The development of atypical hepatectomies requires a selective embolization adapted to the surgical planning.

P. Chabrot, MD, PhD (✉) • L. Boyer, MD, PhD
Department of Radiology, University Hospital of Clermont-Ferrand, Clermont-Ferrand, France
e-mail: pchabrot@chu-clermontferrand.fr; lboyer@chu-clermontferrand.fr

V. Vidal, MD, PhD
Department of Radiology, Assistance Publiqùe-Hôpitaux de Marseille, Marseille, France

L. Poincloux, MD
Department of Gastroenterology, University Hospital of Clermont-Ferrand, Clermont-Ferrand, France

L.T. Dung, MD
Department of Radiology, Viet Duc University Hospital, Hanoï, Viet Nam

G. Gahide, MD, PhD
Department of Radiology, Sherbrooke University Hospital, Sherbrooke, QC, Canada

P. Perreault, MD
Department of Radiology, University of Montreal Hospital Center, Montréal, QC, Canada

P. Chabrot, L. Boyer (eds.), *Embolization*,
DOI 10.1007/978-1-4471-5182-1_8,

8.2 Relevant Radiological Anatomy

Initial CT and ultrasound findings as well as arteriography allow the definition of the puncture target as well as the evaluation of the intrahepatic portal distribution. The identification of the portal distribution is an essential prerequisite for an embolization. In the modal distribution, the portal vein divides into a left branch (segments 2, 3, and 4) and a right branch which gives anterior sectorial branches (segments 5 and 8) and posterior sectorial branches (segments 6 and 7).

On a frontal view, the right posterior branch most frequently runs out medially in comparison to the right anterior branch; a left anterior oblique view allows a better depiction of this medial course.

The variations are frequent:

- Convergence of the right anterior branch with the left branch (13 %)
- Portal trifurcation (9 %)
- Separated affluence of segmental branches 6 and 8 (7 %)

8.3 Technique

- Ideally, the procedure takes place using general anesthesia or conscious sedation. But this procedure is frequently undertaken using a local anesthesia in association with the administration of morphine-based *drugs* that are delivered just prior to the injection of the embolization agent.
- To our knowledge, there is no consensus concerning systematic antibiotherapy, except for patients who have drained bile ducts.
- The percutaneous transhepatic approach is the most frequently used, even if the percutaneous transjugular routes [1] or ileocolic surgical approach [2] can also be used. The access can be ipsi- or contralateral to the target segments, depending upon the anatomy, the extension of the tumor, the type of resection planned, and the embolization agent used. The complication rates are comparable for these two different approaches.
  - *Using an ipsilateral approach,* puncture of a right portal branch is performed. Puncture of the FLR is avoided with this approach which however exposes to the theoretical risk of seeding if the puncture goes through the tumor. The catheterization of the right portal branches is more difficult and requires the use of angulated catheters [3]. The risk of migration of embolization agents is increased and final portography cannot be performed.

  The puncture of a distal right branch a 22-gauge Chiba needle is undertaken under ultrasound guidance. This allows the insertion of a long introducer sheath in the right portal branch. The access can be secured with a second security guidewire in either the portal or the splenic vein.

  Following the portal vein embolization, the parenchymal tract can be embolized by coils, absorbable gelatin sponge (our preference), or glue.

- *Contralateral approach* consists of puncturing a left peripheral portal branch, through the parenchyma that will be conserved. This approach allows a more direct access to the right branches and a greater choice of occlusion agents (embolizing with the flow). However, it exposes the FLR to puncture complications.

Access to segment 4 implies a puncture above the Rex recess. Under ultrasound guidance, a subxiphoid puncture allows for a peripheral access, most frequently in segment 3, using a 22-gauge needle, followed by the insertion of a 5 Fr introducer sheath after cannulation of the portal trunk with a catheter and a 0.035 hydrophilic guidewire. The length of the catheterized segment, the direct access to the right portal vein, and the willingness to minimize the diameter of the introducer sheaths incite to not insert any other security guidewire (as with the ipsilateral approach).

- The portal vein is catheterized to allow the global opacification through a diagnostic catheter (20 cm^3, 10 cm^3/s) on frontal and oblique views (most frequently left anterior), completed by selective right and left portal injections (12 cm^3, 6 cm^3/s) allowing the identification of each segment. Manometry allows the detection of a portal hypertension in cirrhotic or post chemotherapy patients, which generally constitutes a contraindication.

In the case of extended right hepatic resection, the chronology of the embolization of the segment 4 and the choice of embolization agent depend on the approach site.

- *Via a contralateral approach,* segment 4 is embolized just after the right branches, thus allowing an easier individualization due to the flow redistribution.

According to the technique described by De Baere et al. [4, 5], embolization is often achieved using a cyanoacrylate-based glue. Cannulation of the right branches is achieved with a selective 4 or 5 Fr catheter and a hydrophilic guidewire. The distal extremity of the introducer sheath must be placed as close as possible to the right segmental branches, in order to allow a safe retrieval of the catheter if needed. Injection of contrast agent under fluoroscopy allows an estimation of the flow and thus determines the dilution of cyanoacrylate and Lipiodol® (classical cyanoacrylate/Lipiodol® ratios = 1/2 or 1/3). The catheter must be flushed with a glucose solution, and then the glue is injected by using a stopcock and “Luer-Lock” syringes (cf. Chap. 1). The injection speed must be neither too slow, to avoid the formation of isolated aggregates, nor too fast, in order to avoid reflux towards the catheter and untargeted zones. After that, the volume of the catheter lumen is flushed by a 5 % glucose solution in the embolized branch, before catheterizing the remaining segmental branches. After a control opacification, the segment 4 branch is eventually catheterized and embolized. If the flow or the catheterization conditions are not safe enough to use glue, microparticles and/or coils or plugs may be used.

- *Via ipsilateral approach,* the embolization of segment 4 will take place before the right branches, to limit the risk of migration of the embolization agent when handling catheters. According to the Madoff technique [6], the embolization is achieved using microparticles and coils progressively delivered into each segmental branch. The cannulation of segment 4 vein is achieved using a 4 or 5 Fr diagnostic catheter and a microcatheter. Microparticles of increasing size are injected, in order to obtain an adequate distal embolization (we start with spherical 300 μm particles). Once a complete stagnation has been obtained, the catheter is carefully flushed in order to avoid a reflux of particles towards the left liver, and the embolization is completed by the deployment of micro-coils. The microcatheter is retrieved, and a control injection confirms that the exclusion is satisfactory. The right branches are cannulated after exchanging the catheter for a Simmons or Chuang reverse curve catheter, thus allowing access to each segmental branch; the branch which has allowed this transhepatic approach is the last occluded. Microparticles are injected according to the same increasing caliber progression, completed by the proximal deployment of coils. An opacification of the portal vein is then performed. A transhepatic tract embolization is not systematic [7].

- *Embolization Agents:* In order to obtain an optimal hypertrophy, embolization must be as complete as possible. The development of intrahepatic shunts observed after surgical ligations has led us to associate distal and proximal embolization agents. Glue and association of coils and particles are most widely used.

  - *Gelfoam* is not used alone, but may complete some procedures.
  - *Glue:* The mixture n-butyl cyanoacrylate (NBCA)/Lipiodol is most often used. The glue allows a rapid and durable occlusion for a limited cost, but its use requires some expertise. The dilution and the rate of the injection have to be adapted to the portal flow, evaluated by a manual injection of contrast medium. There is an increasing risk of migration during the procedure: the slowing down of the flow in the right branches increases the risk of a reflux towards the left. Careful attention must therefore be paid when embolizing the last segments. Small-sized fragments can remain at the distal extremity or in the inner lumen of the catheter and can migrate during the retrieval of the catheter or during the injection. In order to limit these secondary migrations, the distal extremity of the introducer sheath is directed into a target branch, thus allowing the retrieval of the distal extremity of the catheter (or microcatheter) and of eventual glued fragments outside of left portal branches. Similarly, the distal extremity of the catheter is maintained in a target branch before being flushed with a glucose solution to exclude the volume of the catheter lumen.
  - *Coils and Spherical Microparticles:* Microparticles allow a progressive and controlled distal embolization. The association with coils allows a more proximal embolization with a lesser risk of reflux. Many authors use 300–500 μm calibrated particles at first, and then 700–900 μm, followed by coils.
  - *Plugs:* Coils can be replaced by AVP occluder® if intrahepatic catheterization allows the use of sufficiently large catheters. These agents, which can be

initially repositioned, allow a fast occlusion. The advances in introduction profiles and the availability of a wider choice of plugs have led to a larger use of AVP for this indication.

No matter what embolization agent is used, the occlusion must be as complete as possible, so as to favor the compensating hypertrophy, but at the same time taking care to preserve the first centimeters of the right portal branch to permit its clamping without mobilizing the embolization agent during surgery.

8.4 Results

8.4.1 Immediate Technical Results

- The rate of immediate technical success as reported in literature is very high: 187/188 in a retrospective multicenter European study and 1,086/1,088 in a meta-analysis [7, 8].
- No deaths have been reported in these two series [7, 8].
- The complication rate, which varies between 1 and 6.5 %, includes transitory liver failure, especially among cirrhotic patients, no matter what the CHILD score is. Portal thrombosis remains rare (between 0.2 and 0.5 %). Bleeding, notably at the puncture site (1 %), is often limited to a subcapsular hematoma discovered at follow-up CT, which most of the time does not require any further treatment. The migration of embolic agents has also been described, but it remains most frequently infra clinical, no matter what the embolization agent is (glue or coils) [7, 8].

8.4.2 Hepatic Volume and Operability

- The hypertrophy obtained varies with respect to the embolic agent used and the sustainability of the occlusion, the existence of an initial parenchymal affection (steatosis, inflammation, cholestasis, and fibrosis), or of comorbidities, notably diabetes (in that case, insulin acting like a growth cofactor for liver regeneration).

  De Baere [5] has documented considerable differences of hypertrophy between cyanoacrylate and temporary agents.

  In the absence of underlying chronic liver disease, a constant increase of 8–25 % is reported, limited to 6–20 % in cases of preexisting cirrhosis; a 20 % failure rate (no hypertrophy of the left lobe) is observed in these latter cases.

  Smallest remaining parts of the liver are subject to most consistent hypertrophy, thus leading some authors to consider that there is not inferior limit of initial FRL volume for portal embolization.

- Surgery takes place after a 2- to 5-week interval, after evaluation of the liver hypertrophy and possible interval tumor progression.
  The surgical operability rate after an embolization is between 80 and 90 %. In case of an insufficient hypertrophy or of an intra- or extrahepatic tumor progression, surgery can be contraindicated (6.4–33 %) [7, 9–11].
- Several authors have evoked the role of embolization in intrahepatic tumor growth [12–14]. Growth mechanisms remain rather unknown, implying cellular factors (modifications of membranes after embolization), hormone factors (cytokines and growth factors), and hemodynamic factors via increase of arterial perfusion [15].

8.5 Indications

8.5.1 Indications

Initially indicated before resections of colorectal metastases, portal embolization indications have been extended to HCC and cholangiocarcinomas. The hypertrophy obtained is conditioned by the existence of the underlying liver disease (cirrhosis).

The indications must take into account the preoperative volumetry. The FLR to total liver ratio (FLRR) is defined as (FLR volume-tumor in the FLR)/(total liver volume-total tumor volume) [5].

- Developed in normal underlying liver: portal embolization is recommended when FLRR is <25–30 %.
- Cirrhosis or diabetes: FLRR <40 %.
- If dilation of bile ducts: FLRR <40 %, + prior drainage of the bile ducts.

8.5.2 Contraindications

- Embolization is only proposed before hepatectomy: patients with distant metastases or lymph node involvement are not candidates for resection.
- However, some patients with bilateral hepatic involvement can benefit from combined treatments [21, 22].
- A tumor invasion of the portal vein and a portal hypertension with portosystemic shunt are absolute contraindications.
- Coagulation disorders and renal insufficiency are relative contraindications.

8.5.3 Therapeutic Associations

- With bilateral lesions, treatment for a tumor on the FLR (radiofrequency, surgery) is first carried out, before performing embolization followed by hemihepatectomy.
- Encouraging results have been reported in the treatment of HCC by combining intra-arterial chemoembolization and preoperative portal embolization. The hypertrophy of the FLR, the tumor necrosis, and the survival are greater in the combined treatment group in comparison to the portal embolization group.
- An interval of 1–3 weeks between arterial chemoembolization and portal embolization has been advocated in order to reduce the risk of parenchymal necrosis, which constitutes a limit to this strategy [16–18].
- Data concerning an eventual interruption of a neoadjuvant chemotherapy, especially in case of colorectal metastases, are controversial: favorable for some authors [19, 20], it could slow down hypertrophy for others.

Key Points

- Indication: volumetry, causal hepatopathy, and comorbidities (diabetes).
- Morphological evaluation and operating planning mandatory.
- Bile duct drainage if necessary.
- Approach and occlusion agents depend on anatomy, operator experience, and material.
- Embolization as complete as possible, sparing the FLR.
- Glue: 3 at-risk situations:
  - Slow flow rate
  - Fragments coming from the extremity of the catheter
  - Fragments coming from the internal lumen of the catheter
- A free vein segment must be preserved for clamping.
- Embolization of segment 4: to prepare for an enlarged hepatectomy
  - At first by ipsilateral approach
  - At the end by contralateral approach
- Surgery between 2 and 5 weeks after reevaluation of:
  - Hypertrophy
  - Tumor staging

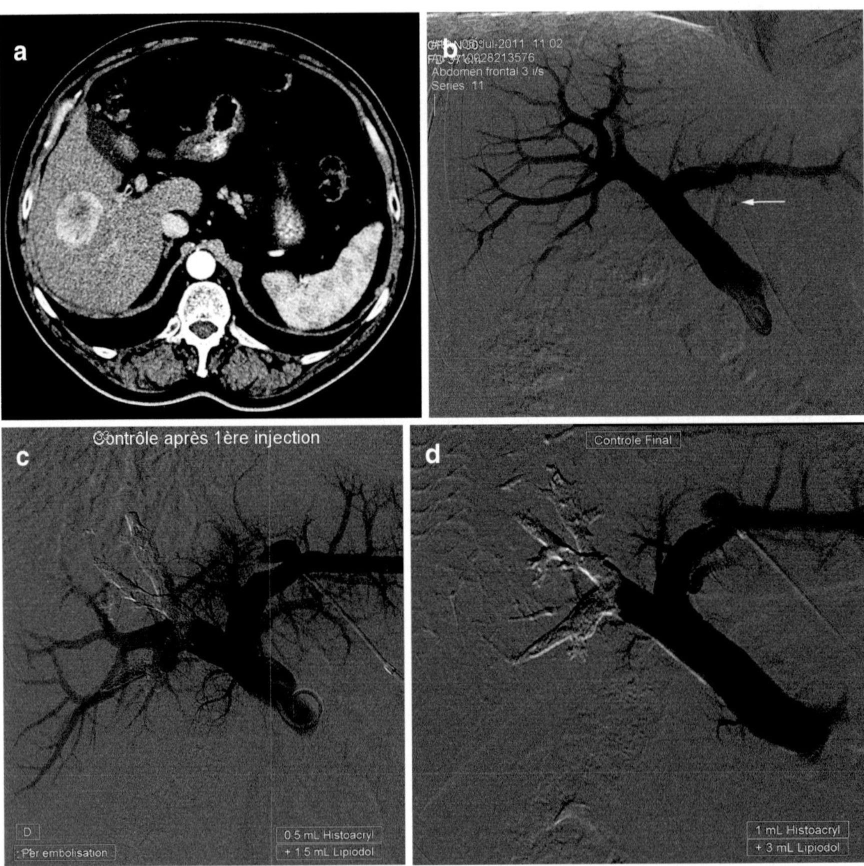

Fig. 8.1 68-year-old M, bifocal HCC (2 lesions of 3 cm diameter) on healthy liver; a right hepatectomy has been planned. The hepatic volumetry analysis led to plan a preop right portal branch embolization. (**a**) CT, arterial phase: segment IV tumor (the second tumor was located in segment VII). (**b**) Transparietal left portal vein puncture: note the end of the introducer sheath (*arrow*) and a pigtail catheter in the portal vein trunk. (**c**) Intermediate control after exclusion of anteromedial segmental branches, using a Histoacryl + Lipiodol emulsion. (**d**) Last control after exclusion of the posterolateral branches (pigtail catheter in the portal vein)

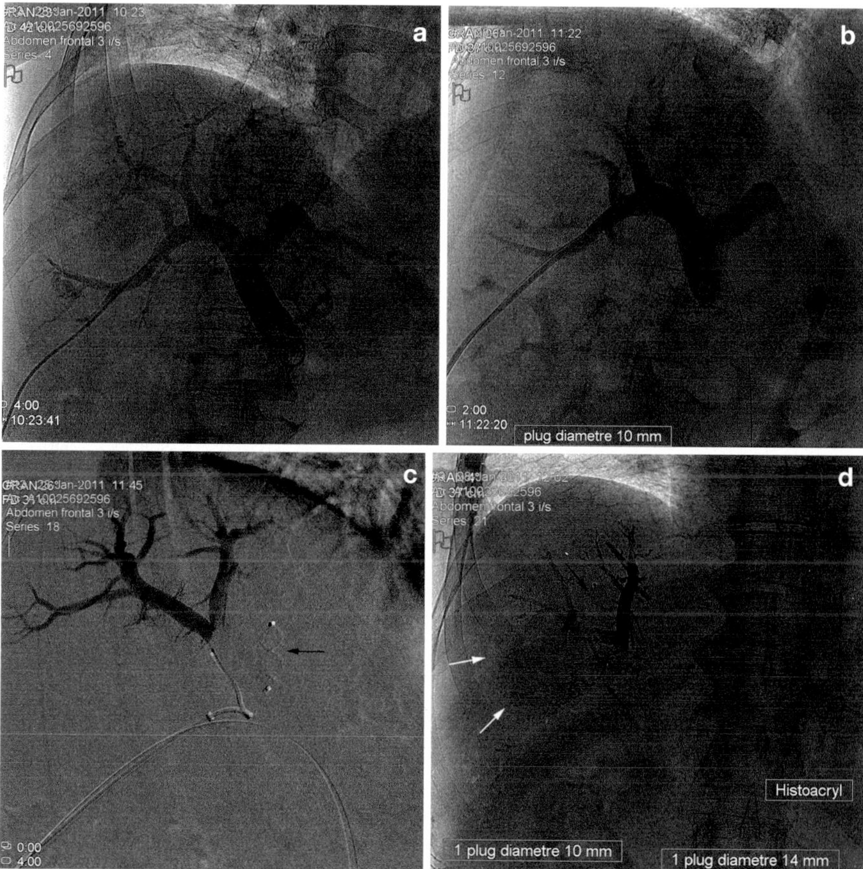

Fig. 8.2 Sgt VI 5 cm HCC, a right lobectomy has been planned, after a TACE session first, and then a portal embolization 2 m later. (**a**) Transparietal puncture of the right portal vein, decided because the access to the left portal vein was ultrasonically considered too difficult. (**b**) Control portography after exclusion by AVP of the segment IV portal branch, arising from the right portal vein. Note the security GW beside the introducer sheath in the portal vein. (**c**) Selective catheterization of the segment VIII branches (Mikaelsson catheter): occlusion with glue (Histoacryl) (*arrow:* AVP previously delivered in the segment IV branch). (**d**) Plain film (without any ICM injection) after introducer sheath retrieval: occlusion with an AVP of the posterolateral branch (with this ipsilateral access, a final portography was impossible). Note the spontaneous radio-opacity of Histoacryl-Lipiodol emulsion used to occlude the segment VIII branches; AVP: *black arrow*; intratumoral retention of Lipiodol, consequence of the previously performed TACE (*white arrows*)

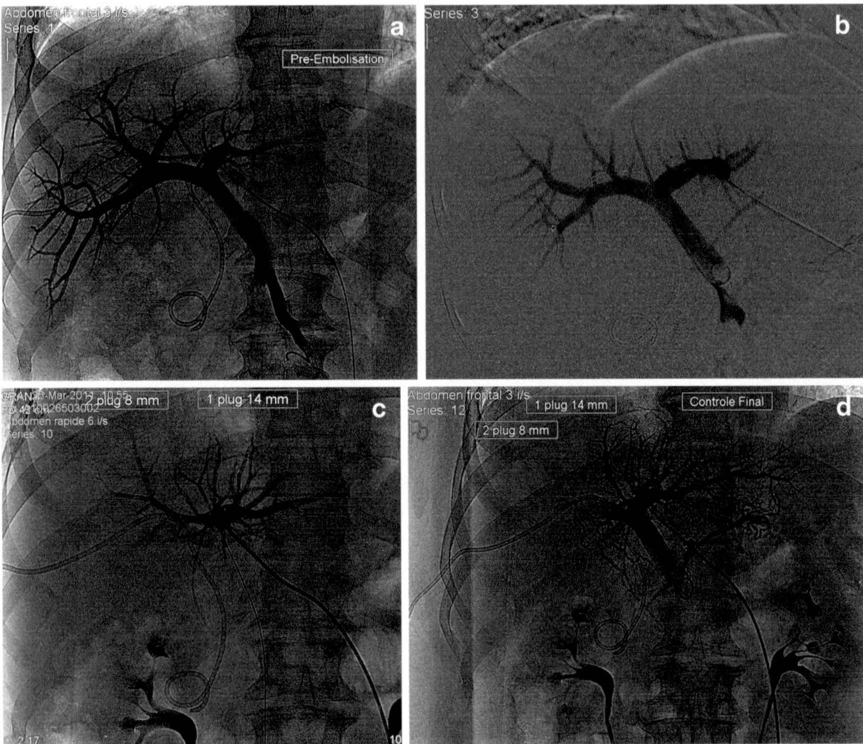

Fig. 8.3 Klatskin 3 B cholangiocarcinoma: a right lobectomy has been decided, preceded by a right portal vein preoperative embolization. An internal–external biliary drain has also been installed. (**a**, **b**) After a transparietal left portal vein puncture: portography (frontal (**a**) and oblique (**b**) views), via a pigtail catheter in the portal vein. (**c**) Sheath injection in the left portal branch: occlusion with an AVP of the right lobe branches. Note the remaining GW in the portal vein. (**d**) Last control portogram, after AVP exclusion of the segmental IV branch

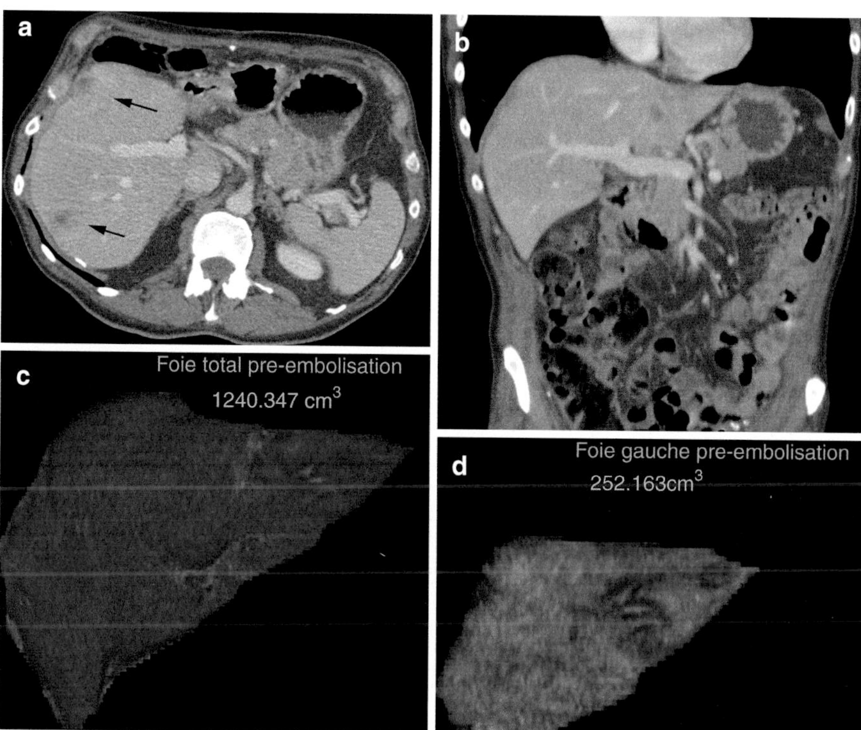

Fig. 8.4 50-year-old W, sigmoid cancer with synchronous liver metastases. First, the following have been performed: a colic resection and preop radiofrequency ablation of left liver metastases. A right hepatectomy is then planned. (**a**) Pre-embolization CT, portal phase: metastases (*arrows*). (**b–d**) CT frontal reconstruction and hepatic volumetry. The volume of the left lobe is limited: FLR is evaluated as 25 % of this healthy liver volume. (**e**) Transparietal portography (right portal branch access; pigtail catheter in the portal vein, GW in the paramedian sector to guide the AVP release). (**f**) Control opacification via the introducer sheath after the release of a 16 mm diameter AVP in the right portal vein. (**g–i**) CT 3 w later: correct position of the plug in the right portal vein; more than 50 % induced liver hypertrophy. (**j–l**) CT 6 m after right hepatectomy

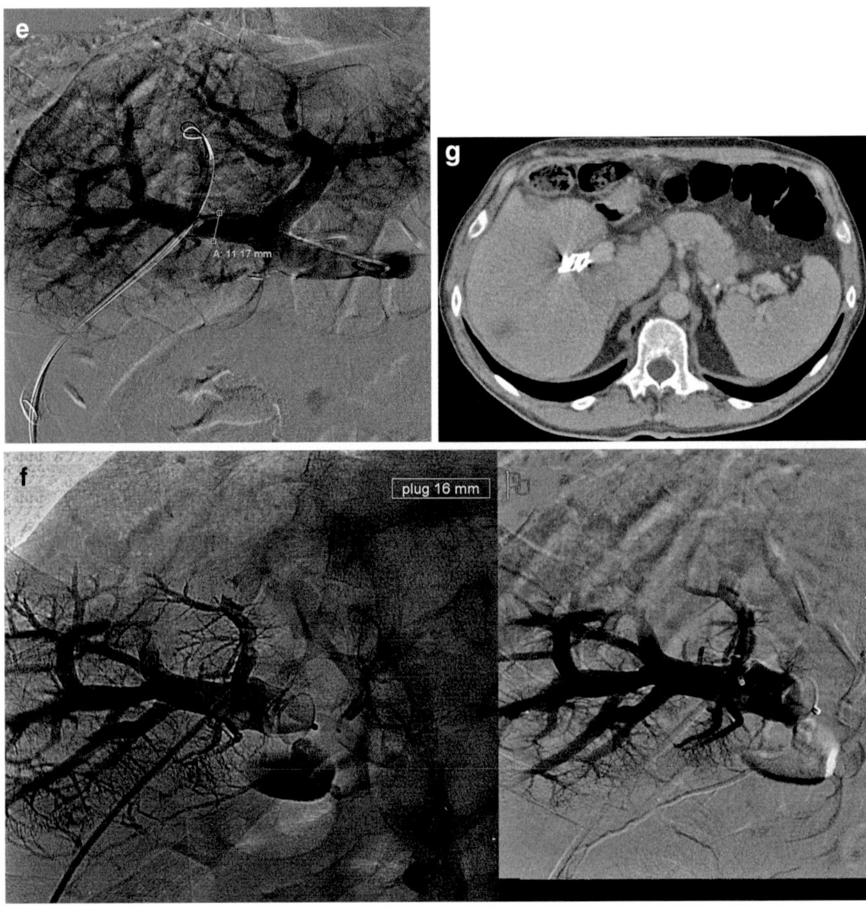

Fig. 8.4 (continued)

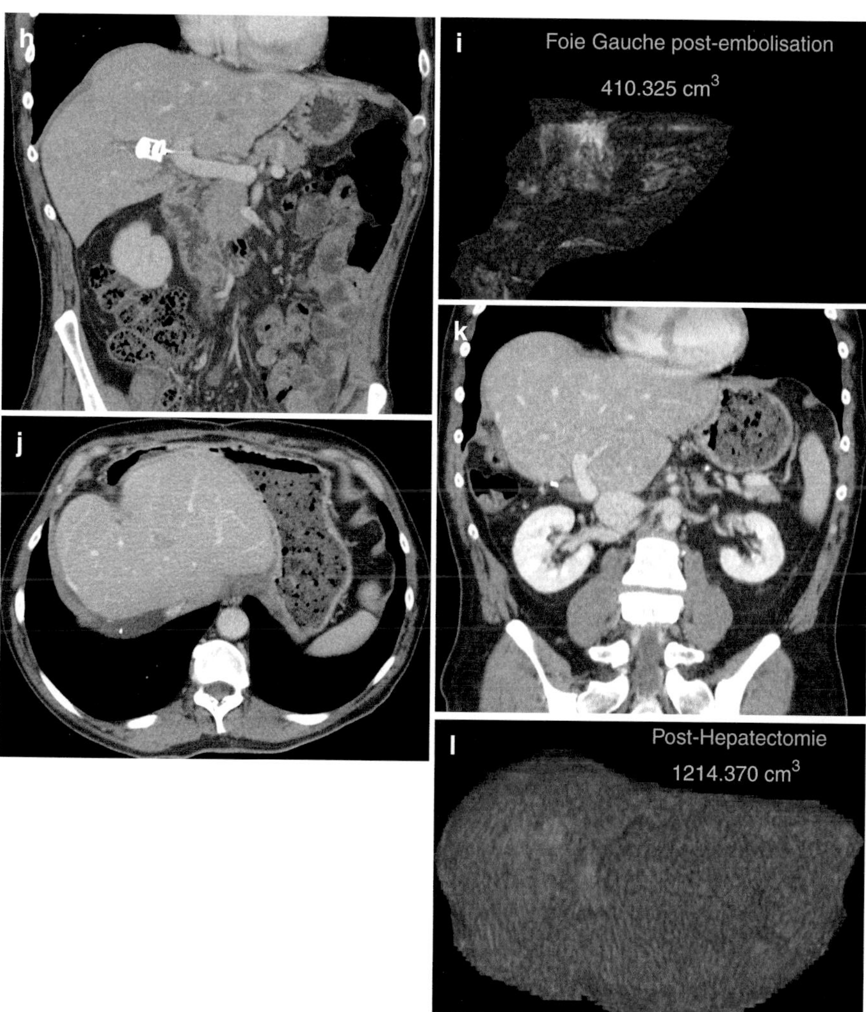

Fig. 8.4 (continued)

References

1. Perarnau JM, et al. Transjugular preoperative portal embolization (TJPE) a pilot study. Hepatogastroenterology. 2003;50(51):610–3.
2. Tsuge H, et al. Right portal embolization before extended right hepatectomy using laparoscopic catheterization of the ileocolic vein: a prospective study. Surg Laparosc Endosc. 1994;4(4):258–63.
3. Gibo M, et al. Percutaneous ipsilateral portal vein embolization using a modified four-lumen balloon catheter with fibrin glue: initial clinical experience. Radiat Med. 2007;25(4):164–72.
4. de Baere T, Denys A, Madoff DC. Preoperative portal vein embolization: indications and technical considerations. Tech Vasc Interv Radiol. 2007;10(1):67–78.
5. de Baere T, et al. Preoperative portal vein embolization for extension of hepatectomy indications. Hepatology. 1996;24(6):1386–91.
6. Madoff DC, et al. Transhepatic portal vein embolization: anatomy, indications, and technical considerations. Radiographics. 2002;22(5):1063–76.
7. Di Stefano DR, et al. Preoperative percutaneous portal vein embolization: evaluation of adverse events in 188 patients. Radiology. 2005;234(2):625–30.
8. Abulkhir A, et al. Preoperative portal vein embolization for major liver resection: a meta-analysis. Ann Surg. 2008;247(1):49–57.
9. Azoulay D, et al. Resection of nonresectable liver metastases from colorectal cancer after percutaneous portal vein embolization. Ann Surg. 2000;231(4):480–6.
10. Hemming AW, et al. Preoperative portal vein embolization for extended hepatectomy. Ann Surg. 2003;237(5):686–91, discussion 691–3.
11. Imamura H, et al. Preoperative portal vein embolization: an audit of 84 patients. Hepatology. 1999;29(4):1099–105.
12. Barbaro B, et al. Preoperative right portal vein embolization in patients with metastatic liver disease. Metastatic liver volumes after RPVE. Acta Radiol. 2003;44(1):98–102.
13. Elias D, et al. During liver regeneration following right portal embolization the growth rate of liver metastases is more rapid than that of the liver parenchyma. Br J Surg. 1999;86(6): 784–8.
14. Kokudo N, et al. Proliferative activity of intrahepatic colorectal metastases after preoperative hemihepatic portal vein embolization. Hepatology. 2001;34(2):267–72.
15. de Graaf W, et al. Induction of tumor growth after preoperative portal vein embolization: is it a real problem? Ann Surg Oncol. 2009;16(2):423–30.
16. Aoki T, et al. Sequential preoperative arterial and portal venous embolizations in patients with hepatocellular carcinoma. Arch Surg. 2004;139(7):766–74.
17. Ogata S, et al. Sequential arterial and portal vein embolizations before right hepatectomy in patients with cirrhosis and hepatocellular carcinoma. Br J Surg. 2006;93(9):1091–8.
18. Yamakado K, et al. Long-term follow-up arterial chemoembolization combined with transportal ethanol injection used to treat hepatocellular carcinoma. J Vasc Interv Radiol. 1999; 10(5):641–7.
19. Covey AM, et al. Combined portal vein embolization and neoadjuvant chemotherapy as a treatment strategy for resectable hepatic colorectal metastases. Ann Surg. 2008;247(3): 451–5.
20. Goere D, et al. Chemotherapy does not impair hypertrophy of the left liver after right portal vein obstruction. J Gastrointest Surg. 2006;10(3):365–70.
21. Liu H, Zhu S. Present status and future perspectives of preoperative embolization. Am J Surg. 2009;197:686–90.
22. Jaeck D, et al. A two-stage hepatectomy procedure combined with portal vein embolization to achieve curative resection for initially unresectable multiple and bilobar colorectal liver metastases. Ann Surg. 2004;240(6):1037–49, discussion 1049–51.

Suggested Reading

Denys A, Bize P, Demartines N, Deschamps F, De Baere T. Quality improvement for portal vein embolization. Cardiovasc Intervent Radiol. 2010;33:452–6.

Madoff DC, et al. Transhepatic portal vein embolization: anatomy, indications, and technical considerations. Radiographics. 2002;22(5):1063–76.

Part V
Situations and Strategies: Abdomen and GI Tract

Chapter 9
Splenic Arterial Embolizations

Pascal Chabrot, Marie-Aude Vaz Tourret, Rémy Guillon, Anne Ravel, Denis Pezet, Jean-Marc Garcier, and Louis Boyer

9.1 Background

Advances in catheterization techniques have led to the broadening of the indications of splenic artery embolization. Although their indications are yet to be completely established in hematology, splenic embolizations are valuable as a programmed procedure in treating vulnerable patients affected by pseudoaneurysms, aneurysms, hypersplenism, as well as splenic traumas in an emergency setting.

The potential impact of these embolizations on hemostasis, the pancreas, and infectious state, as well as eventual painful consequences, makes pain management mandatory, during and after the procedure, in collaboration with anesthesiologists and referring physicians.

9.2 Relevant Radiological Anatomy

The splenic artery provides the arterial vascularization of the spleen. It is a terminal branch of the celiac artery (which originates from the ventral part of the aorta at T12 level immediately downstream the median arcuate ligament of the diaphragm).

P. Chabrot, MD, PhD • M.-A. Vaz Tourret, MD • A. Ravel, MD • L. Boyer, MD, PhD (✉)
Department of Radiology, University Hospital of Clermont-Ferrand, Clermont-Ferrand, France
e-mail: lboyer@chu-clermontferrand.fr; pchabrot@chu-clermontferrand.fr

R. Guillon, MD
Department of Radiology, Clinique Saint Roch, Montpellier, France

D. Pezet, MD, PhD
Department of Abdominal Surgery,
University Hospital of Clermont-Ferrand, Clermont-Ferrand, France

J.-M. Garcier, MD, PhD
Department of Anatomy and Radiology,
University Hospital of Clermont-Ferrand, Clermont-Ferrand, France

P. Chabrot, L. Boyer (eds.), *Embolization*,
DOI 10.1007/978-1-4471-5182-1_9, © Springer-Verlag London 2014

It is located at the upper edge of the corporeo-caudal part of the pancreas and terminates into superior and inferior lobar branches, at the level to the tail of the pancreas, or at the level of the splenic hilum, or between both of them. Each lobar branch then divides into 2–5 segmentary branches and then subsegmentary ones. The superior lobar artery provides the main splenic arterial vascularization; the inferior lobar artery courses to the left gastroepiploic, anastomosed with the right one, and provides the vascularization of the greater gastric curve.

The splenic artery gives off branches feeding the left part of the pancreas: the dorsal pancreatic artery (in 78 % of the cases, located behind the pancreatic isthmus), the great pancreatic artery, and an average of four little pancreatic branches.

The splenic vein originates at the confluence of five to six branches emerging from the dorsal splenic hilum and is caudal to the arterial branches. It then courses transversally to the left, along the posterior face of the pancreas. Most often it receives the lower mesenteric vein, before joining with the upper mesenteric vein to form the portal trunk.

It receives the short veins of gastric origin, the left gastroepiploic vein, and a number of little pancreatic veins.

9.3 Techniques

- Embolization is carried out under the usual strict aseptical conditions.
  - For splenic parenchyma exclusions, it is recommended to give a short-lasting antibiotic prophylaxis treatment before the procedure, in order to prevent post-splenectomy septicemia, which can occur days after. Some authors carry out preventive antibiotherapy using penicillin up to 1 year after embolization in case of beta-thalassemias. Patients must be informed of their vulnerability to pneumococcal infection: should a fever occur, an antibiotherapy using Oracillin must be undertaken immediately, and the patient must consult his physician as rapidly as possible.

    A few days before the embolization for hypersplenism or hematological conditions, an antipneumococcal vaccination is systematically administered by some authors. We do not carry out preventive pneumococcal and hemophilus vaccination in case of partial embolization. When the embolization is carried out in order to facilitate a splenectomy, the vaccination is always given 1–2 weeks before the intervention.
  - In the cases of aneurysm and false aneurysm exclusions, antibiotic prophylactic treatment is given only to weak patients with a high infectious risk. Pneumococcal vaccinations and other antibiotic preventive measures are not prescribed, except if a splenectomy is planned secondarily or in case of a massive splenic parenchyma infarction.

- Analgesia
  - Post-embolization pain observed with parenchymal embolizations may require an epidural anesthesia at T4 level or an intravenous injection, just before the embolization or during the procedure directly into the catheter which is placed in the splenic artery, just before the embolus unloading.

    We then use the association of analgesics and morphinics given either by a syringe pump or better still self-administered by the patient (patient-controlled analgesia). This treatment takes place for at least 3 days, depending on the pain and the infarction extent. This analgesia is important as it limits respiratory inhibition and therefore left pleuro-parenchymal complications.
  - For exclusions of arterial trunk lesions, a simple premedication is sufficient in adults. Antalgics are then administered upon demand, taking into account the extent of splenic parenchyma infarction and eventual complications.

- Femoral access is commonly used.
- The procedure begins with a global opacification of the aorta, followed by selective injections of the superior mesenteric artery (with assessment of portal venous return), celiac trunk, then splenic artery, in order to visualize the size, the course of the splenic artery, and the location of the principal collateral branches.

The catheter is then positioned at the level of the splenic artery trunk in case of proximal lesion; it is positioned very distally if part of the splenic parenchyma has to be excluded, in order to spare the branches feeding the pancreas.

Depending on the sinusitis found, it may be possible to use a microcatheter, introduced into a stable selective guiding catheter. In this case, a continuous wash by physiological saline must be put in place.

- Embolic agents: the choice of the technique (embolization agent and site) varies with the indications. Both absorbable and nonabsorbable materials can be used.

Proximal agents (coils, plugs, or balloons) allow occlusion of the splenic artery. They bring about little change with respect to the splenic parenchyma as long as the collateral branch network is not affected.

If the goal is to destroy part of the spleen's parenchyma, then some intraparenchymal branches must be occluded and the splenic artery must be blocked as distally as possible, beyond the gastric and pancreatic efferent branches.

In case of partial parenchymal embolization, whenever possible, our preference goes out to the exclusion of the lower part of the spleen, so as to reduce the risk of pleural effusion or subphrenic collection.

- Intraoperative quantification of excluded parenchyma: intraoperative echography, 3D-angio, cone beam "CT-like" imaging technique.
- The hemostasis at the puncture site must be carefully controlled, especially in cases of thrombocytopenia; small caliber introducer sheaths and eventually closure devices must be used.

- Follow-up: The clinical tolerance depends on different factors: the size of the spleen, the importance of the parenchymal exclusion, the underlying clinical condition, the embolization agent used, and the quality of the analgesia.

The collaboration between clinicians, anesthesiologists, and vascular radiologists is of utmost importance.

In our team, parenchymal embolizations normally require a 4–6 days hospitalization; this can be longer for large spleens.

Normally we carry out a CT or MRI on day 8 and 1 month after the procedure in case of parenchyma embolizations and 1 month and 1 year after in case of aneurysm treatment.

9.4 Technical Results

9.4.1 *Success and Failure*

Selective catheterization of the splenic artery trunk is usually feasible, but tortuosities can make the exercise very difficult, especially in older patients.

An ultra-selective catheterization up to the splenic hilum is not always feasible notably in emergency situations even with a microcatheter.

9.4.2 *Biological Follow-Up*

Long-lasting biological modifications are observed when the embolization affects more than 50 % of the splenic parenchyma.

- *In adults*, up until the end of the second week, *leukocytes* increase by a factor of three times their normal rate. Then they diminish up to the third month, followed by an increase. A stabilization is noted from the fourth month onwards (the basic rate increased by an average of 1.3–2).

In adults the *platelets'* curve is quite similar, with a peak after 2 weeks (base rate multiplied by 4): consequence of the suppression of the platelet sequestration, possibly induced by a splenic unloading, but can also have for origin the improvement of transfusion efficiency and an increase of platelet life. Then there is a decreasing oscillating pattern up to the third month and then finally a stabilization (basic rate is multiplied by 2 or 3 on average). Sometimes this effect lasts for up to 5–6 years after the embolization.

- *In children,* the *hyperleukocytosis* period is prolonged. The peak takes place between 4 and 6 days after the procedure. The rate remains above 10,000/mm^3 between 9 and 21 days (13.6 days on average). For the *platelets,* the peak occurs between 6 and 13 days. It can be important (up to 1,000,000/mm^3) before returning to a normal rate after several months.

The *red blood cells* increase significantly up to 2 months after the procedure, and then they start to stabilize out after the ninth month.

- *Liver Function*: inconstant but significant increases in levels of prothrombin, albumin, and cholesterol after the first year means an improvement of the liver function. A transitory increase in the bilirubin is also found in the first week.

For aneurysm exclusions and truncal splenic-artery pseudoaneurysm exclusions, there is no major modification in the blood count, except in cases of important splenic infarction or sepsis. But the amylasemia must be monitored in order to detect a pancreatitis.

9.4.3 Morphological Follow-Up

- After a parenchymal embolization, a transitory splenomegaly has been observed (110–140 %) during the first 2 weeks; this edematous-necrotic phase leads to a risk of a rupture for a period of about 4 weeks. Then there is a decrease in the volume of the spleen which lasts from 6 to 21 months, corresponding to necrotic resorption. The infarcted zones (which are not contrast enhanced) disappear after 2–4 months. The decrease in the volume of the spleen can even continue after the disappearance of these necrotic zones.

In children, regeneration of the splenic parenchyma (from a few days to several months afterwards) may be observed, without any recurrence of the previous lesion or hypersplenism.

During follow-up, it is possible to see air on CT or ultrasound scans: this corresponds to anaerobic metabolism. This gas collected in the infarcted tissues can spread to the other parts of the parenchyma. These images are normally seen during the first month and then disappear after a few months. They must not be interpreted as a sign of an infection.

The volume of the infarcted parenchyma seems to be correlated with the risk of splenic and/or portal vein thrombosis, which must be checked for on the early follow-up CT scan on day 8. In the case that embolization exposes to extensive parenchymal infarction, then sequential embolizations in two or three sessions would be the best choice. In case of portal thrombosis, an anticoagulant treatment must be given.

In practice, the efficacy of the parenchymatous embolizations must be judged with respect to the biological results and not to spleen size: the biological results can be very acceptable even though the volume of the spleen remains considerable.

- During exclusions of truncal arterial lesions, small hypodense parenchymal areas may be seen at different times after injection on CT. These are small infarction foci induced by the migration of the emboli. The excluded aneurysm must not be enhanced.

9.4.4 Complications

The mortality rate after complete splenic parenchymal embolization is probably not negligible.

The persistence of a fraction of functional parenchyma allows the preservation of the spleen's immunological functions.

The experience of the team carrying out the procedure as well the ongoing care given after is without any doubt essential in reducing the morbidity. One can observe:

- Nonspecific technical complications (hematoma at the puncture site, catheterization complications, vascular dissections or spasms, contrast agent adverse effects)
- Minor complications: post-embolization syndrome, which is very frequent and often resolved after 2–5 days: asymptomatic splenic vein thrombosis, pain, fever, left pleuro-pneumopathy, slight pancreatitis (abdominal pain and amylasemia increase), and ileus. A very strict aseptic environment plus an adapted prophylactic antibiotic treatment and sedation limits the occurrence of these complications.
- Major complications
  - Vascular: migration of the occlusive agent, pseudoaneurysm rupture, and splenic and portal vein thrombosis.
  - Splenic: hematoma (0.7 %), infection (1.4 %), collection of splenic lysis or cyst, and splenic rupture. Post-embolization abscesses can be treated by a percutaneous drainage.
  - Abdominal: pancreatitis (2.9 %) and gastric ulcer.
  - Thoracic: left pneumopathy (0.7 %) and pleural effusion (7.1 %).

These complications are observed with massive splenic infarctions, affecting more than 80 % of the splenic vasculature. An embolization of 90 % of the parenchyma usually always leads to the formation of abscess. Thus, the embolization should be interrupted after a 50–60 % occlusion of the vascular network (and if the biological results are insufficient, the embolization can be repeated 15 days to 1 month later).

Biological glues are more likely to cause pancreatic ischemia.

The risk of an extensive infarction (with all its complications) when large spleens are embolized must make one discuss an alternative therapeutic sequence: arterial embolization, rapidly followed by a laparoscopic splenectomy.

9.5 Indications

9.5.1 Traumatisms of the Spleen

Splenic traumatisms can bring about both sub- and trans-capsular parenchymal damages, with formation of arterial wounds, arteriovenous fistulas, or intraparenchymal pseudoaneurysms. Surgery was the treatment of first intention in the past.

Presently, a conservative nonsurgical approach is often indicated in patients who are hemodynamically stable: this can correspond to a simple attentive supervision or to an arterial embolization which provides the hemostasis of the traumatic lesions, thus avoiding hemorrhagic delayed ruptures (which prognosis is very severe). Patient selection is the key step.

9.5.1.1 Indications and Technique

The advantage of embolization is to preserve the splenic functions by conserving the vitality of a part of the parenchyma, but the vital prognosis is to be preserved at first.

- A systematic angiography advocated by some authors to help to select patients who can benefit from an embolization cannot today be recommended. The fundamental criteria to be discussed when considering an embolization are the hemodynamic stability and the CT-scan pattern: AAST grade [1] (see Appendix 9.1), blush (active contrast extravasation) false aneurysms, and arteriovenous fistula. The extravasation may be intraparenchymal, subcapsular, or intraperitoneal.
  - According to most of the authors, patients suffering from a hemorrhagic shock and/or showing signs of peritonitis must benefit from emergency explorative surgery, while for the hemodynamic stable patients the normal conservative treatment is the standard. Hagiwara [2] has recently suggested to widen the embolization indications to hemodynamically unstable patients responding to vascular filling and having high AAST scores (4 and 5), but this is contested by some other authors.
  - Besides surgical indications, all traumatic splenic lesions with a blush on the CT scan, or for some, having only an abundant hemoprotein, must undergo a selective arteriography, generally followed by an embolization. This arterial blush observed on CT is of positive predictive value, but it is only found in 93 % of the cases on arteriography [3]. In cases of arteriovenous fistula or posttraumatic false aneurysm, embolization is also indicated.

A strict clinical and radiological surveillance is necessary for AAST grade 1 (in which a blush is rarely visible), thus allowing an intervention in case of bleeding.

AAST grade 2 without any blush on CT needs also surveillance for a number of authors; in case of a blush, an arteriography/embolization must be carried out.

Arteriography must be carried out for grades 3 and 4, irrespective of whether there is a blush or not.

For grade 5, there is no consensus. We recommend, as do so a number of other authors, a surgical intervention.

  - The "Bhaltimore" codification has been proposed by Marmery et al. [4] (Appendix 9.2), in order to take into account vascular lesions along with the splenic anatomical damages which determine the AAST classification. In that way, patients needing a surgical approach or embolization, that is to say with blush and/or false aneurysm and/or posttraumatic arteriovenous fistula (Baltimore grade 4), would be better identified within spleen-traumatized patients.

- Also there is no consensus on embolization technique, proximal or distal. For all the authors, neither method is exclusive. The distal embolization, technically more difficult, gives a safer intraparenchymal hemostasis and at the same time conserving the spleen's immunological functions.

For proximal embolization, the positioning of coils and the choice of their diameter size are fundamental; this embolization is supposed to stop the arterial bleeding, by diminishing the flow and the arterial pressure. Notably it has been proposed for high-grade traumas without extravasation. But it can lead to a situation of an incomplete hemostasis and a delayed re-bleeding (where re-embolization may be difficult). Proximal embolization may be inefficient in the case of AVF, due to remaining perfusion via collateral branches.

In our team, as first-line treatment, we try to carry out distal embolizations by using microparticles (firstly 300–700 diameter microns, then 900–1,200 μm); if it fails, we carry out a proximal embolization (coils, even Amplatzer occluders). In the case of a pseudoaneurysm or of AVF, a distal embolization is our initial choice, with or without additional proximal embolization.

9.5.1.2 Results SFICV 2007 (Recommendations [5])

- In more than 90 % of the cases, embolizations of an active bleeding are a technical success.
- The failures are the consequences of catheterization difficulties or bleeding recurrences.
- Complications have been noted in about 5 % of the cases, notably with partial splenic necrosis and abscesses (which come about more frequently after distal than proximal embolization).

We have noted lower morbidity when the embolization is carried out within 24 h after the trauma.

- If one compares in intention to treat the nonsurgical treat strategy versus the surgical strategy:
  - The global mortality is identical (5–10 %).
  - Complications are less important and the duration of the hospital stay is shorter with the nonoperative approach.
  - Splenectomy rates vary from 26 to 43 % for the surgical management approach while 12–15 % for the nonoperative strategy; thus, embolization performed in case of active arterial blush, and systematically for high lesional grades, would grant a global splenectomy gain of 7–19 %.

9.5.2 Arterial Trunk Lesions: Aneurysms and Pseudoaneurysms (See Also Chap. 11: Aneurysms of Visceral Arteries)

Aneurysms and pseudoaneurysms of visceral arteries are classically rare: 1 % of aneurysms for visceral arteries in autopsy series, among which 60 % splenic arterial aneurysms. These lesions are diagnosed more frequently today, due to detection on US, CT, and MRI.

The surgical treatment consists of a ligation, sometimes associated with a pancreatic or splenic resection, especially for pseudoaneurysms. The death rate for these operations is 1.3 % for aneurysms and 16 % for pseudoaneurysms.

9.5.2.1 Technique

A selective catheterization is necessary in order to try and preserve the collateral vessels and therefore sparing the spleen and if possible the pancreas. This catheterization may be difficult; therefore, microcatheters can be used.

Coils are most often used; care is given to preserve the splenic vascularization by the collateral vessels. They can be either directly placed inside the aneurysm ("packing") or it can be placed at the level of its neck. Packing must be avoided in case of false aneurysm. An occlusion balloon can be temporarily positioned upstream and inflated, thus reducing the flow and securing the procedure. When there is no neck, we use either the Moret's remodeling technique (unloading of coils which are protected by an inflated balloon before the opening) or larguable balloons. One can still implant a bare stent and then unload the coils through the meshes using a microcatheter. One can also carry out the equivalent of a ligature-exclusion by "sandwiching" the aneurysm with some coils disposed upstream and downstream; a downstream reinjection by means of the collateral pathway can happen in the case of a simple upstream occlusion ("closing the back door"). The association of Gelfoam + coils can be useful to treat large aneurysms and pseudoaneurysms.

A surgical bypass can precede an embolization.

The coverage of the aneurysmal segment by a covered stent can also theoretically be envisaged, knowing that the progression of a long and therefore rigid stent graft can be difficult given that this artery is often tortuous. The angled path at the origin of the celiac trunk and the splenic artery is also a technical difficulty. Multilayer stents (flow diverters) ensure a modulation of the flow, thus maintaining the patency of the collateral vessels; they can probably be used in the splenic artery.

Glues and Onyx have been used to treat aneurysms of visceral arteries, but necessitate an excellent technical expertise.

False aneurysm must not be treated in the same manner.

A thrombin injection can be proposed to treat visceral false aneurysms, especially when endovascular access is not possible (false aneurysms fed by small arteries which are impossible to catheterize).

9.5.2.2 Indications

- In case of rupture: the configuration of the lesions, the experience, and the 24/24 availability of the medical staff can make endovascular treatment possible in some cases. An upstream temporary balloon occlusion allows the limitation of blood loss before the exclusion of the ruptured aneurysm.

- Other situations: arteriography is necessary for the therapeutic indications and for the choice of endovascular or surgical techniques, but it only shows arterial lumens and therefore must always be used in association with CT (which up until now is our preference) or MRI.

When it is feasible, endovascular treatment is proposed as the first-line treatment for aneurysms and false aneurysms of the splenic artery, because of its limited morbidity and spleen sparing.

- All false aneurysms must be treated.
- Symptomatic aneurysms must be treated.
- According to the academic recommendations of the AHA, the treatment for rupture prevention concerns: aneurysms of 2 cm and more in women of childbearing age, in case of portal hypertension, or in patients awaiting hepatic transplantation (class I, evidence level B); the treatment of visceral aneurysms of more than 2 cm in older women and in men is "probably indicated" (class IIa, level B).

In practice, due to low morbidity-mortality rate of the endovascular techniques, some authors have recommended to lower the 2 cm threshold, taking into account the diameter of the parent artery and defining the critical threshold as twice the diameter of this artery. Aneurysms of 20 mm or less can be so treated, notably in young patients, women in childbearing age wishing to be pregnant, and in cases of an obvious size increase on successive imaging.

After treatment an imaging control is necessary, especially in cases of false aneurysms, in order to eliminate the reperfusions, which are not exceptional. We carry out a systematic CT control at 1 month and 1 year so as to ensure the sustainability of the exclusion and the decrease in size of the lesion.

- When a therapeutic abstention is indicated (small aneurysms), follow-up imaging is mandatory. In the absence of precise recommendation, we usually suggest an annual imaging follow-up by ultrasound, CT, or MRI.

To conclude, there are some nuances in the therapeutic indications, and alternative treatments must have been explained before any procedure.

9.5.2.3 Results

Published series are limited. When it is technically feasible, the endovascular treatment has a primary technical success in 60–90 % of the cases, with reduced morbidity.

9.5.3 Hypersplenism

Hypersplenism is defined as an association of a pancytopenia (anemia, leukopenia, thrombocytopenia), of a splenomegaly, and of a rich bone marrow, resulting from a portal hypertension (PHT). It occurs for a variety of reasons, but most often the consequence of cirrhosis, usually also complicated by bleeding of esophageal varices.

9.5.3.1 Technique

In case of a hypersplenism secondary to segmental PHT (in particular due to thrombosis or compression of the splenic vein), a proximal arterial occlusion can be used so as to reduce the collateral circulation originating from the splenic network.

In the case of a PHT due to intrahepatic block, a proximal occlusion of the splenic artery will only have a temporary effect due to the importance of the collateral vascular network. Therefore, the embolization must be distal and parenchymal.

For some authors, the embolization agent must be absorbable: they consider that the other agents give no extra advantage with respect to Gelfoam. We often use gelatin to complete an embolization with small size microparticles (250–500 μm). It has been recommended to impregnate the Gelfoam with an antibiotic solution (penicillin G 1,000,000 UI/100 ml, or cefazolin 500 mg/100 ml, gentamicin 80 mg/100 ml). A small balloon catheter may be inflated upstream to avoid the reflux of the embolization agent.

The extension of the infarction is monitored with fluoroscopy and must be stopped when two thirds of the splenic parenchyma has been excluded, without exceeding the 80 % threshold, thus avoiding major complication. It is interesting in this context to obtain cone beam "CT-like" images during the procedure. When the flow in the splenic artery slows down, it can be considered that the embolization has covered 70–80 % of the parenchyma. There is maybe a relationship between the recurrence of hypersplenism after embolization and the percentage of the embolized parenchyma: no recurrence is observed above 50 %, whereas between 30 and 50 % there are limited effects on hypersplenism.

Taking into account the severity of the complications when embolization concerns more than 80 % of the parenchyma, it must therefore be carried out between 60 and 80 %.

9.5.3.2 Indications and Results

The indications for a splenectomy are usually the size of the spleen (discomfort of the patient) and hypersplenism refractory to blood transfusions, as a palliative treatment. But the immune functions of the spleen, and therefore the consequences of a splenectomy, must be kept in mind before carrying out surgery, even more so in those patients who are somewhat weak.

There is only very few data available comparing surgery and partial embolization.

Hypersplenism being a consequence of PHT, it is the main indication for an arterial embolization of the parenchyma of a nontraumatic spleen.

Besides the biological effects of the embolization which have already been discussed, the embolization allows preservation of the spleen, without excluding the possibility of a distal splenorenal shunt. With respect to the PHT, the embolization can also contribute to a better control of the gastric and esophageal varices and of the congestive gastric mucosa (which is a non-negligible source of bleeding in case of PHT).

Gastroesophageal bleedings found in children, as a consequence of hypersplenism secondary to Gaucher's disease, intrahepatic biliary duct atresia, and portal vein thrombosis, can also be treated by splenic embolization.

A partial embolization is recommended for a splenomegaly with a platelet count inferior to 40,000/mm^3.

Even though a post-embolic syndrome is commonly observed, morbidity remains limited if the technical recommendations have been respected (aseptic conditions, appropriate antibiotics, and partial necrosis of the splenic parenchyma <80 %). The frequency of complications (splenic abscesses, respiratory, and edemato-ascitic decompensation) seems correlated with infarction extent.

In this way hypersplenism can be controlled, and the bleeding consequences of PHT are limited. If necessary, the procedure can be repeated later in case of recurring symptoms. Embolization constitutes an alternative treatment to surgery, especially in children. It can also be an additional treatment, helping to maintain efficient doses of thrombocytopenic medications (interferon, immunosuppressors, chemotherapy, etc.).

9.5.4 Hematological Diseases

9.5.4.1 Autoimmune Thrombocytopenic Purpura (AITP)

In chronic AITP (at least a 6-month evolution), a treatment must be carried out; splenectomy, with its 1 % mortality rate, is an option. Embolization is an alternative treatment to surgery and to corticotherapy.

Technically the procedure must be carried out according to the same modalities as for a hypersplenism. It is generally well tolerated because the spleen volume remains limited.

The rate of success is comparable to that of the splenectomies (71–83 % after 6 months). The procedure can be repeated. The percentage of the infarcted parenchyma isn't correlated to the success rate.

9.5.4.2 Myeloproliferative Diseases

Myeloproliferative diseases are frequently responsible for important splenomegalies, which can be symptomatic by their volume and cause anemia, thrombocytopenia, and hyperleukocytosis.

A splenectomy is often carried out during the late stage of the disease; its mortality rate is 15–18 %.

Embolization must be carried out according to the same modalities as that of a hypersplenism.

It helps to reduce hypersplenism and to improve the comfort of the patient. The expected reduction in volume following embolization is lower for tumoral spleens than that of congestive or normal spleens.

Embolization can be used either as a first-line treatment or preoperatively, taking place less than 24 h before surgery so as to diminish its inherent risks: the occlusion of the splenic artery allows the reduction of the splenic mass and the perioperative bleeding and to increase platelet count before a splenectomy.

9.5.4.3 Thalassemia

At the ultimate stage of the disease, most of the patients develop a hypersplenism which increases blood transfusional needs and the iron burden.

A splenectomy reduces significantly the transfusional needs. But patients with thalassemia who have had a splenectomy are even more candidate to postsplenectomy infections (50 % during the 3 following years, with a mortality rate of 33 %). Moreover, after a splenectomy they lose a relatively healthy site for storing iron.

Therefore, a partial splenic embolization is considered as an alternative to a splenectomy, with the objectives of reducing blood transfusional needs and at the same time preserving the splenic function. The effects of spleen embolization seem sustainable if the initial embolization concerns more than 50 % of the spleen parenchyma. However, little is known about the side effects of partial embolization related to the excretion and the evolution of the iron distribution in the body. To our knowledge, it has not yet been shown that the remaining splenic parenchyma in thalassemic patients, in which immune functions are limited, is enough to protect them against infections.

9.5.5 Other Indications

- An embolization can be proposed to hemodialyzed patients in case of pancytopenia and splenomegaly and also in kidney transplant patients who do not withstand immunosuppressors.
- Splenic embolization has also been recommended for patients with hypersplenism and cytopenia induced by chemotherapies.
- Preoperative embolizations can be carried out, before laparoscopic splenectomies for tumors, hypersplenism, and in patients at surgical risk such as Jehovah Witness patients who refuse blood transfusions. They can also be performed in case of very large spleens at risk of post-embolization arterial infarction.
- Spontaneous hemoperitoneum: nontraumatic splenic ruptures, occurring as complications of infections (paludism, infectious mononucleosis), pancreatitis, congenital cysts, metabolic diseases (amyloidosis, Gaucher's disease), hemopathies (leukosis, lymphoma), tumors (hemangiomatosis, angiosarcoma, metastasis), or peliosis.

Key Points

- Partial parenchymal splenic embolization allows the preservation of the spleen immunologic functions.
- An embolization of 50–70 % of the parenchyma ensures hematological effects and reduction of hypersplenism which are comparable to a surgical splenectomy, but with a lower morbidity rate.
- The splenic abscess which complicates the parenchymal infarction is the main complication; it can be prevented using a strict aseptical environment during the procedure, plus antibiotherapy and prophylactic pneumococcal vaccine.
- In case of spleen trauma, indications are best defined by a perfect radiosurgical cooperation, hemodynamic stability, and CT-scan data (AAST stage, blush). An embolization can be carried out in hemodynamically stable patients, presenting with a pseudoaneurysm, an AVF, a stage 2 AAST with a blush on CT, and for AAST stages 3 and 4, with or without a blush. We recommend whenever it is possible an immediate distal embolization. Stage 5 AAST requires surgery in our opinion on the other hand.
- Embolization is of great interest, on the one hand, for weak patients affected by pseudoaneurysms and/or having hypersplenism and, on the other hand, to treat splenic artery aneurysms, with good results and low morbidity.
- The exact indications of this technique in hematology (autoimmune thrombocytopenic purpura, myeloproliferative diseases, thalassemia) remain to be more clearly specified.

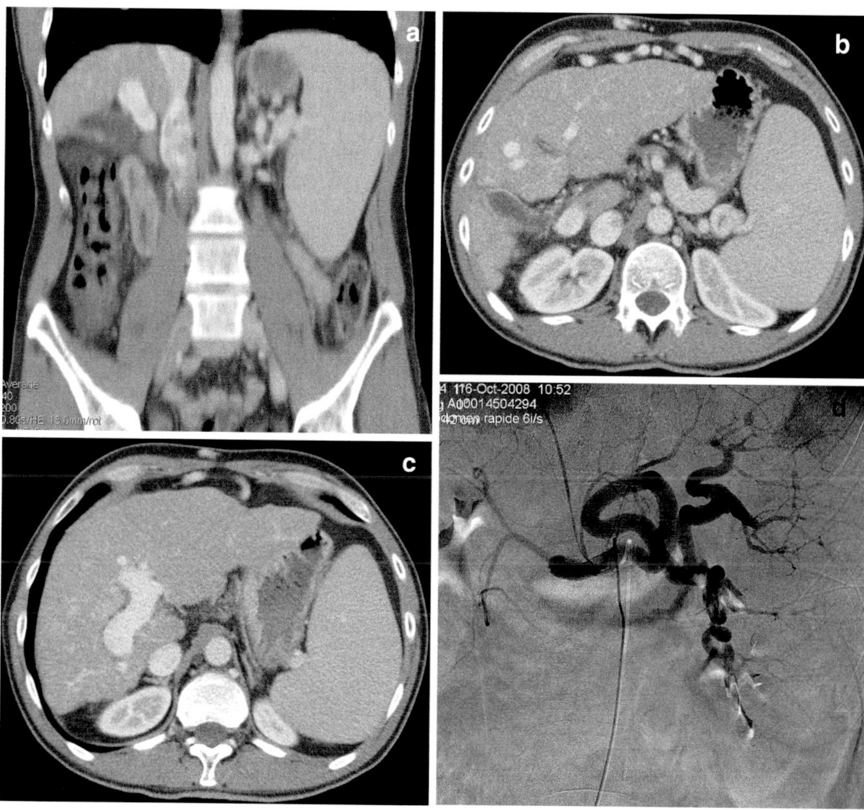

Fig. 9.1 Liver cirrhosis, consequence of a nodular regenerative hyperplasia, complicated by hypersplenism with thrombopenia (platelets 28,000 G/l), and bleeding esophageal varices. A restoration of the platelet count is researched. (**a**) CT frontal reconstruction: splenomegaly. (**b**) Splenomegaly, large splenic vein. (**c**) Large diameters of portal vein and its branches. (**d**) Celiac trunk (CT) selective angiogram: large and sinuous splenic artery. (**e**) Distal splenic A hyperselective catheterization (microcatheter): modal pattern in bifurcation; microaneurysms. (**f**) Hyperselective catheterization of the lower terminal branch, which has been occluded with microparticles, and then catheterization and occlusion of the lower branch of the superior terminal branch. At the end of this procedure, 4 cm^3 of 300–500 μm diameter particles, and then 3 cm^3 of 500–700 μm diameter, and finally 1 cm^3 of 900–1,200 μm diameter have been injected, in order to observe a considerable slowing of the flow in these branches. (**g**) The upper pole of the spleen has not been embolized. (**h**) CT, 1 month later: 60–70 % devascularization of the splenic parenchyma. During the immediate follow-up: moderate fever (38 °C), limited pleural effusion, and platelet count progressively arising (from 28×10^3 to 109×10^3 G/l) without any pancreatic enzymes movement

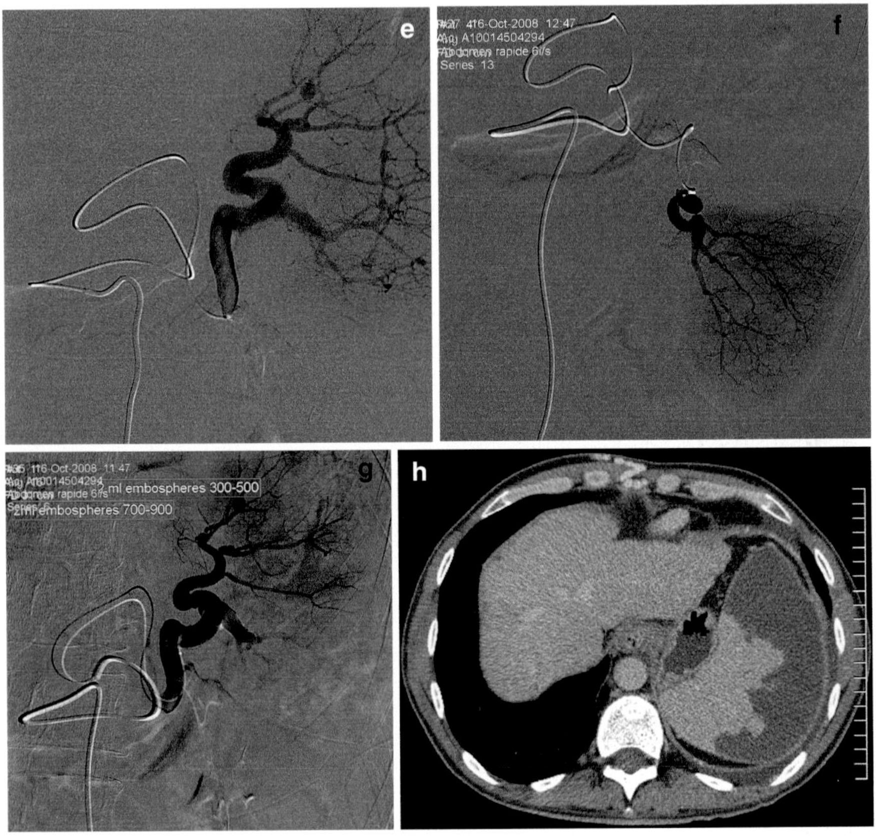

Fig. 9.1 (continued)

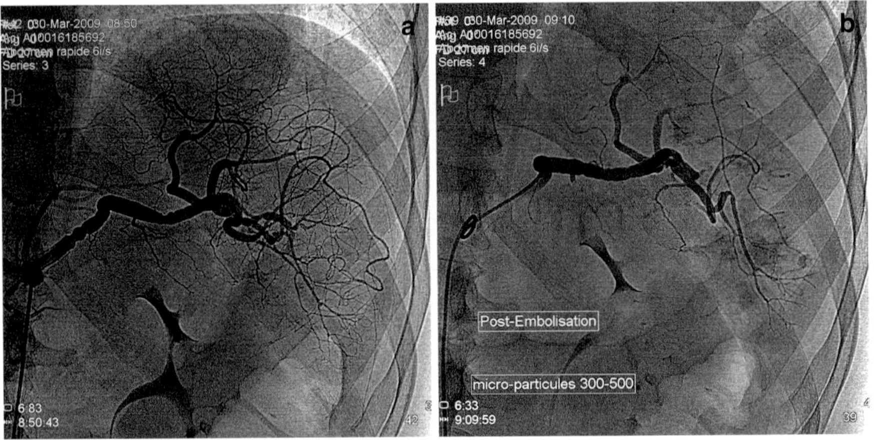

Fig. 9.2 45-year-old M, HCC on VHC cirrhosis, waiting for hepatic transplantation, with a iatrogenic thrombopenia (antiviral treatment). The association of a splenic embolization to a TACE has been proposed. (**a**) Splenic A selective angiogram: moniliform and large splenic A, splenomegaly. (**b**) Control angiogram after a partial embolization of the lobar inferior branch of the splenic A (microparticles, 300–500 μm 3 cm^3 and then 700–900 μm 1 cm^3)

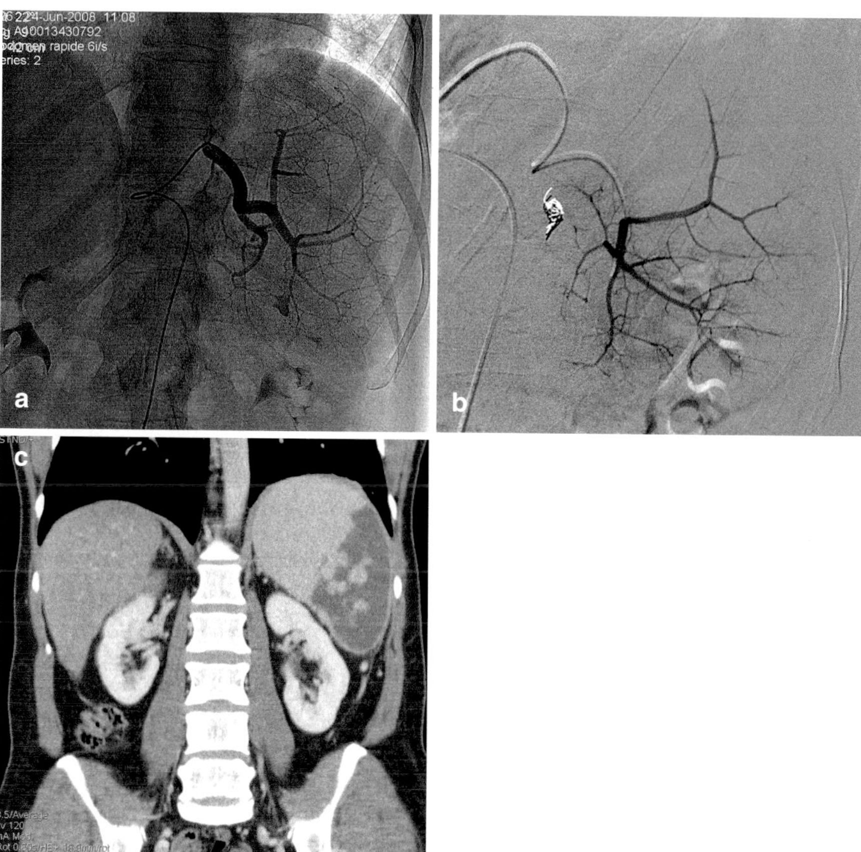

Fig. 9.3 Alcoholic and post-HVC cirrhosis, with hypersplenism and thrombopenia (platelets 16,000 G/l). (**a**) Selective catheterization of the splenic A. (**b**) After exclusion (microparticles + coils) of the inferior lobar branch of the splenic A, the remaining functional splenic parenchymal volume looks important. A complementary embolization of a part of the superior lobar A parenchyma was decided: hyperselective angiogram of this territory before embolization. (**c**) No clinical adverse event during the first month follow-up; platelets 81,000 G/l

Appendix: AAST Classification (Spleen) [1]

Grade[a]	Injury type	Injury description	AIS
I	Hematoma	Subcapsular <10 % surface area	2
	Laceration	Capsular tear <1 cm parenchymal depth	2
II	Hematoma	Subcapsular, 10–50 % surface area; intraparenchymal, <5 cm in diameter	2
	Laceration	Capsular tear, 1–3 cm parenchymal depth that does not involve a trabecular vessel	2
III	Hematoma	Subcapsular, >50 % surface area or expanding; ruptured subcapsular or parenchymal hematoma; intraparenchymal hematoma ≥5 cm or expanding	3
	Laceration	>3 cm parenchymal depth or involving trabecular vessels	3
IV	Laceration	Laceration involving segmental or hilar vessels producing major devascularization (>25 % of the spleen)	4
V	Hematoma	Completely shattered spleen	5
	Laceration	Hilar vascular lesions that devascularize spleen	5

AIS Abbreviated Injury Scale
[a]Advance one grade for bilateral injuries up to grade III

Appendix: "Baltimore" Classification of Spleen Traumas [4]

Grade	1	2	3	4a	4b
Subcapsular hematoma	<1 cm	1–3 cm	>3 cm		
Intraparenchymal hematoma	<1 cm	1–3 cm	>3 cm		
Laceration	<1 cm	1–3 cm	>3 cm	Shattered spleen	
Other lesions			Capsular tear	Active intraparenchymal and subcapsular splenic bleeding, splenic vascular injury	Active intraperitoneal bleeding

References

1. Tinkoff G, et al. American association for the surgery of trauma organ injury scale I: spleen, liver, and kidney, validation based on the National Trauma Data Bank. J Am Coll Surg. 2008;207(5):646–55.
2. Hagiwara A, et al. Blunt splenic injury: usefulness of transcatheter arterial embolization in patients with a transient response to fluid resuscitation. Radiology. 2005;235(1):57–64.
3. Hagiwara A, et al. Nonsurgical management of patients with blunt splenic injury: efficacy of transcatheter arterial embolization. AJR Am J Roentgenol. 1996;167(1):159–66.

4. Marmery H, et al. Optimization of selection for nonoperative management of blunt splenic injury: comparison of MDCT grading systems. AJR Am J Roentgenol. 2007;189(6):1421–7.
5. Thony F, Gaubert JY, Varoquaux A. Embolisations en urgence. In: Vernhet H, editor. Recommandations de bonnes pratiques en radiologie vasculaire interventionnelle. SFICV Ed and Paris; 2007.

Suggested Reading

Guillon R, Garcier JM, de Fraissinette B, et al. Embolisation de l'artère splénique: techniques, indications et résultats. Feuill Radiol. 2001;41(1):31–9.

Maillard M, Novellas S, Baudin G, et al. Anévrisme de l'artère splénique: diagnostic et thérapeutique endovasculaire. J Radiol. 2010;91:1103–11.

Matsumoto T, Yamagami T, Terayama K, et al. Risk factors and clinical course of portal and/or splenic vein thrombosis after partial splenic embolization. Acta Radiol. 2009;50:617–23.

Petermann A, Chabrot P, Cassagnes L, et al. Embolisations spléniques pour hypersplénisme par hypertension portale: 18 patients. J Radiol. 2012;93(1):30–6.

Thony F, Gaubert JY, Varoquaux A. Embolisations en urgence. In: Vernhet H, editor. Recommandations de bonnes pratiques en radiologie vasculaire interventionnelle. sous la direction de H Vernhet 2007. SFICV; 2007.

Van Der Vlies CH, Van Delden OM, Punt BJ, et al. Literature review of the role of ultrasound, computed tomography, and transcatheter arterial embolization for the treatment of traumatic splenic injuries. Cardiovasc Intervent Radiol. 2010;33:1079–87.

Chapter 10
Gastrointestinal Tract Arterial Hemorrhages

Louis Boyer, Denis Pezet, Grégory Favrolt, Isabelle Brazzalotto, and Pascal Chabrot

10.1 Background

GI tract hemorrhages are frequent and can be potentially serious: if the bleeding spontaneously stops in about 80 % of the patients, it reoccurs in about one quarter of them, increasing mortality and morbidity, particularly in older patients. The quality of the multidisciplinary care is therefore essential, and the radiologist plays an important role in the diagnosis (the CT being of major importance) and in the treatment.

Gastroduodenal ulcers, esophagitis and gastritis, Mallory-Weiss syndrome, and venous bleeding due to portal hypertension (PHT) are the main causes of upper hemorrhages. Bleeding from the papilla (hemobilia: spontaneous, traumatic, or iatrogenic after an endoscopic sphincterotomy and from pancreatic origin: false aneurysms, tumors) is another severe acute non-variceal upper GI hemorrhage causes, for which embolization can be indicated. We will not discuss here the endovascular care for venous hemorrhagic complications due to PHT (TIPS: transjugular intrahepatic portosystemic shunt and embolization of PHT varices: see Chap. 24).

L. Boyer, MD, PhD (✉) • P. Chabrot, MD, PhD
Department of Radiology, University Hospital of Clermont-Ferrand, Clermont-Ferrand, France
e-mail: lboyer@chu-clermontferrand.fr; pchabrot@chu-clermontferrand.fr

D. Pezet, MD, PhD
Department of Abdominal Surgery, University Hospital of Clermont-Ferrand, Clermont-Ferrand, France

G. Favrolt, MD
Department of Radiology, Clinique de Fontaine, Dijon, France

I. Brazzalotto, MD
Department of Anesthesia, University Hospital of Clermont-Ferrand, Clermont-Ferrand, France

P. Chabrot, L. Boyer (eds.), *Embolization*,
DOI 10.1007/978-1-4471-5182-1_10, © Springer-Verlag London 2014

The main causes of lower gastrointestinal bleedings are diverticular disease (diverticula of the right colon are less frequent than those of the left colon, but they bleed more frequently), angiodysplasia (predominantly on the right colon, malformative or more frequently acquired, essentially in patients over 50 years), and tumors but also the causes of upper GI tract hemorrhages. Other causes are inflammatory diseases of the GI tract, colonic ischemia, Meckel's diverticulum, intestinal and colonic ulcers caused by nonsteroidal anti-inflammatory drugs, as well as traumatic rectal ulcers or ulcers due to fecal impaction and hemorrhoids.

Esogastroduodenal endoscopy must be performed first; it allows to distinguish upper GI hemorrhages (80 % of the cases) from the lower GI bleeding with respect to the duodenojejunal flexure. In case of upper hemorrhages, it often allows to carry out immediate local treatment. An esogastroduodenal endoscopy must also be carried out in cases of lower hemorrhages (all the more so given that the hemorrhage is made up of totally or partially digested blood); hence, at the same time, a colonoscopy is necessary, which is frequently only partial and therefore frequently gives poor diagnosis results. The choice of the optimal method for the diagnosis and the initial care of acute lower GI bleeding has not yet been formally established.

An immediate three-phase CT scan must be carried out during the acute episode of bleeding for all of the hemorrhages whose origin has not been determined by endoscopy. Iodine contrast medium must be injected at a high flow rate (4 ml/s). CT is able to visualize GI hemorrhages with a flow rate of at least 0.3 ml/mn. An extravasation (density of 100 uH or more, which does not exist before injection but appears in the arterial phase, and spreads to the portal phase) allows the diagnosis and localization of the hemorrhage. This extravasation is almost never seen in case of hemorrhages of venous origin. The visualization of a lesion (tumor, polyp, vascular malformation, aneurysm…) also allows a highly reliable diagnosis of the hemorrhagic topography. However, noncomplicated diverticula don't have a localizing value.

However, bleeding is detected by MDCT only in about half of the cases because of an insufficient blood flow during the CT exploration. If GI tract hemorrhage persists or reoccurs and initial CT was normal, then CT must be repeated. The minimal flow required to depict a hemorrhage on an arteriography is 0.5 ml/mn: theoretically there is no need to carry out an arteriogram should the CT be negative.

Arteriography in emergency cases is today indicated as a first step of embolization, after a multidisciplinary concertation, in patients that are clinically unstable or in case of important repeated bleedings whose origin has been located.

As in some other teams, in our group severe nontraumatic GI tract hemorrhages that are hemodynamically unstable remain however indications for emergency angiography should diagnostic/therapeutic endoscopy fail.

10.2 Relevant Radiological Anatomy

Three visceral ventral branches of the abdominal aorta contribute to the arterial vascularization of the GI tract: the celiac artery (CA), the superior mesenteric artery (SMA), and the inferior mesenteric artery (IMA). The first two can sometimes originate from a common celio-mesenteric trunk. These three arteries are anastomosed.

- CA (see Chaps. 6 and 9): it originates from the ventral part of the aorta at the level of T12 and branches into left gastric, splenic, and common hepatic arteries. The latter ends by dividing into gastroduodenal and proper hepatic arteries. In this way, the CA ensures the arterial feeding of the stomach and the duodenum, as well as the liver, the bile ducts, the pancreas, and the spleen.
- The SMA originates from the aorta at the level of L1, at less than 15 mm from the origin of the CA, immediately above the renal arteries. Its initial track is sagittal, forming with the aorta the aorto-mesenteric angle (in which are found the left renal vein, the third duodenum, and the pancreatic uncus). The territory of the SMA extends from the duodenojejunal flexure to the middle third-inferior third of the transverse colon.
- Its right branches supply the colon (2–3 branches: right colic artery, inconstant medium colic artery, and ileocolic artery, which fan out in the terminal ileum, the cecum, and to the lower part of the ascending colon). The left branches of the SMA go to the small intestine: the jejunal arteries (4–6) originate downstream the duodeno-pancreatic arcades and upstream the ileocolic artery; the ileal arteries (8–12) originate then downstream. These arteries divide into an ascending branch and a descending branches, which form a peripheral arterial arcade on the mesenteric edge of the small intestine, from which originate the vasa recta.

  The SMA is anastomosed to the CA via the pancreatico-duodenal arcades (and the gastroduodenal artery) and with the IMA via the marginal artery (transverse colon).
- The IMA originates from the aorta approximately at the level L3 and has an oblique inferior and lateral course to the left. It ensures the vascularization of the left third of the transverse colon, of the descending colon, of the sigmoid, and of the rectum: the left colic artery courses towards the left colic angle, and then three sigmoid arteries can originate from the same common trunk. These arteries make up a peripheral arterial arcade. The IMA terminates into the upper rectal artery, which courses vertically and divides into two branches.

The IMA is anastomosed with the SMA via the marginal artery (transverse colon).

The rectal arterial vascularization is ensured by the superior rectal artery, the middle rectal arteries (visceral branches of the internal iliac arteries), and the inferior rectal arteries, which originate from the internal pudendal arteries.

An anastomosis occurs therefore at the level of the rectal walls between the IMA and the hypogastric arteries.

10.3 Techniques

- A large venous access is mandatory so as to allow a massive vascular filling and/or resuscitation should it be required, as well as sedation. We do not give antibiotics.

- Most frequently a femoral approach, with a 4 or 5 Fr introducer sheath, is used. Quality of the femoroiliac vessels and the ostia of CA, SMA, and IMA (stenosis?) have already been assessed by CT.
- A urinary catheterization allows optimal exploration the pelvic arterial branches by voiding the bladder.
- After a global aortography, selective injections are performed into the CA, the gastroduodenal artery, and if necessary in other branches and then into the SMA and IMA. If there is the slightest doubt, complementary selective injections into other visceral collateral branches are performed. The hypogastric arteries are also catheterized in the case of hemorrhage the lower GI tract.

Late acquisitions must be performed, so as to depict tardive low contrast extravasations. To avoid artifacts due to peristalsis, one must change the subtraction masks and sometimes use nonsubtracted images. The administration of Glucagon ® or Buscopan ® can be helpful in reducing peristalsis.

Injection of vasodilators, anticoagulants, or even fibrinolytic drugs has been advocated in case of negative angiographies.

If an endoscopy took place immediately before the angiography and showed some evidence of bleeding, it could be interesting to mark the area with a hemostatic clip. Persistence of colonic distension (immediately after endoscopy) is helpful for the colic wall analysis on arteriography.

The predictive factors of the visualization of an active hemorrhage on angiography are clinical signs of active bleeding (hypotension, tachycardia…), transfusion of more than three packed cell units per 24 h, active bleedings shown by endoscopy, and a bleeding flow of 0.5 ml/mn or more.

On angio, the extravasation of the contrast agent is the only direct sign. The indirect signs (not specific of bleeding) are dilatations of arterial lumens (false or true aneurysms), vascular irregularities, "stop" pattern of the lumen (non-opacification of arterial lumen downstream), arteriovenous and arterio-portal fistulas, hyperemia (colitis), neovascularization (tumors), and arteriolar hypervascularization (mostly seen with angiodysplasias, in which a dense opacification and a late washing of the draining vein are also seen).

A superselective catheterization and the use of automatic injector may be necessary so as to reveal an active bleeding.

- When an extravasation is seen, the main goal is to exclude the bleeding source. A covered stent maintains vessel patency, but the diameter of the bleeding artery is frequently limited, making the navigation of the stent graft difficult, and its long-term patency is uncertain. In most cases, the exclusion of the bleeding source by embolization is the only possible option. Coils are preferred, due to the precision of delivery and also because of the low risk of induced GI ischemia. In case of hemorrhagic shock, the arterial diameter is reduced due to vasoconstriction: an oversizing is mandatory when choosing the size of the coils. In some conditions such as coagulation disorders, other embolization agents can be used.

Embolization must always be as selective as possible, especially for lower GI hemorrhages, using if necessary coaxial microcatheters and microcoils. If particles are used, they must be injected slowly, so as to avoid any reflux.

If embolization is either impossible or inefficient, positioning a coil in the hemorrhagic area or leaving in situ a microcatheter for injection of saline solution or methylene blue solution will be able to help the surgeon after patient transfer to the operating room.

10.3.1 Upper Hemorrhages

Upper Hemorrhages and Especially Gastroduodenal and Splenic Arterial Bleedings:

The bleeding source has to be excluded both upstream and downstream ("sandwich" coiling), so as to avoid all persistent feeding from downstream collateral vessels that reverse the blood flow. After an embolization via the CA, a control injection of the SMA is necessary, so as to check that there is no persistent collateral feeding of the bleeding. Symmetrically, an embolization in the territory of the SMA must be controlled by an opacification of the CA, so as to make sure that there is no reinjection from collateral branches ("closing the back door").

In spite of these precautions and even though embolization was technically well performed, rebleeding can be seen in approximately 30 % of the cases, due to the fact that there is an extensive arterial vascularization network of the stomach and the duodenum: another embolization is nevertheless possible and can be then carried out. This rebleeding is seen more frequently in cases of hemostasis disorders, and when only coils have been used, suggesting the use of particles in case of gastric and cardiac bleedings, with or without associated coils.

The risk of induced ischemia after an embolization of upper GI tract bleeding is limited, so the gastroduodenal artery can be occluded without fear of any adverse effects.

In case of gastritis or hemorrhagic diffuse duodenitis, and when a bleeding of gastric or of duodenal origin is shown by the endoscopy but not found on the angiography, we complete the occlusion with absorbable gelatin sponge.

10.3.2 Lower Hemorrhages

There are fewer collateral vessels and therefore all embolizations must be superselective (if possible at the arcade or vasa recta levels), with microcatheters and microcoils. If particles are used, a diameter of at least 300 μm must be chosen. The injection must be given slowly. This superselective embolization has supplanted vasopressin infusion, a fastidious technique which has inconstant results, and can lead to ischemic complications.

Once a technical success has been achieved, we retrieve the introducer sheath 12–24 h later in order to be ready for a new catheterization should early rebleeding occur. The vital parameters, blood count, gastric tubes, and stools are closely monitored, as well as abdominal palpation. If the etiologic investigation had not been completed, then it should be done.

10.4 Indications

10.4.1 Upper Hemorrhages

Endoscopic treatment of duodenal or gastric ulcers is considered as the first-line treatment. However, the following conditions make up the most frequent indications for embolizations:

- Bleeding ulcers refractory to endoscopic treatment
- Recurrences after multiple endoscopic treatments
- Bleeding following surgery for ulcers

Nowadays surgery is generally performed if endoscopic and endovascular treatments fail. Embolization, which points out bleeding site, is less invasive, repeatable, and better tolerated in weak patients. In case of hemostasis failure when using endoscopic treatment on a bleeding duodenal ulcer, the lack of visualization of an angiographic extravasation leads many authors embolize nonetheless the territory of the gastroduodenal artery. The negative predictive factors are lateness of the embolization, transfusion of more than six packs of red blood cells, and the rebleeding which occurs after duodenal ulcer surgery.

Embolization is also the first-line treatment for:

- False aneurysms and hemorrhaging pseudocysts complicating a pancreatitis
- Bleeding true aneurysms
- Hemobilia of tumor, traumatic, or iatrogenic origin, postoperative or after endoscopic sphincterotomy

10.4.2 Lower Hemorrhages

- Bleeding diverticula: Embolization avoids a high-risk emergency surgery; because of its efficiency, it is for some teams a frequent indication (Weldon).
- In case of the suspicion of aortoenteric fistula, embolization is not a good treatment option.
- Bleeding caused by inflammatory GI diseases, tumors, and angiodysplasias are not good indications for an embolization, even if in some circumstances it can be useful in postponing emergency colectomy and preparing patients for elective surgery.

10.5 Results

10.5.1 Upper Hemorrhages

In 1997 Drooz reported for the SIR, embolization success rates ranging from 62 to 100 %.

Long-term clinical success can be seen in 50–80 % of the cases.

Rebleeding is seen in about 30 % of the patients, among which some can benefit from a new embolization. Rebleeding is favored by hemostasis disorders and seems to occur more frequently when the embolization is tardive and when coils have been used alone. It requires inpatient post-procedural monitoring.

In case of embolization of true or false aneurysms complicating an acute pancreatitis, success rates of more than 90 % have been reported. But during pancreatitis, there may be recurring hemorrhages: embolization does not solve the ongoing evolution of the inflammatory lesions.

10.5.2 Lower Hemorrhages

In a meta-analysis pooling 15 recent publications (309 patients), Weldon described a technical feasibility for superselective embolizations in 82 % of the cases and an achievement of hemostasis in 95 %.

Due to the limited anastomotic network, rebleedings are less frequent than that observed for the upper hemorrhages: Weldon observed a rebleeding during the 30 days following the embolization in 21 % of the cases (of which 45 % occurred at the original bleeding site which had been embolized). During these 30 days, rebleeding seems to occur far more frequently in non-diverticular causes (45 %) than for hemorrhagic diverticula (15 %).

10.5.3 Complications

Recent data estimated that the global major and minor complication rates are less than 10 %.

Besides nonspecific problems such as iodine contrast medium tolerance, renal failure, or complications related to the puncture site or the endovascular navigation, one must keep in mind the risks of liver infarct when a portal occlusion already exists, splenic infarct when the splenic artery is occluded, and lastly the risk of intestinal ischemia.

In older data, the intestinal ischemic complications were seen in more than 15 % of the patients; these complications, in recent papers, are around 5 %. When embolizing upper GI hemorrhages, this risk must be considered, should the patient have history of serious atheroma and/or surgical or irradiation of the region. The risk of inducing an ischemia after an embolization of the vasa recta in case of a colic bleeding remains limited: 2 % of serious complications requiring surgery (stenosis, infarction) and 10 % of moderate ischemic complications, ranging from transitory pain to asymptomatic stenosis.

Key Points

- Cooperation between radiologists, gastroenterologists, and surgeons
- 80 % spontaneous cessation of the bleeding, but severity in older patients with recurrences (25 %)
- Upper endoscopy = reference + coloscopy in case of lower hemorrhage
- If the origin of the bleeding is not established by endoscopy: emergency CT; if normal CT and recurring or persisting hemorrhage: CT should be repeated
- Arteriography: for an emergency embolization in clinically unstable patients, after fibroscopy ± CT
- Tardive arteriographic acquisitions; threshold flow rate of bleeding for detection = 0.5 ml/mn (≠ MDCT: 0.3 ml/mn)
- Preferentially: coils, with slight oversizing (vasoconstriction in case of hemorrhagic shock)
- Superselective embolization is reliable and safe: 50–80 % of long-term clinical results for upper hemorrhages; feasibility for lower hemorrhages: 82 %
- Upper hemorrhages: recurrences ≈ 30 %: the refeeding by the anastomotic network has to be excluded ("closing the back door")
- Lower hemorrhages: risk = intestinal ischemia (2 %)
- Gastroduodenal bleeding ulcers: embolization if endoscopic treatment fails
- Lower hemorrhages: embolization avoids high-risk emergency surgery

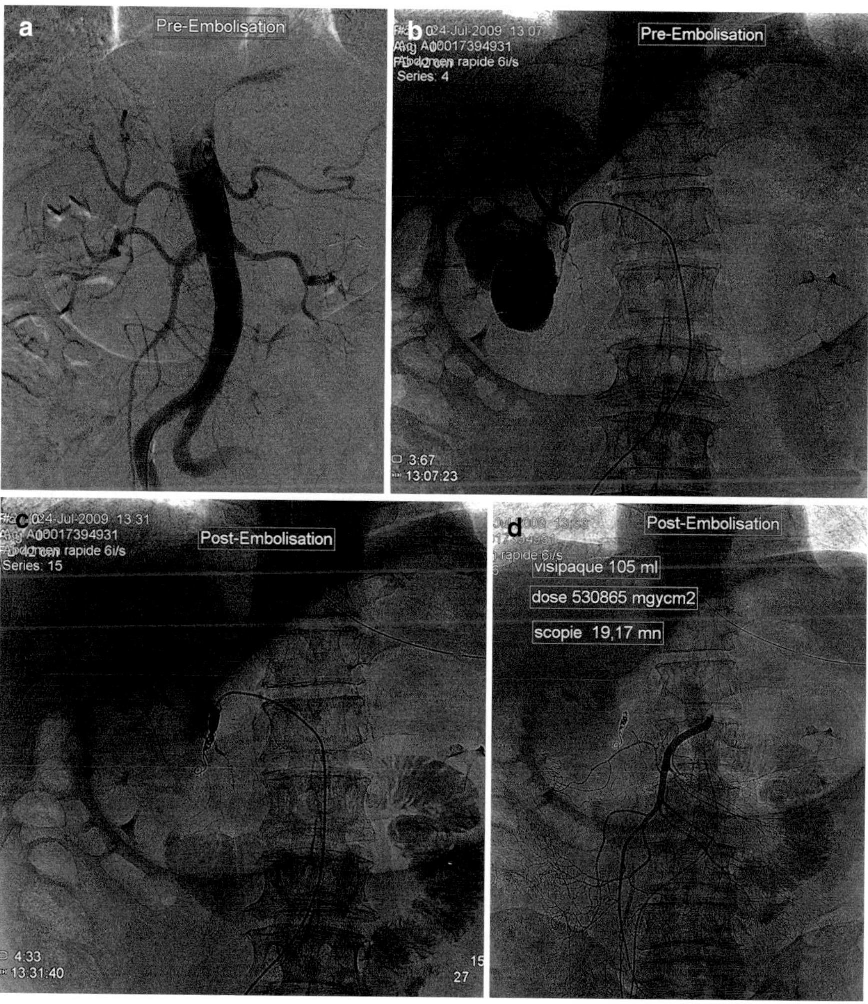

Fig. 10.1 Massive hematemesis, complication of a pancreatic adenocarcinoma. Upper endoscopy showed an active bleeding of the second duodenum: an arteriography has been performed in emergency. (**a**) Aortography: modal anatomical arterial pattern of the splanchnic arteries; no evident blush. (**b**) Selective catheterization of the CT and then of the common hepatic artery. The injection near the ostium of the gastroduodenal artery shows a massive extravasation in the second duodenum, meaning a severe arterial erosion. (**c**) Control opacification after coils occlusion of the gastroduodenal A, just upstream of the extravasation. (**d**) Injection of the SMA to verify that there is not any "back door" reinjection via the duodeno-pancreatic arcades

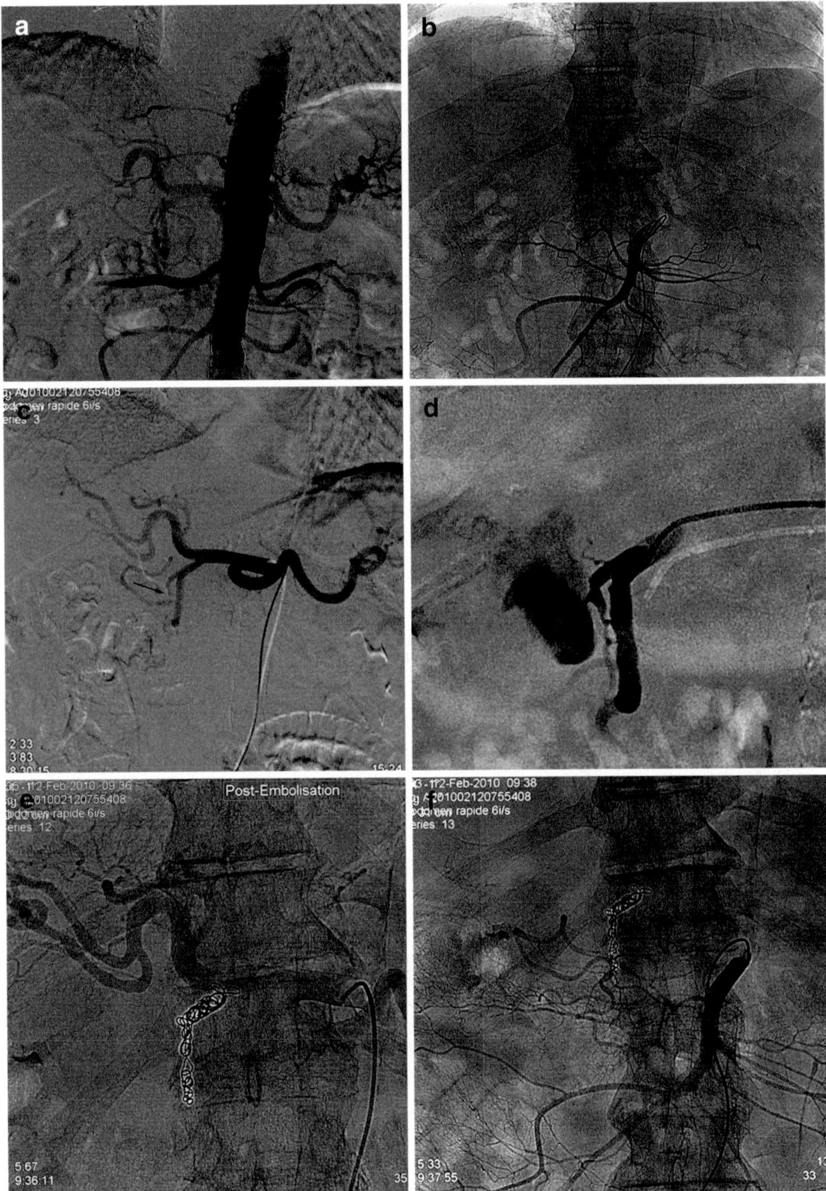

Fig. 10.2 78 years old M, GI tract hemorrhage considered as the consequence of a duodenal bulb ulcer. Hemodynamic shock and general status led in emergency to an arteriography, in order to embolize if possible an arterial bleeding. (**a**) Aortography: normal anatomy of the splanchnic arteries; diffuse atheroma. (**b**) Selective injection of the SMA: no extravasation. (**c**) Selective injection of the CT: note the variation of diameter of the superior and posterior duodeno-pancreatic arcades (*arrow*). (**d**) Hyperselective gastroduodenal A injection: massive duodenal extravasation from the previous noted abnormal segment, corresponding to an arterial erosion by the bulbar ulcer. (**e**) CT control opacification after coils exclusion of this abnormal artery and of the upstream gastroduodenal artery. (**f**) Last SMA control injection to be sure of no "back door" reinjection

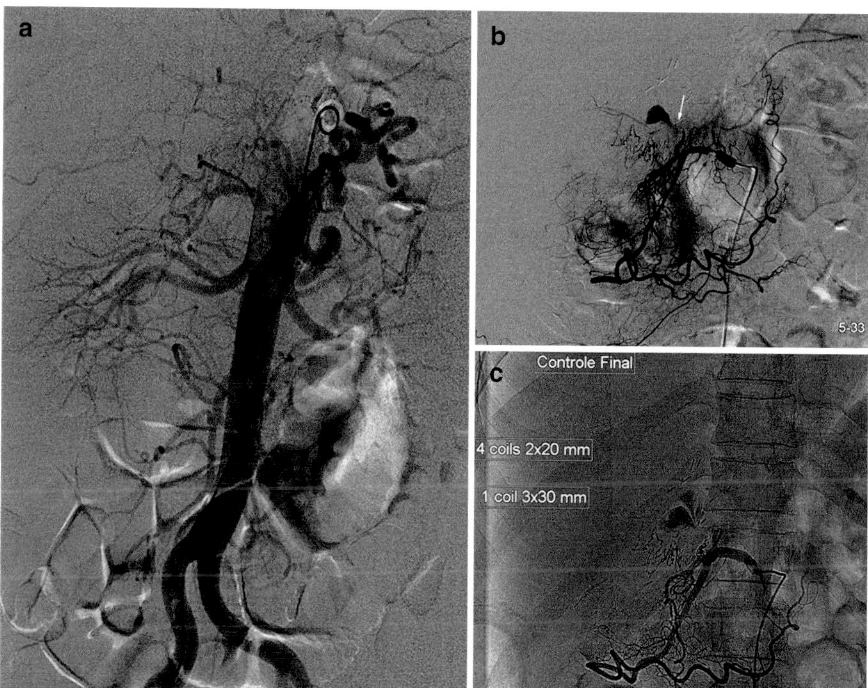

Fig. 10.3 Immediate follow-up after an hepatic segmentectomy with a bilio-digestive anastomosis to treat an ischemic choledochal stenosis, 3 years after a left hepatectomy (metastasis resection). Fibroscopies didn't conclude to precise the site of a low flow bleeding. (**a**) Aortography: sinuous splenic artery; not any hypervascularization or blush. (**b**) Selective common hepatic A injection: initial variation of the lumen diameter (*black arrow*): spasm, irregular thin segment (*white arrow*), and extravasation from the duodeno-pancreatic arcade. (**c**) Control angio after exclusion by coils

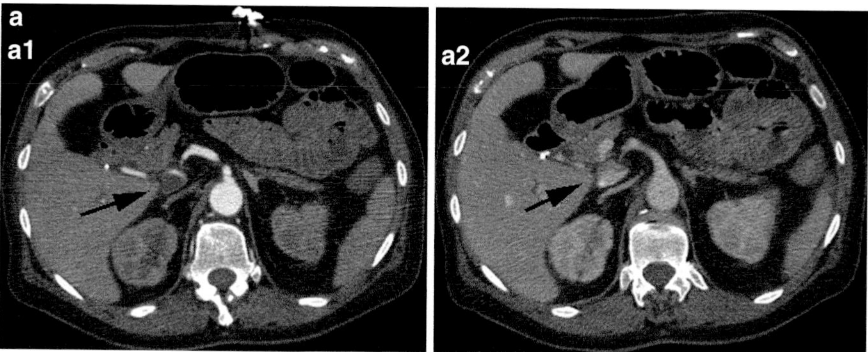

Fig. 10.4 71 years old M, chronic lymphoid leukemia, upper and lower GI tract bleeding. (**a**) Blush at the level of the dilated third duodenum; note the collapsed vena cava. (**b**) Massive bleeding from a thin proximal branch of the right hepatic A, collateral of the SMA. (**c**) Control angio after exclusion by coils

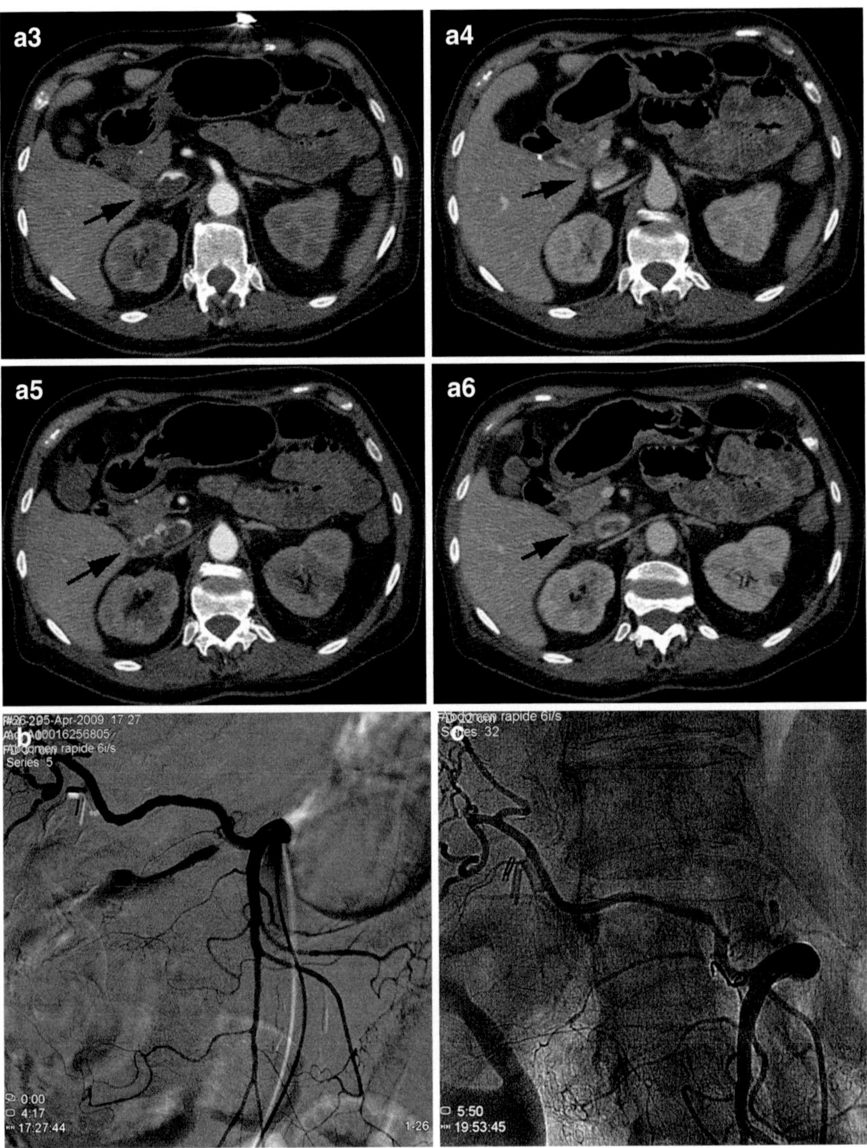

Fig. 10.4 (continued)

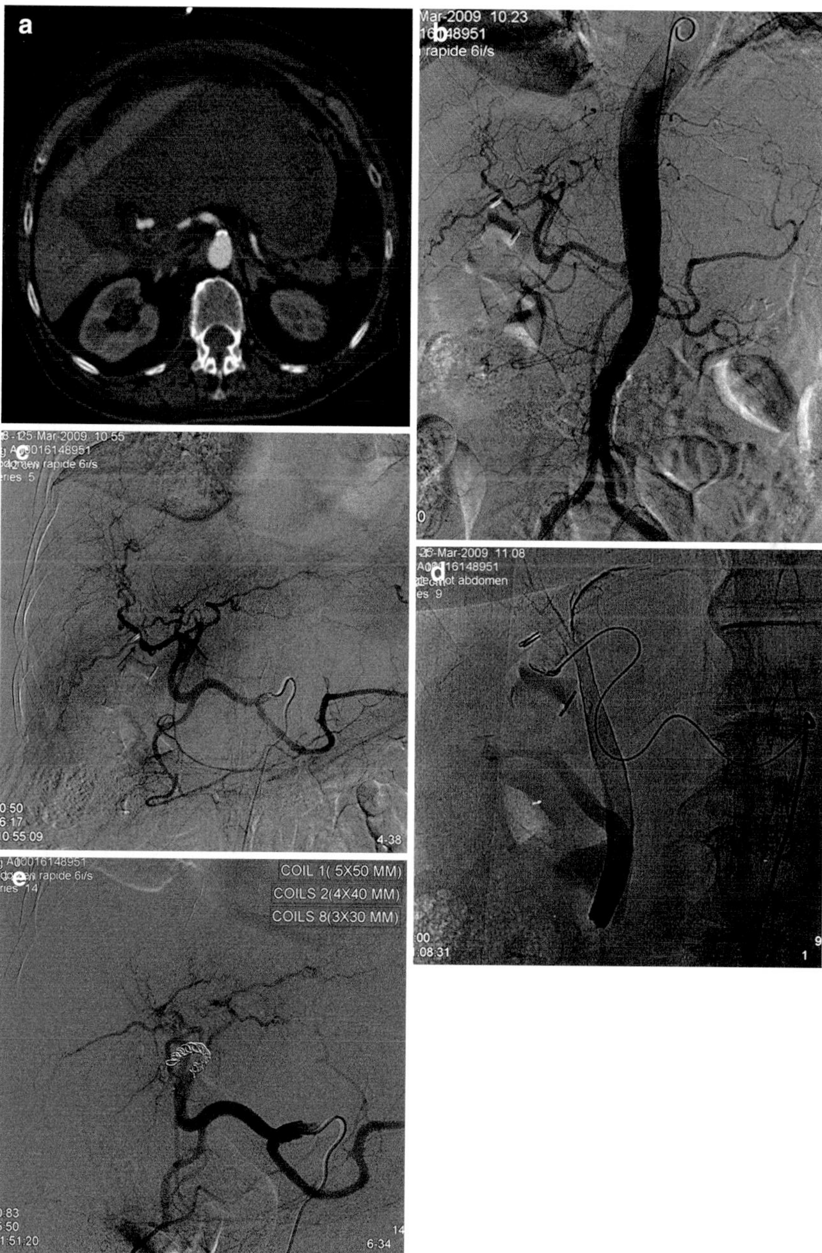

Fig. 10.5 78 years old, cholecystectomy, and then surgical redux at D7 because of a gallbladder space hematoma. But the day after, hemorrhagic shock again. (**a**) CT in emergency: very large gallbladder space hematoma. (**b**) Aortography: normal arterial anatomy; stretching of the splenic artery, consequence of this voluminous hematoma; diffuse atheroma. (**c**) Selective injection of the CT: note a variation of the right hepatic A lumen (*arrow*). (**d**) Right hepatic artery injection: opacification of the biliary duct, consequence of an arterio-biliary fistula. (**e**) Coils upstream of the arterial lesion

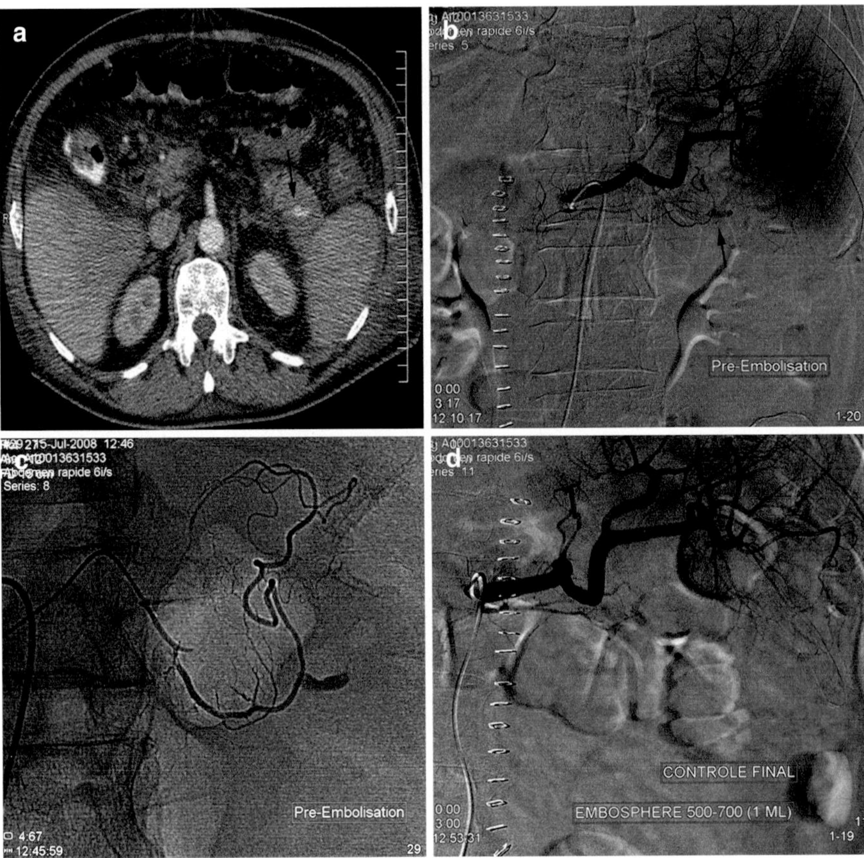

Fig. 10.6 Necrotico-hemorrhagic acute pancreatitis, complication of a chronic pancreatitis in a 70 years old alcoholic M, during the immediate follow-up of a colic surgery. (**a**) CT arterial phase: caudal pancreatic blush (*arrow*). (**b**) Selective injection of the splenic A: extravasation from pancreatic arterial branches (*arrow*). (**c**) Hyperselective catheterization. (**d**) Splenic A injection control after microparticles embolization (500–700 μm diameter)

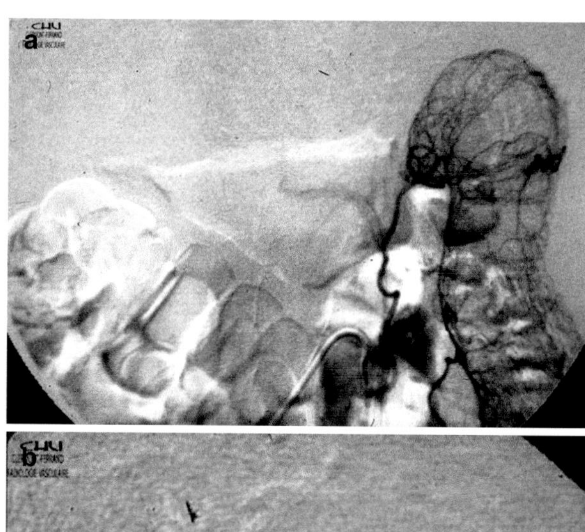

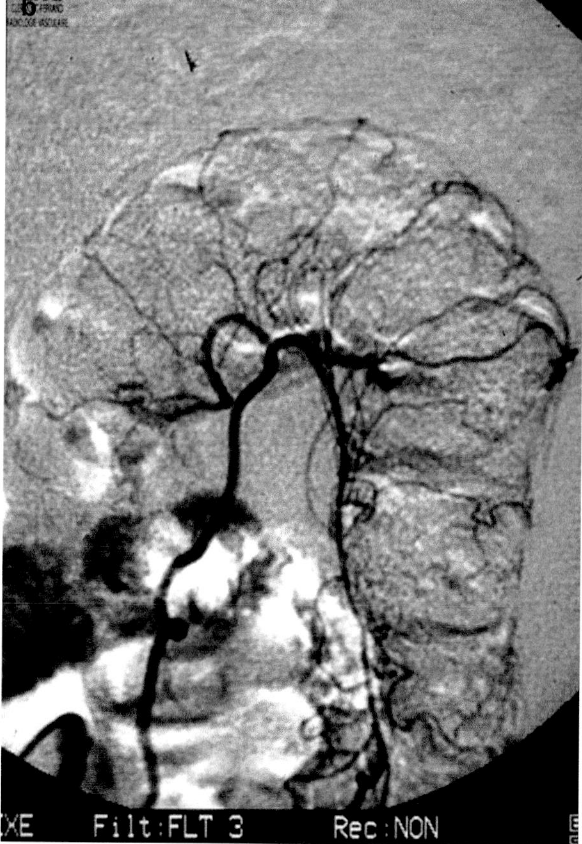

Fig. 10.7 Moderate lower GI tract hemorrhage; coloscopy: suspicion of a left colic angle arterial lesion. Arteriography performed immediately after fibroscopy and before complete colic exsufflation. (**a**, **b**) Hyperselective catheterization of the left colic artery, terminal branch of the IMA; vascular lake, typical of angiodysplasia, which was excluded with coils

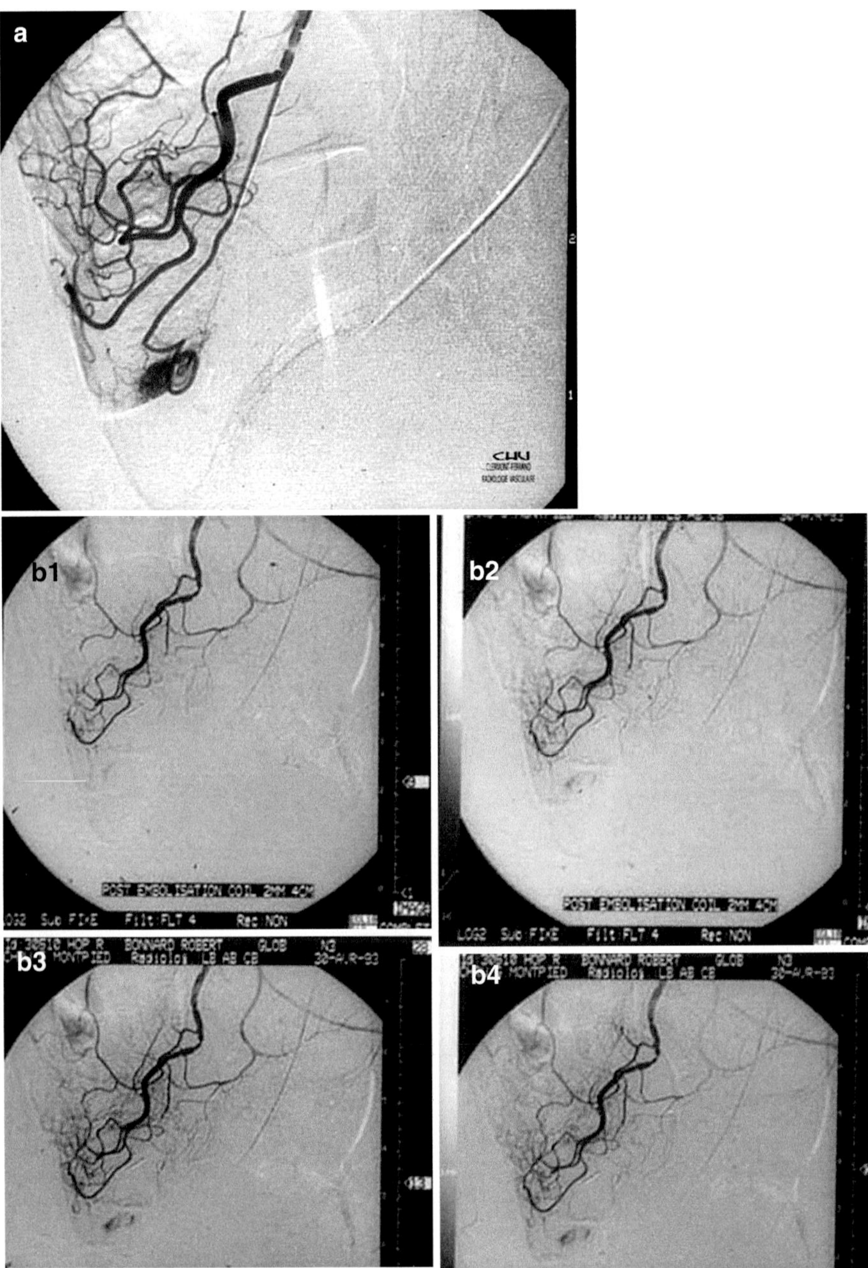

Fig. 10.8 17 years old M, recurrence of a lower GI tract hemorrhage; the check up after the first bleeding episode (1 year before), showed on arteriography an AVM, but the spontaneous stop of bleeding in this teenager led us to a therapeutic abstention. (**a**) Selective catheterization of ileo-bicaeco-colo-appendicular artery (terminal branch of the SMA): extravasation from the AVM. (**b1**–**b4**) Distal arterial coils occlusion: AVM exclusion

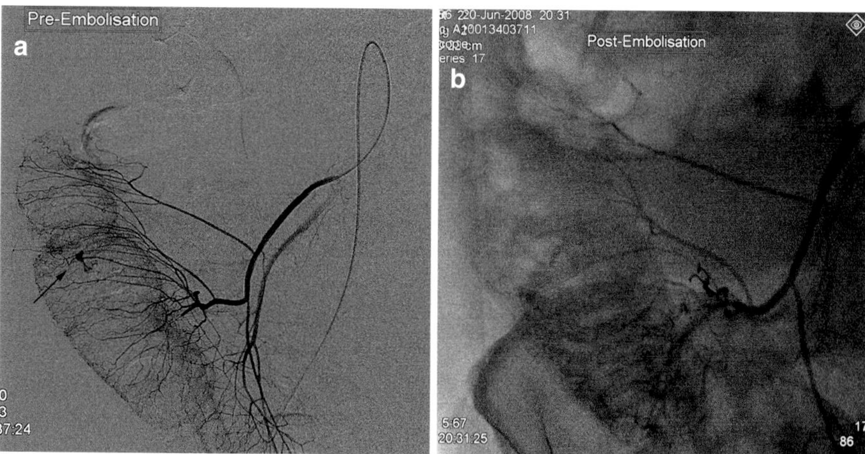

Fig. 10.9 Mild severe lower GI tract hemorrhage in a 63 years old cirrhotic M; a perforated gastric ulcer was surgically treated 7 weeks before. Upper fibroscopy was normal. The coloscopy showed a bleeding coming from the right colon. Surgery was considered as not possible by the anesthesiologist. (**a**) Ileo-bicaeco-colo-appendicular artery selective injection: extravasation in the ascending colon, near the vasa recta. (**b**) Control angio after distal coils exclusion (microcatheterization)

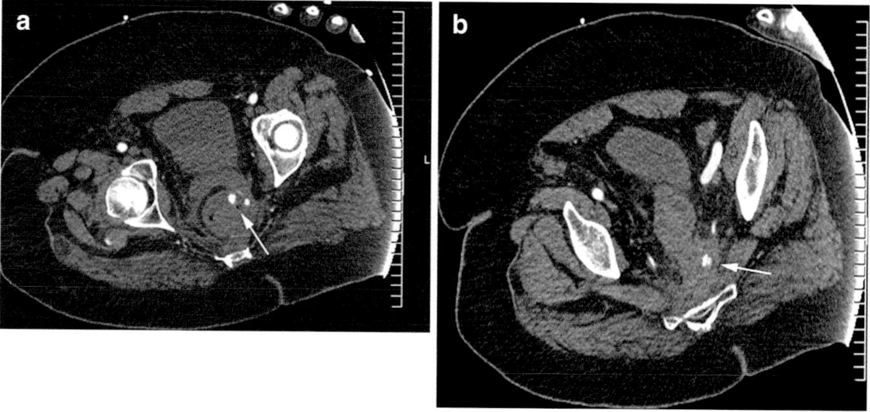

Fig. 10.10 Known advanced rectum cancer; lower GI tract active hemorrhage, hemodynamically unstable. (**a**, **b**) CT: spontaneously hyperdense colorectal lumen (*arrows*) (consequence of the bleeding). (**c**) Selective injection of the left hypogastric A via a right femoral access (cross over): massive extravasation. (**d**) Control opacification after coils exclusion

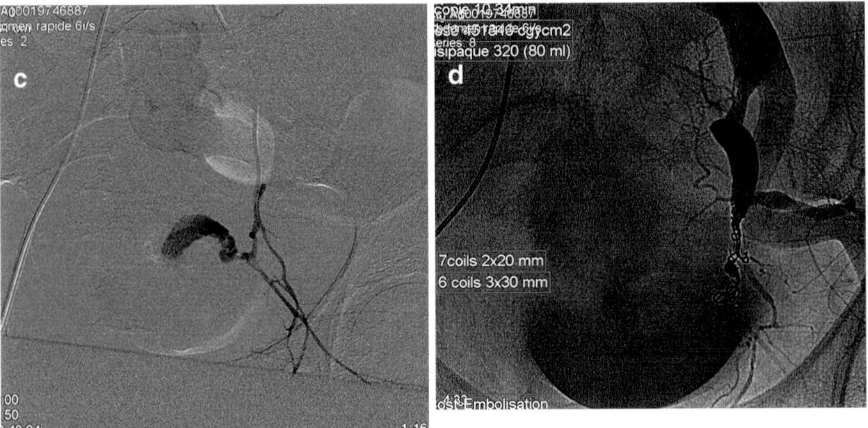

Fig. 10.10 (continued)

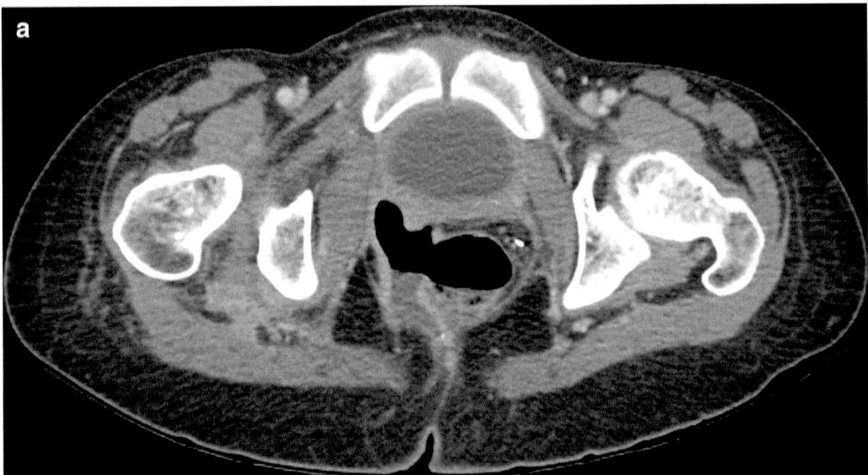

Fig. 10.11 T 4 N3M 0 rectum cancer: surgery (resection), irradiation, and IV chemotherapy. Painful pelvic abscess 4 m later. (**a**, **b**) Pelvic fistulas; presacral and gluteal abscesses. On the scanner trolley, sudden abundant rectorrages and hemorrhagic collapsus: complementary CT scans 10 mn later showed intense abscess and GI lumen enhancements, but no real blush. Nevertheless, the patient was led in emergency to the angio suite (**c**–**f**). (**g**, **h**) Diffuse iliac and splanchnic arterial vasoconstriction. Massive extravasation from the right hypogastric A (early and late phases). (**g**, **h**) Anterior trunk of the right hypogastric catheterization, from the left femoral puncture site (cross over). (**i**) Control angio after coils embolization (**j**)

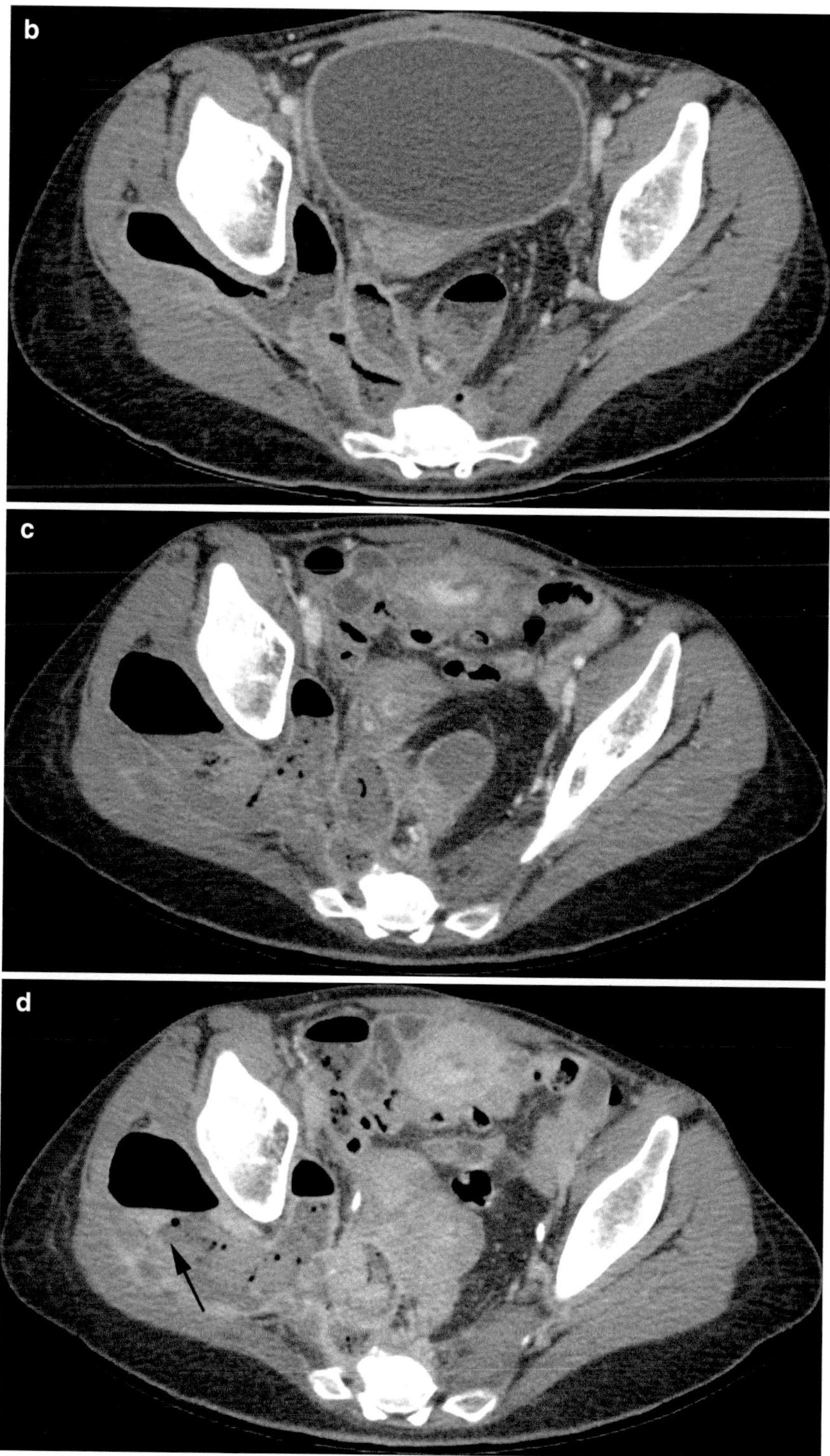

Fig. 10.11 (continued)

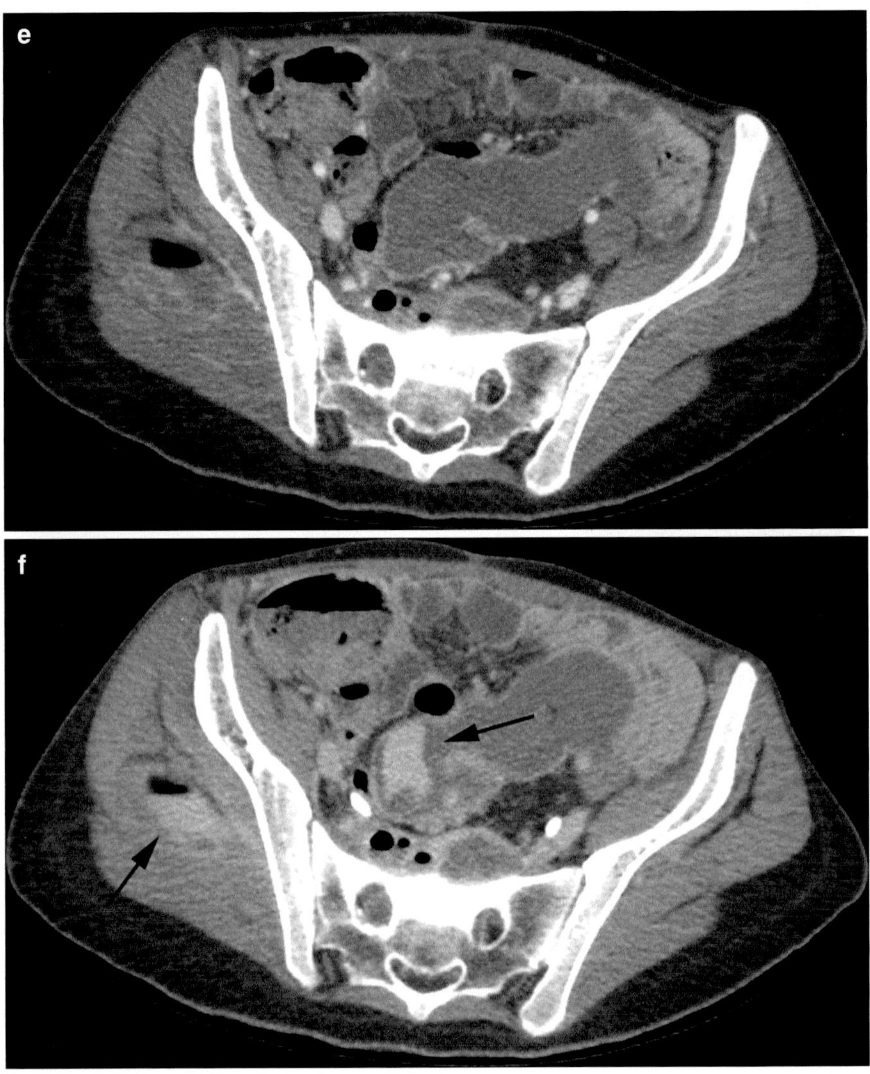

Fig. 10.11 (continued)

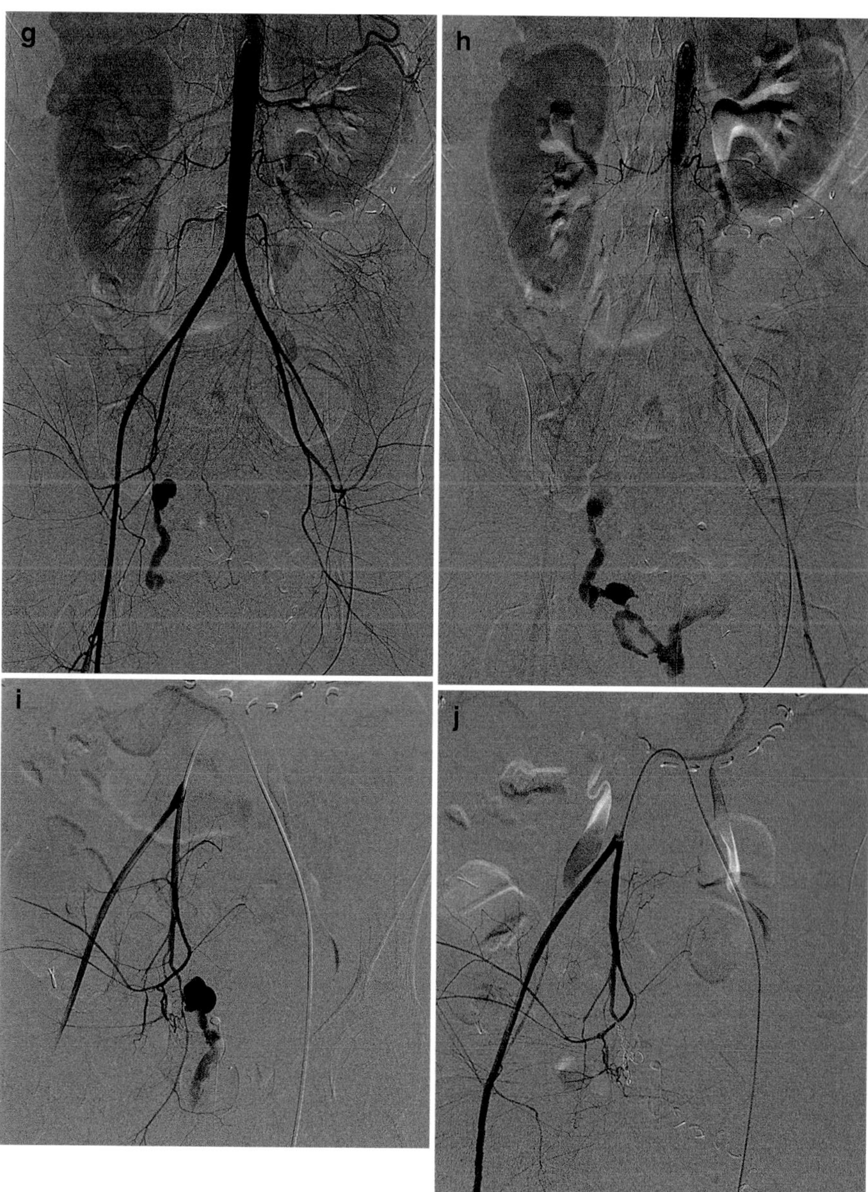

Fig. 10.11 (continued)

Suggested Reading

Drooz AT, Lewis CA, Allen TE, et al. Quality improvement guidelines for percutaneous transcatheter embolization. Society of Interventional Radiology Standard of Practice Comittee. J Vasc Interv Radiol. 1997;8:889–95.

Ernst O. Hémorragies digestives. In: E Schouman Claeys et P Taourel (editor), Imagerie TDM et IRM des urgences non traumatiques. Paris:SFR; 2008.

Ichiro I, Shushi H, Akihiko I, Yasuhiko I, Yasuyuki Y. Empiric transcatheter arterial embolization for massive bleeding from duodenal ulcers : efficacy and complications. J Vasc Interv Radiol. 2011;22:911–6.

Kamaoui I, Milot L, Pilleul F. Hémorragies digestives basses aiguës : intérêt de l'imagerie. J Radiol. 2010;91:261–9.

Loffroy R, Guiu B, D'Athis P, et al. Arterial embolotherapy for endoscopically unmanageable acute gastroduodenal hemorrhage : predictors of early rebleeding. Clin Gastroenterol Hepatol. 2009;7:515–23.

Loffroy R, Rao P, Ota S, et al. Embolization of acute non-variceal upper gastrointestinal hemorrhage resistant to endoscopic treatment: results and predictors of recurrent bleeding. Cardiovasc Intervent Radiol. 2010;33:1088–100.

Weldon DT, Burke SJ, Sun S, Mimura H, Golzarian J. Interventional management of lower gastrointestinal bleeding. Eur Radiol. 2008;18:857–67.

Chapter 11
True and Pseudoaneurysm of Visceral and Renal Arteries

Louis Boyer, Amr Abdel Kerim, Antoine Petermann, Mickaël Fontarensky, and Pascal Chabrot

11.1 Background

The incidence and natural history of visceral artery aneurysms (VAAs) are not well known, with a reported incidence of renal artery aneurysms (RAAs) of 1–3 % and about 1 % in autopsic series for all visceral arteries aneurysms, among which the splenic artery (SA) is the most commonly affected (60 %), followed by the hepatic artery (HA) (20 %).

Pseudoaneurysms (lack of a complete arterial wall) can develop after trauma (sometimes iatrogenic) or as a complication of pancreatitis. Mycotic (infectious) pseudoaneurysms are rare and usually affect the proximal segment of the superior mesenteric artery (SMA) in a context of endocarditis. The wall of true aneurysm is sometimes calcified and well defined, whereas pseudoaneurysms appear as foci of intense arterial enhancement adjacent to an artery and surrounded by a thrombus or hematoma; they are adjacent to or developed within a pseudocyst in case of pancreatitis. Nevertheless, there are no formal radiological criteria to distinguish a true from a pseudoaneurysm. The latter diagnosis depends mainly on the associated context of pancreatitis, trauma, or infection.

True VAAAs are often constitutional or of dysplastic origin. Their frequency is not well known, yet not increased in patients with aortoiliac aneurysm. Celiac artery (CA)

L. Boyer, MD, PhD (✉) • A. Petermann, MD • P. Chabrot, MD, PhD
Department of Radiology,
University Hospital of Clermont-Ferrand,
Clermont-Ferrand, France
e-mail: lboyer@chu-clermontferrand.fr; pchabrot@chu-clermontferrand.fr

A.A. Kerim, MD
Department of Radiology,
University of Alexandria,
Alexandria, Egypt

M. Fontarensky
Department of Radiology, University Hospital of Clermont-Ferrand,
Clermont-Ferrand, France

P. Chabrot, L. Boyer (eds.), *Embolization*,
DOI 10.1007/978-1-4471-5182-1_11,

occlusion usually predisposes to aneurysms of the duodeno-pancreatic arcades, due to the gradual increase in the flow supplying the hepato-gastro-splenic vascular bed via the SMA. The VAAs and RAAs are more frequent among multiparous women. The incidence of SA aneurysms is particularly higher in patients with portal hypertension.

These lesions are rare, and their evolution is insidious. Circumstances of discovery of VAAs might be in an emergency setting when ruptured (more often with VAAs rather than with RAAs) with severe hemorrhagic shock, notably in late pregnancy with SA aneurysm rupture. Other clinical settings are mass effect, hematuria or hypertension with RAAs, hemobilia with HA aneurysms, mesenteric ischemia in cases of SMA aneurysms complicated with dissections, or thrombosis. But only 20 % of VAA are symptomatic, while 80 % remain silent and discovered incidentally during routine radiological examination.

11.2 Relevant Radiological Anatomy

- CA and SMA: see Chaps. 6 and 7 (HA), 9 (SA), and 10 (GI Tract Arterial Bleedings)
- RA: see Chap. 13

11.3 Techniques

- When aneurysmal exclusion exposes to a risk of infarction with significant tissue necrosis, a short preprocedural prophylactic antibiotherapy is advised. Antipneumococcal vaccination is associated in cases of SA aneurysm.
- When treatment takes place in the setting of aneurysmal rupture, blood transfusions and resuscitation are needed. Collaboration with an anesthesiologist is essential in these meticulous endovascular procedures that often last for a long time, and require a calm and immobile patient.
- Standard femoral artery access and sedation.
- A thorough diagnostic angiography guided by cross-sectional imaging data, for a global vascular assessment and notably for the origin of the aneurysm. It is essential to identify the patency of the arterial and venous systems. Precise knowledge of angio-architecture is mandatory for therapeutic planning. Rundback classification is used for RAAs (see Chap. 13).

11.3.1 Parent Artery Occlusion

Usually there is renal parenchyma loss in cases of RAAs, due to the end artery vasculature. When percutaneous procedure exposes to extensive renal ischemia, then surgical treatment appears to be an appropriate alternative.

In case of visceral artery true or pseudoaneurysms, "sandwich" occlusion of the parent artery should be performed proximally and distally to the aneurysm (equivalent to a surgical exclusion ligation) to avoid distal supply via collaterals (a downstream reinjection via the anastomotic network can occur if only a simple upstream occlusion is performed: "closing the back door"). Coils or vascular plugs can be used, if necessary, in conjunction with liquid agents or particles, to achieve an effective treatment when distal downstream occlusion with coils is not feasible.

11.3.2 Dense Packing with Coils While Keeping the Parent Artery Patent (Packing)

Simple coil occlusion is appropriate for aneurysms with a narrow neck. The most challenging technical issue is the placement of the first caging and the last finishing coils (that should not protrude into the parent artery). An occlusion balloon may be temporarily inflated upstream, slowing the flow and thus securing the procedure.

For wider-neck aneurysms, other techniques can be used, including bare stent-assisted coiling (stent placement followed by positioning of coils through its interstices), larguable balloons, and balloon remodeling (Moret's technique: coiling under protection of a temporarily inflated balloon positioned in front of the aneurysmal neck). Glues or Onyx can also be used but necessitate an excellent technical expertise.

Pseudoaneurysms must not be treated with this packing technique, due to their higher risk of rupture.

11.3.3 Injection of Thrombin

Proposed to treat visceral pseudoaneurysms, especially for those of which an endovascular embolization is not feasible, as in case of pseudoaneurysms developed on small vessels not amenable to catheterization.

11.3.4 Covered Stents Placement

"Endo bypass" provides another means to exclude VAAs from the circulation, especially when the parent artery shows large diameter. The use of covered stents is precluded when the sac is located near a bifurcation (making a branch sacrifice inevitable as in RAAs), or when the parent artery is markedly tortuous (as in SA), as the rigid profile of the stent graft will not allow their navigation to the distal target segment. The risk of endostent thrombosis is not negligible, notably in arteries with limited caliber, making the use of a platelet anti-aggregation therapy mandatory.

The introduction of multilayered stents ("flow diverter," which allow a flow modulation) has widened the indication of endovascular treatment of VAAs located near collateral, as they produce progressive thrombosis of the aneurysmal sac while preserving the patency of the side branches. These stents are validated in neuroradiology and still under evaluation for the aorta; a case report was reported concerning the RA [1].

To summarize, the following can schematically be proposed:

- Saccular aneurysms with narrow neck: packing
- Saccular aneurysms with wide neck: balloon remodeling, stent-assisted coiling, or placement of multilayered or covered stent
- Fusiform aneurysms: parent artery occlusion (ideally "sandwich")
- Fusiform aneurysms with maintained patency of the parent artery: stent-assisted coiling, placement of covered or multilayered stents, or surgical bypass (hepatorenal, splenorenal, aortovisceral, etc.) followed by endovascular occlusion

11.4 Results

To date, the few case reports and small series published do not allow firm conclusions regarding the efficacy and potential complications of endovascular treatment of VAAs.

Success can be expected in 60–90 % of cases, with few complications including technical failure, accidental migration of emboli, and preprocedural aneurysmal rupture (especially in cases of pseudoaneurysms). In this latter case, inflation of an occlusion balloon upstream proximal to the aneurysm can prevent a hypovolemic shock, and hemostasis can then be ensured with parent vessel occlusion. Treatment of SA aneurysms can lead to extensive splenic infarction and episodes of pancreatitis (its management is discussed in Chap. 9). Treatment of SMA aneurysms may induce ischemic complications that justify preprocedural heparinization. Exclusion of HA aneurysms is usually well tolerated, except in cases of portal vein thrombosis (notably after severe traumatic liver injury) or in cases with history of previous hepatobiliary surgery, especially after biliary anastomosis and hepatectomy.

Post-embolization follow-up with imaging is advised, particularly in case of pseudoaneurysms, to detect recanalization and to evaluate the residual perfusion downstream of the treated aneurysm. In our group, strict follow-up by cross-sectional imaging is performed after 1 month and 1 year to ensure the durability of the occlusion and the decrease in lesion size.

11.5 Indications

11.5.1 In Case of Ruptured Aneurysms

The mortality rate following open surgery is high (at least 25 %). Endovascular treatment can be proposed on first intention according to the aneurysmal architecture, experience and availability of the operators. Temporary upstream inflation of balloon proximal to the aneurysm will limit blood loss until complete exclusion of the ruptured aneurysm is obtained.

11.5.2 In Unruptured Aneurysms

Active therapeutic management is not always mandatory, and the conservative alternatives must have been discussed with the patient.

Conventional angiography is the gold standard to make a final therapeutic decision and to planify either endovascular or surgical treatments; however, it only delineates the arterial lumen and must always be preceded by a CT (which is our preferred imaging modality) or an MRI.

- Pseudoaneurysms must always be treated without delay, regardless of their size, and endovascular treatment should be proposed in first intention.
- To prevent aneurysm rupture, according to the guidelines of American Heart Association (AHA), elective treatment of VAAs measuring 2 cm or more is:
    - Highly recommended for females in the childbearing period (to be carried out outside of pregnancy), in case of SA aneurysm associated with portal hypertention, or among candidates for liver transplantation. (Class I, level of evidence B)
    - Probably indicated in elderly women and men (Class IIa, level B).

Besides the aneurysmal architecture (location, surrounding branching pattern, size of the neck…) and the condition of the parent artery (diameter, patency, tortuosity, etc.), the cumbersome surgical procedures in usually weak patients, when compared to the satisfactory results obtained with endovascular techniques, have made the latter become the first-line treatment.

The lower estimated morbid-mortality rate of endovascular treatment has encouraged some authors to lower the cutoff value for treatment to less than 2 cm and to consider aneurysmal size as twice or more than that of the parent artery diameter as the threshold of an indication for treatment.

Elective treatment could be suggested for VAA measuring less than 2 cm, especially in young patients, in females in childbearing period desiring to become pregnant, when patients are symptomatic (renal ischemia, hypertension), for aneurysms associated with RA stenosis, in dissecting aneurysms or with distal embolization, for aneurysms increasing in size on follow-up imaging controls, for HA aneurysms in cases of polyarteritis nodosa or fibromuscular dysplasia, and for SMA aneurysm, because of their high potential risk of complications (rupture, thrombosis, and embolism).

When a conservative treatment is indicated, follow-up imaging is mandatory. In the absence of precise recommendation, we usually suggest a yearly imaging follow-up by ultrasound, CT, or MRI.

Key Points

- VAAs are rare lesions, often asymptomatic, discovered either incidentally or following mass effect, hypertension, hematuria (RA), or rupture (with severe prognosis).
- True aneurysms: usually congenital or dysplastic, with higher frequency among multiparous women and in cases of portal hypertension for SA aneurysms.
- Pseudoaneurysms: usually sequel to iatrogenic complications, posttrauma, infection, or pancreatitis.
- Feasibility of endovascular treatment is determined by comparing CT and angiography data.
- Endovascular treatment of VAAs includes selective packing with coils; parent artery occlusion, ideally proximally and distally to the sac (sandwich), and balloon-assisted coiling; implantation of covered or multilayer stent preserving the patency of parent artery; or surgical bypass followed by endovascular occlusion.
- AHA recommendations: all pseudoaneurysms and true aneurysms of 2 cm or more in size in women at the childbearing age or when associated with portal hypertension and in liver transplant candidates in cases of SA aneurysm should be treated.
- Elective treatment of aneurysms less than 2 cm to prevent rupture is justified especially when parent artery is of limited caliber in young patients and/or when they are symptomatic, in case of progressive increase in size, in RA aneurysm associated with RA stenosis, in HA aneurysm (dysplastic or associated with polyarteritis nodosa), and in aneurysms of the SMA.
- Whenever feasible, endovascular treatment is considered as the first-line treatment.
- When conservative management applies, regular periodic monitoring should be done by imaging.

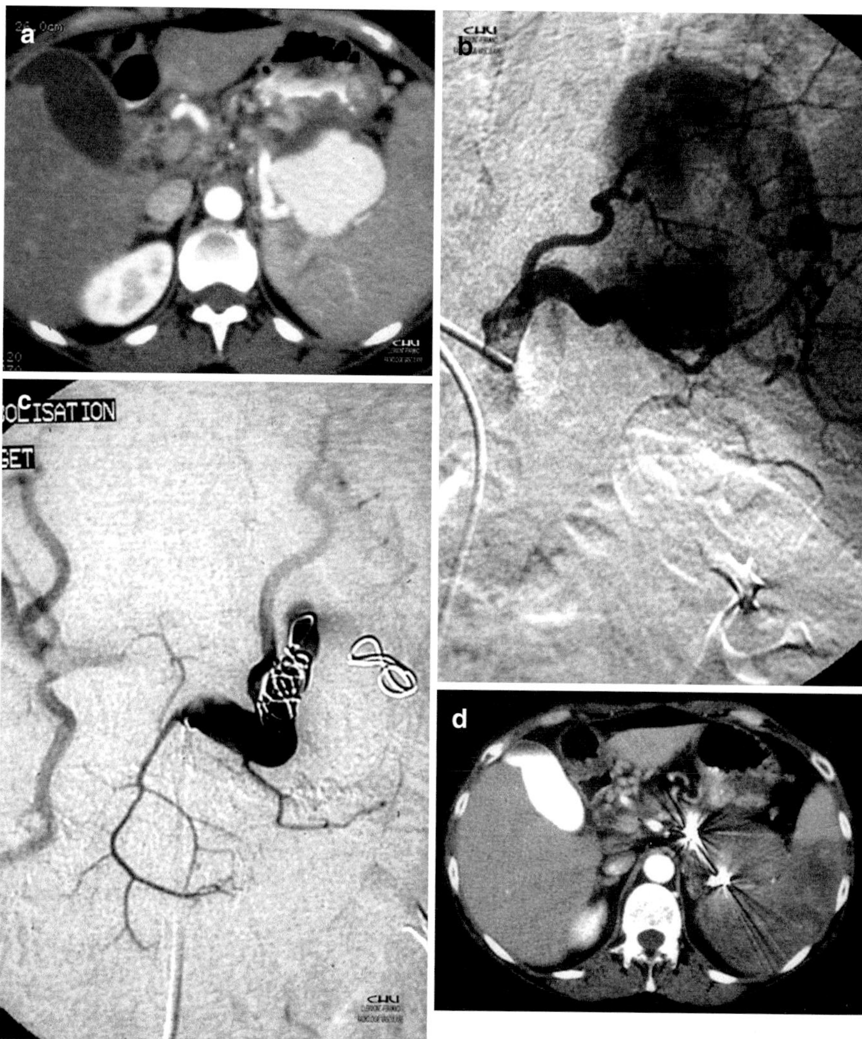

Fig. 11.1 Huge splenic artery false aneurysm opened in a pseudocyst, discovered 6 m after an acute pancreatitis. (**a**) CT: Large pseudoaneurysm opened in a pseudocyst. (**b**) Selective injection of the splenic artery: slow enhancement of this voluminous hilar lesion. (**c**) Coiling upstream of the lesion and immediately downstream of a collateral branch independent of this false aneurysm, feeding the superior pole of the spleen parenchyma. (**d**) CT 1 month later: excluded false aneurysm, large hypodense splenic parenchymous area, but remaining consequent enhanced parenchyma

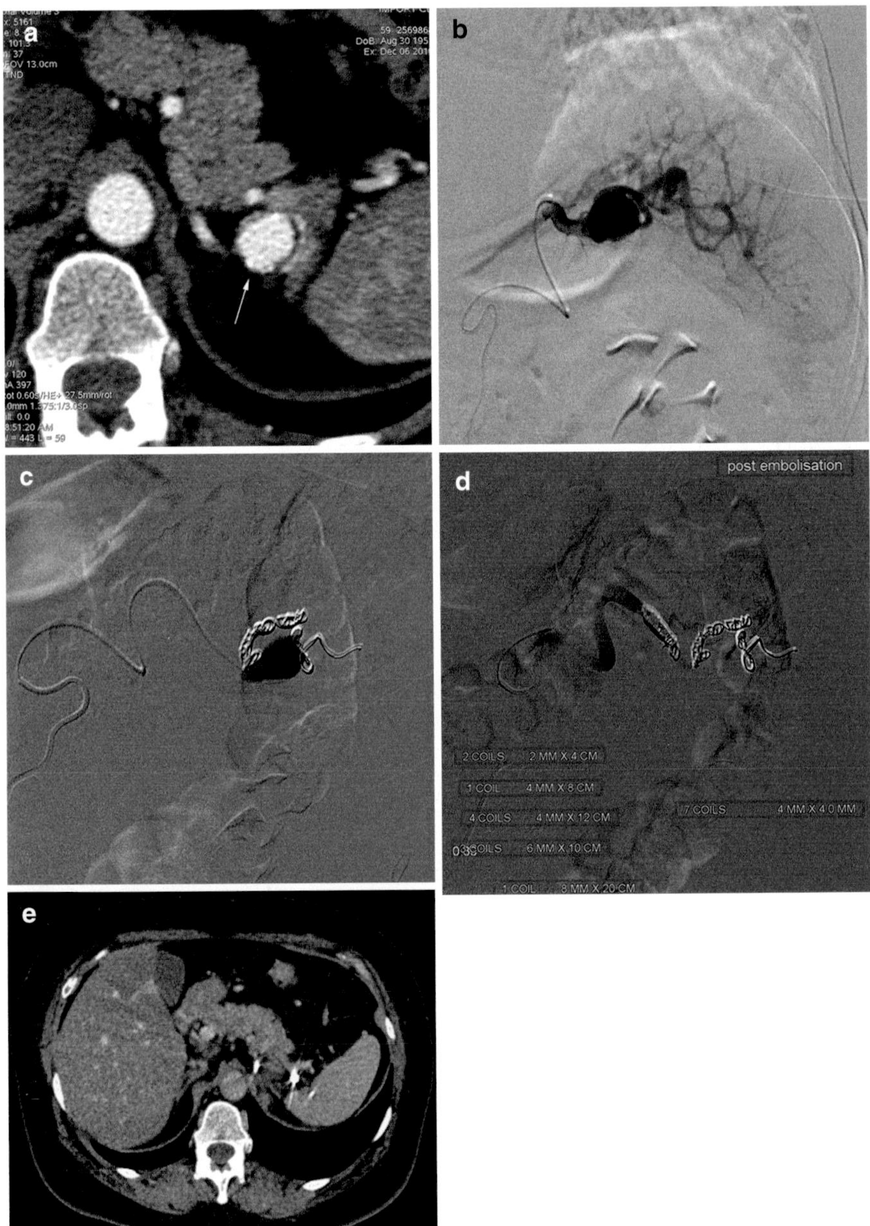

Fig. 11.2 Asymptomatic 18 mm diameter sacciform splenic artery aneurysm. (**a**) CT: diagnosis of a splenic artery aneurysm (*arrow*). (**b**) Hyperselective splenic artery injection (microcatheter): aneurysm, with two efferent branches. (**c**) Catheterization and coiling of the branches downstream to the aneurysm (**d**) and then upstream coiling, leading to a "sandwich" exclusion (upstream + downstream). (**e**) CT 1 m later: correct splenic parenchymal enhancement via the gastric arteries collateral feeding

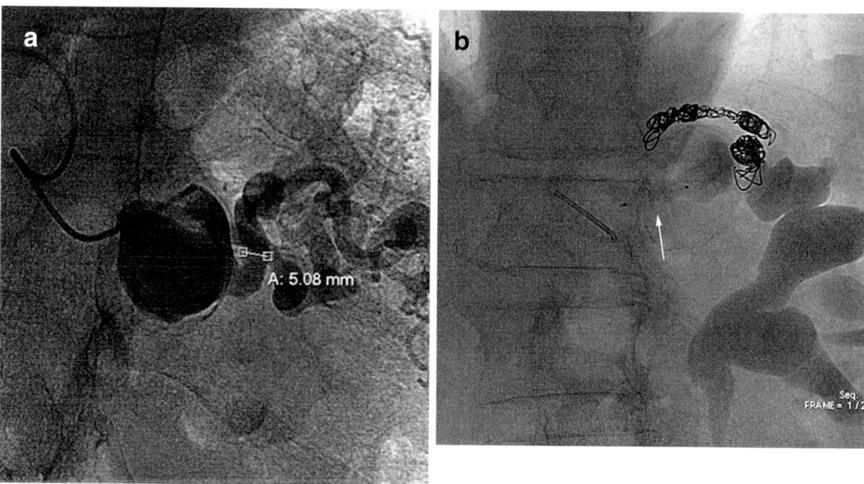

Fig. 11.3 A 65-year-old W, asymptomatic 35 mm truncal SA aneurysm, discovered on a CT. (**a**) Selective SA arteriography: two efferent arteries. (**b**) Control angio after sandwich exclusion: downstream (coiling of two efferent branches) and upstream (truncal AVP, *arrow*)

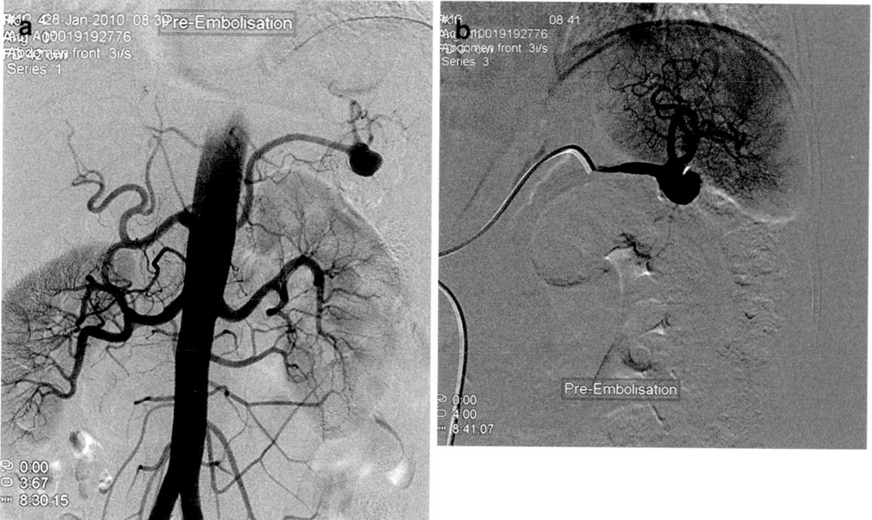

Fig. 11.4 (**a**) Asymptomatic CT diagnosed sacciform SA 30 mm aneurysm: aortography. (**b**) Selective arteriography: large neck aneurysm, located at the end of the SA trunk. (**c**) Control angio after coil packing. (**d**) CT 1 month later: correct splenic parenchyma enhancement

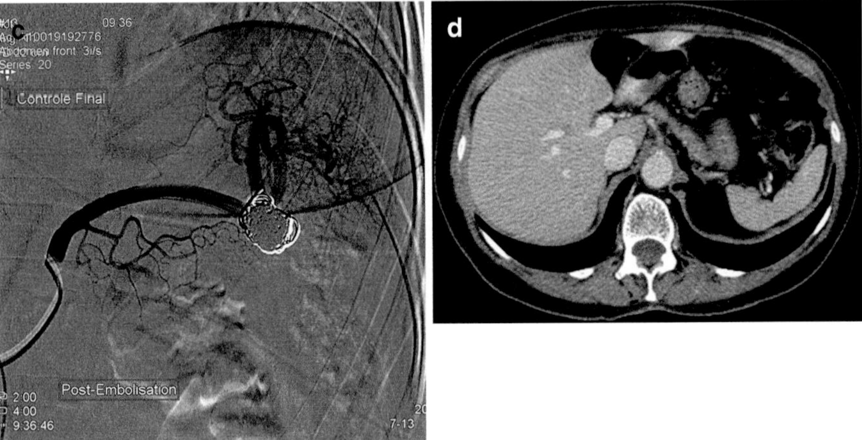

Fig. 11.4 (continued)

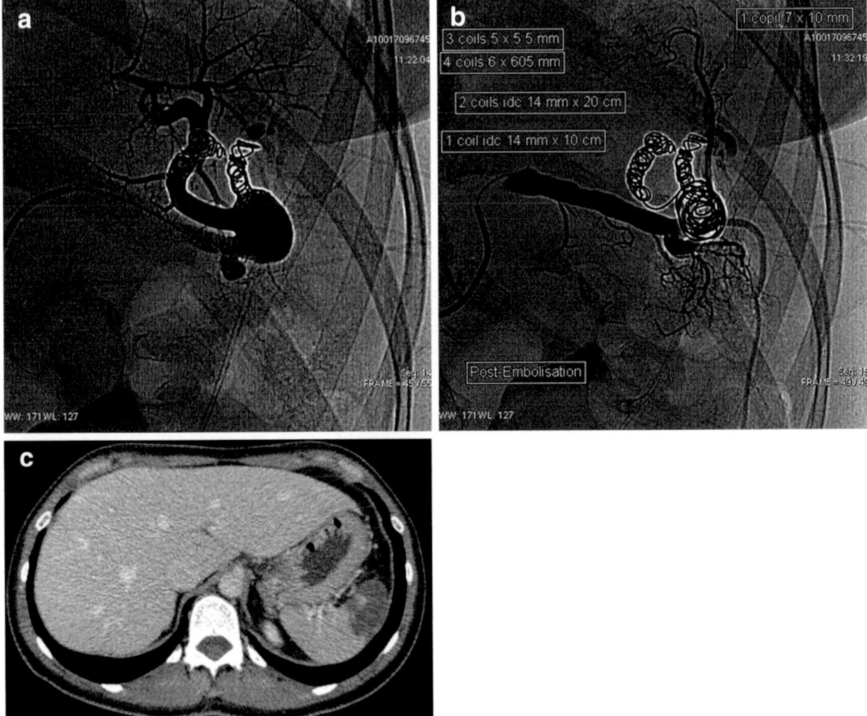

Fig. 11.5 Huge asymptomatic splenic artery aneurysm. (**a**) Efferent branches coil exclusion (**b**) and then packing of the sac. (**c**) CT 1 month later: partial splenic infarction

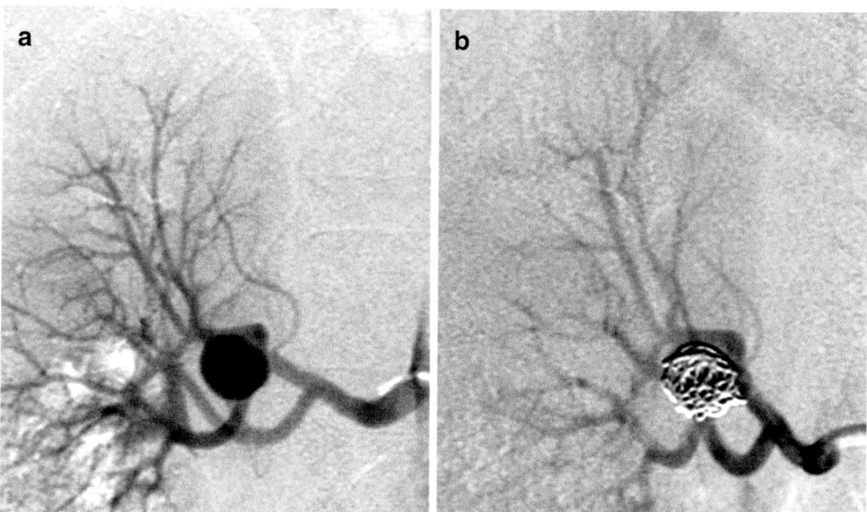

Fig. 11.6 Sacciform aneurysm of the inferior first-order branch of the right prepyelic renal A (Rundback type II). (**a**) Selective arteriography. (**b**) Angiographic control after packing

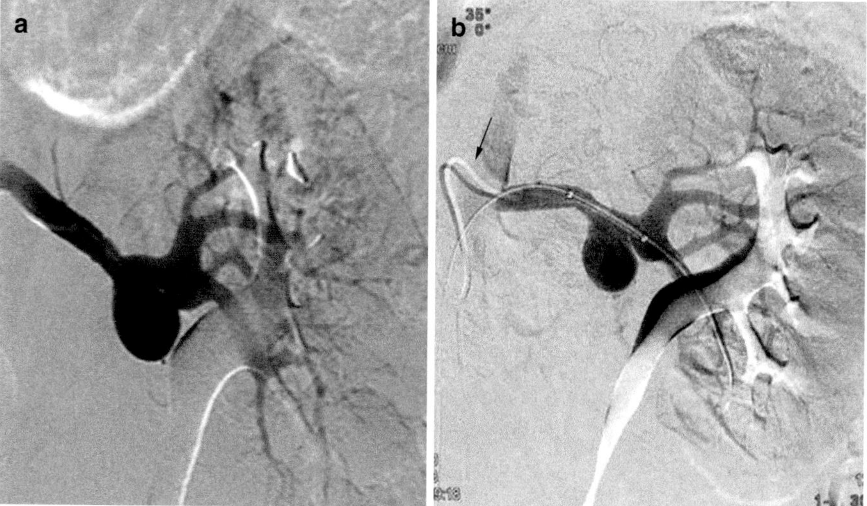

Fig. 11.7 45-year-old W, asymptomatic left RA aneurysm (2 cm), discovered on a US Doppler exploration (**a**) Selective angio: large neck sacciform aneurysm, located at the end of the left RA trunk, (**b**) preprocedural angio before balloon expandable stent grafting: note (*arrow*) a selective catheter beside the coaxial GW carrying the stent graft, and (**c**) control angio: aneurysm excluded, good patency of the pre- and retro-pyelic RA terminal branches

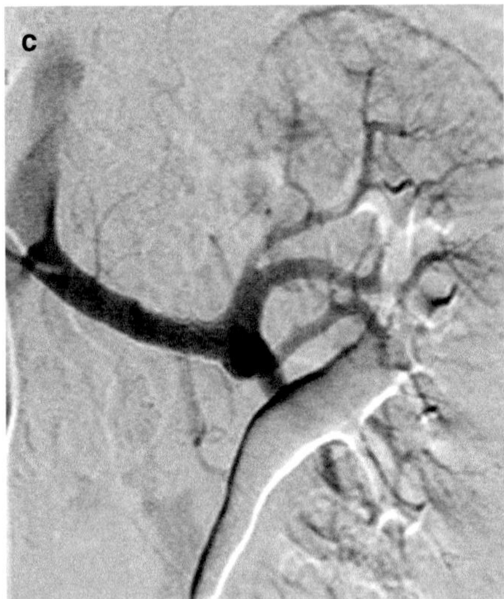

Fig. 11.7 (continued)

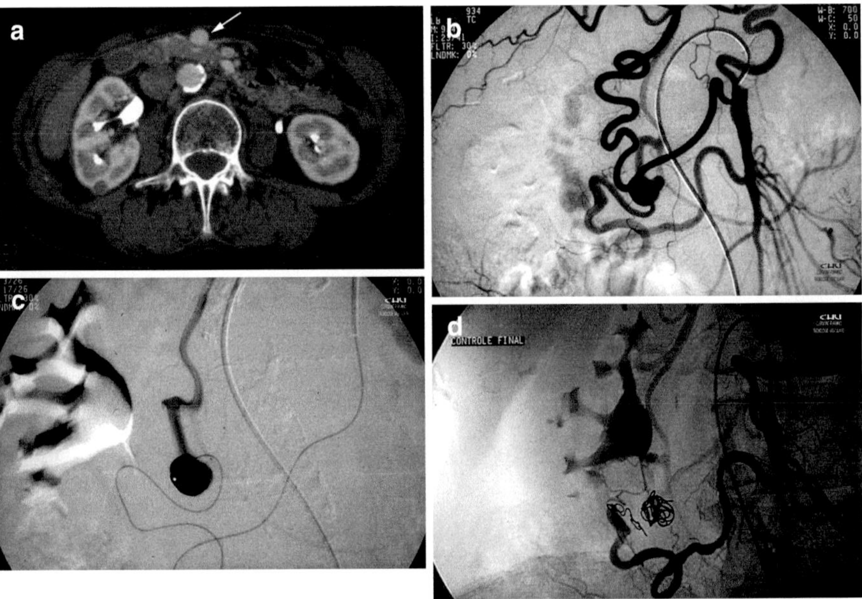

Fig. 11.8 (**a**) Systematic discovery of a splanchnic aneurysm (*arrow*) in an asymptomatic 75-year-old W. An occluded celiac trunk was also seen on CT. (**b**) Selective SMA angio: the aneurysm is located on the duodeno-pancreatic arcades. (**c**) Hyperselective catheterization (microcatheter). (**d**) Control angio after endovascular exclusion (packing + coils upstream of the lesion)

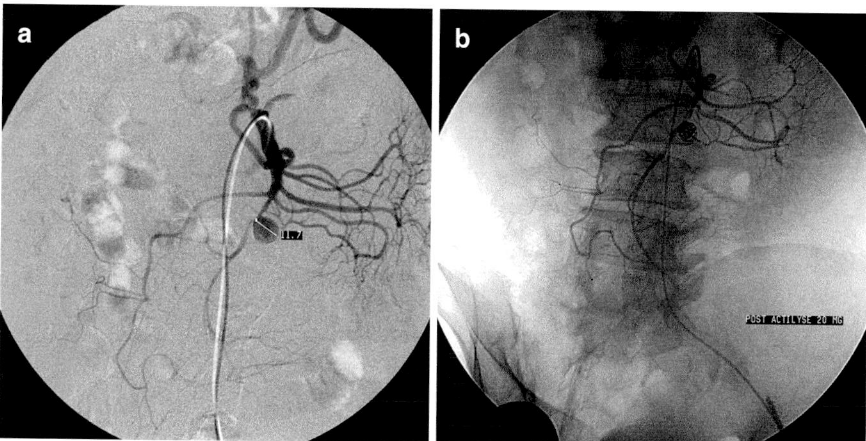

Fig. 11.9 Rendu-Osler Weber's disease; cardiac arrhythmia with anticoagulants. CT to explore abdominal pain: splanchnic aneurysms. (**a**) Selective SMA injection: 12 mm large neck sacciform distal SMA aneurysm, at the level of the ileal branches. SMA diameter at this level measures 4 mm. (**b**) Control angio after bare self-expandable stent deployment and coils packing by microcatheterization through the mesh. A mild intra-stent thrombus required an in situ fibrinolysis (25 mg bolus of rt PA). Heparin anticoagulation was administered during 24 h. And we observed finally a good clinical and technical result

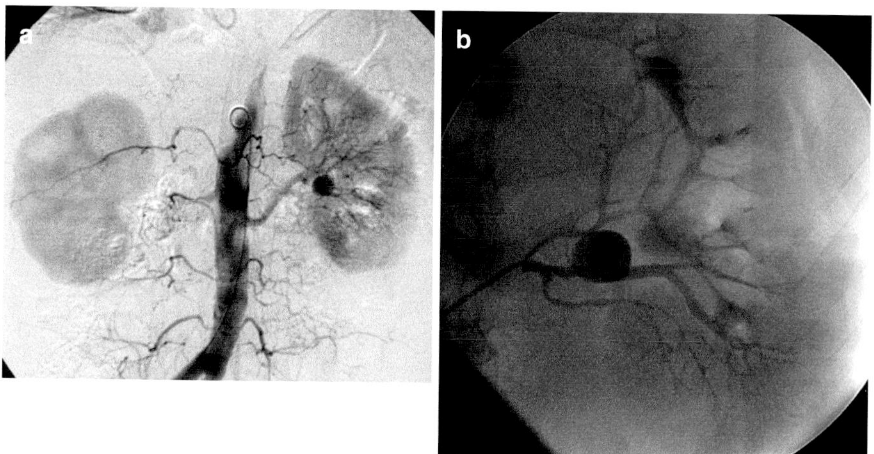

Fig. 11.10 Intrarenal aneurysm discovered on the imaging check up of a hypertensive patient. (**a**) Aortography, late phase: 25 mm aneurysm, with a late wash out. (**b**) Selective intra-arterial injection: the aneurysm depends on a second-order branch, after the prepyelic artery bifurcation. (**c**) Exclusion by packing

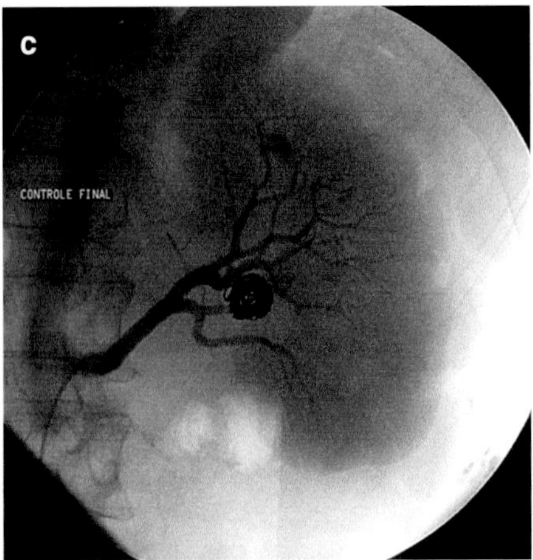

Fig. 11.10 (continued)

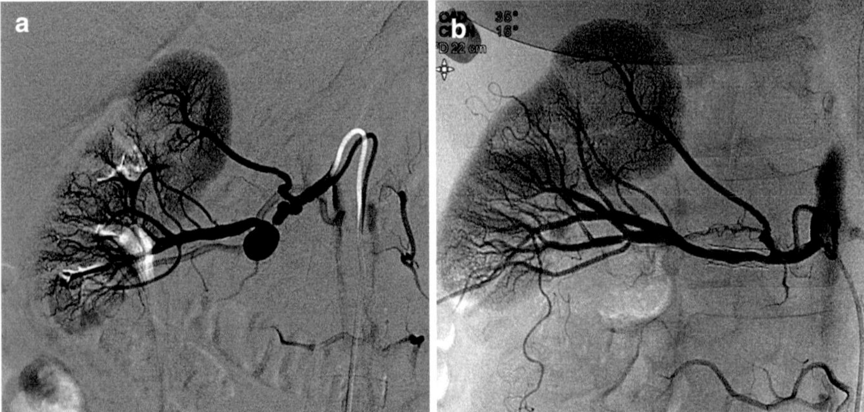

Fig. 11.11 Renovascular hypertension in a 35-year-old W. Duplex Doppler echography has shown a little right kidney, downstream of a severe renal artery stenosis. (**a**) Selective injection of the right renal artery: immediately downstream of the superior polar collateral artery, very severe stenosis and then aneurysm. A dysplasia has been considered. We decide to treat both the stenosis and the aneurysm with a stent graft. (**b**) Control angio 6 m later: the aneurysm is excluded, the stenosis is treated, but a mild endostent hyperplasia is observed

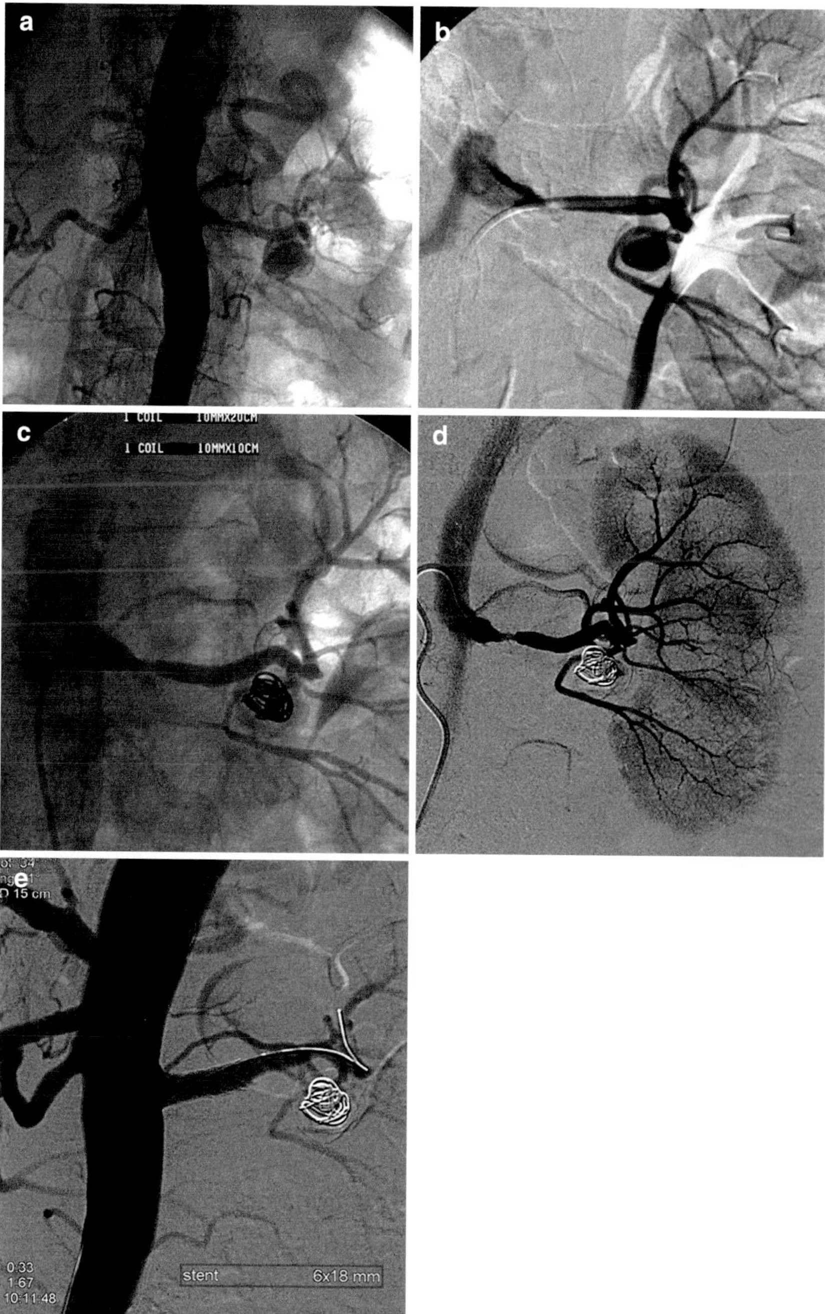

Fig. 11.12 Hypertension, severe left RA stenosis on a duplex Doppler. (**a**) Aortography: severe post-ostial left RA stenosis, but also intrarenal aneurysm. (**b**) Selective injection, downstream of the stenosis: narrow neck aneurysm. (**c**) Aneurysm exclusion by coil packing. (**d**) Control angio 1 m later: the aneurysm is excluded, and the parenchymal lost is limited, so we decided to treat the stenosis. (**e**) Control angio, after angioplasty + stent of the proximal truncal left RA stenosis (remaining trans stenotic GW)

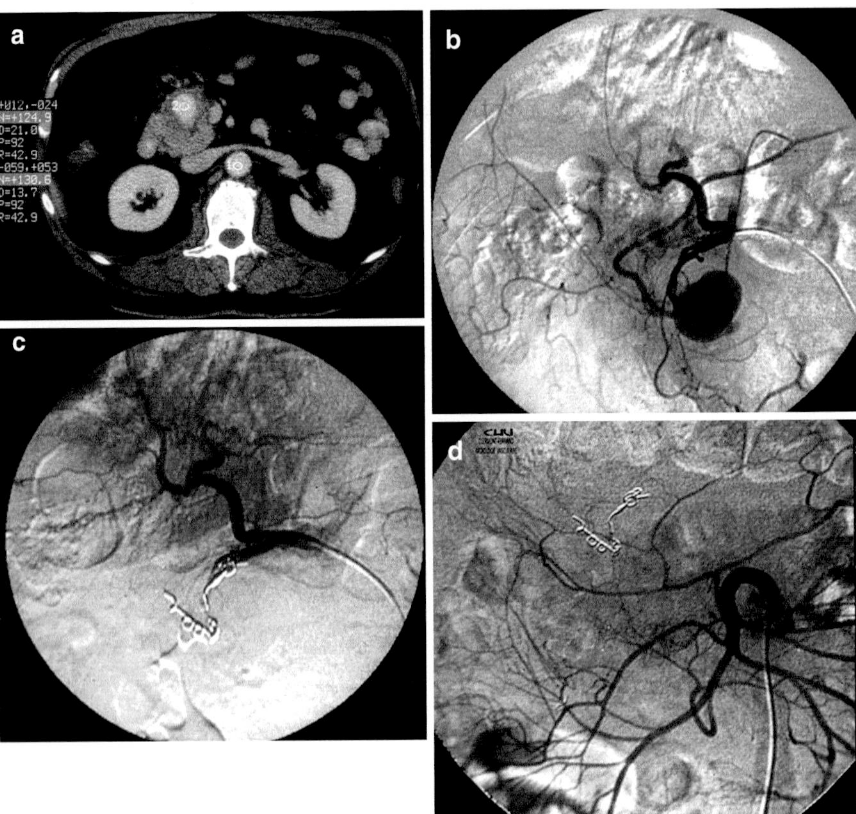

Fig. 11.13 (**a**) Abdominal pain 3 m after an acute pancreatitis: CT, showing a huge intra-pancreatic false aneurysm. (**b**) Selective injection of the common hepatic artery: the aneurysm depends on the duodeno-pancreatic arcades. (**c**) Microcatheterization: coiling upstream and downstream of the false aneurysm. (**d**) SMA injection, to be sure of no "back door" reinjection

Reference

1. Henry M, et al. Treatment of renal artery aneurysm with the multilayer stent. J Endovasc Ther. 2008;15(2):231–6.

Suggested Reading

Hirsch AT, et al. ACC/AHA guidelines for the management of patients with peripheral arterial disease (lower extremity, renal, mesenteric, and abdominal aortic). J Vasc Interv Radiol. 2006;17:1383–98.

Rossi M, Rebonato A, Greco L, Citone M, David V. Endovascular exclusion of visceral artery aneurysms with stent-grafts : technique and long-term follow-up. Cardiovasc Intervent Radiol. 2008;31:36–42.

Chapter 12
Hypogastric Arteries: Aneurysms, Occlusions Before Stent Grafting

Pascal Chabrot, Lucie Cassagnes, Mickaël Fontarensky, Philippe Bourlet, and Louis Boyer

12.1 Background: Two Situations

12.1.1 Occlusions of Hypogastric Arteries Before Endovascular Treatment of Aortoiliac Aneurysms

Occlusions are done to prevent a reinjection of the aneurysmal sac by collateral pelvic circulation via the hypogastric artery (type II endoleak), once the covered stent is positioned in the common and external iliac artery, occluding the hypogastric ostium.

12.1.2 Hypogastric Artery Aneurysms

The iliac aneurysms (common iliac, external iliac, or internal iliac) are defined by an increased diameter, greater than 1.5 times the diameter size of a healthy arterial segment. In practice, this increase in the diameter is considered as aneurysmal above 25 mm.

P. Chabrot, MD, PhD • L. Cassagnes, MD • L. Boyer, MD, PhD (✉)
Department of Radiology, University Hospital of Clermont-Ferrand, Clermont-Ferrand, France
e-mail: lboyer@chu-clermontferrand.fr; pchabrot@chu-clermontferrand.fr

M. Fontarensky
Department of Radiology, University Hospital of Clermont-Ferrand, Clermont-Ferrand, France

P. Bourlet, MD
Department of Radiology, Riom Hospital, University Hospital of Clermont-Ferrand, Clermont-Ferrand, France

P. Chabrot, L. Boyer (eds.), *Embolization*,
DOI 10.1007/978-1-4471-5182-1_12, © Springer-Verlag London 2014

These iliac aneurysms are relatively rare (around 0.03 % in autopsy). However, they are frequent in cases of associated abdominal aortic aneurysms (more than 20 %). Most frequently they concern the common iliac and internal iliac arteries rather than the external iliac arteries; most of them are atheromatous.

The majority of these aneurysms are asymptomatic and discovered during an imaging workup. Other discovery circumstances are the complications they bring about: a mass effect on nervous, urogenital, GI, or venous structures; thrombosis; embolism; or rupture. In the last case, the prognosis is severe (mortality rate of up to 50 % in spite of emergency surgical treatment): so an elective preventive treatment is usually indicated, with a threshold of 3 cm.

12.2 Relevant Radiological Anatomy

The internal iliac (IIA) or hypogastric arteries are terminal branches of the common iliac arteries. The length of the common iliac artery and the position of the iliac bifurcation are variable. The IIA courses posteriorly and medially.

The IIA are voluminous (8–9 mm in diameter), with a length of 4 cm usually.

Most often (57–77 %) they divide into two trunks at the level of the upper part of the greater sciatic notch:

- The posterior trunk gives off several arteries: iliolumbar, superior and inferior lateral sacral (with an intra pelvic parietal supply), and superior gluteal (with an extra parietal pelvic supply).
- The anterior trunk gives off other branches: visceral arteries (umbilical, inferior vesical, middle rectal, prostatic and vesiculo-deferential in men, and uterine and vaginal in women) and extra pelvic parietal arteries (obturator, inferior gluteal or ischiatic, and internal pudendal).

The variations in the way these divisions take place are multiple: only one trunk (≦ 4 %), three trunks (≦ 15 %), four trunks, or more (≦ 3 %), and all these branches can also form a "bouquet" (≦ 2 %). In 90 % of the cases, the division is right/left symmetric.

The absence of IIA is rare (therefore, all these branches originate from the common iliac artery).

There are many anastomoses between parietal or visceral branches of the two hypogastric arteries but also with the external iliac and femoral arteries and with abdominal aorta.

12.3 Embolization Techniques

A bilateral femoral approach allows upstream intermediate aortoiliac opacifications. Generally we prefer to carry out embolizations by a contralateral femoral access, using a long pre-curved sheath.

Most of the procedures take place via a percutaneous access. But stent grafts of larger diameter may require a surgical access or the use of a closure device.

To avoid distal necrotic damage in the territories supplied by the hypogastric branches, coils and plugs should be chosen rather than liquid embolization agents.

12.3.1 Hypogastric Aneurysms

- If the aneurysm is isolated, without any involvement of the external iliac or the primitive iliac artery, and if a proximal neck exists, it is necessary to firstly occlude the efferent branches of the hypogastric artery with coils and to complete with a proximal occlusion of the internal iliac neck, using either coils or Amplatzer vascular plugs. The procedure can have an intermediate phase of packing of the aneurysmal sac.
- In case of an isolated hypogastric aneurysm but without any proximal neck or when confronted with an association of hypogastric and primitive iliac aneurysms with a neck: embolization of the hypogastric branches first using coils and then endobypass of the common iliac artery to the external iliac artery using a stent graft (for the common iliac aneurysms, a proximal neck of at least 15 mm is required).
- Internal iliac aneurysms which develop after a previous aortobifemoral bypass or aorto-bi-external iliac bypass having termino-lateral anastomosis (preserving a retro-hypogastric perfusion: backward flow upstream of the anastomosis): a retrograde puncture downstream to the anastomosis allows a catheterization of the native external iliac artery and of the aneurysm, so as to be able to carry out an exclusion using coils (distal branches in order to avoid reinjections + coils or proximal Amplatzer plug).
- Aneurysm of internal iliac artery after surgery with exclusion of the hypogastric artery: a meticulous assessment of the feeding vessels of the aneurysm is mandatory, in order to detect afferent vessels branching off the external iliac branches or the contralateral hypogastric artery; embolization is then attempted in favorable cases.

However, endovascular navigation up to the aneurysm is not always possible. A CT-guided puncture of the aneurysm has therefore been proposed, in order to carry out a percutaneous occlusion, using either coils or glue.

12.3.2 Embolizations of Non-aneurysmal Hypogastric Arteries, Before the Endovascular Treatment of Aortoiliac Aneurysms Including the Iliac Bifurcation

Truncal occlusions are done using coils or Amplatzer plug, so as to avoid reinjections.

12.3.3 *Follow-up*

After the embolization, a CT scan control is advised after 1 month and then after 1 year (patency? growth of the aneurysmal sac?).

Long-term monitoring of aortoiliac endoprostheses is mandatory.

12.4 Results

A technical success is usual.

Complications at the puncture site are possible, especially when the use of stent graft requires large introducer sheath diameter.

Colic and pelvic ischemic complications are not frequent.

However, the occurrence of buttock claudication has been reported in up to 40 % of the cases. It would be more frequent in case of bilateral embolization. It has also been noted that it would more likely occur in distal occlusions of the hypogastric trunk and its branches. For the majority of the patients, these claudications are transitory; however in some cases they can be permanent.

12.5 Indications

Endovascular techniques (embolization, stent graft) are indicated as the first-line treatment. The choice of the technique depends on the anatomical configuration and the state of the adjacent arteries (aortic bifurcation, iliac bifurcation).

No matter what the indications are, the increased risk of ischemic complication is discussed in the case of bilateral embolization; we therefore prefer in these cases carrying out the bilateral exclusions in 2 steps.

12.5.1 *Hypogastric Aneurysms*

All symptomatic aneurysms (pain, embolism, mass effect, etc.) must be treated.

For most of the authors, when they are asymptomatic, a preventive treatment of the rupture is proposed with a threshold of 30 mm.

12.5.2 Exclusions of Hypogastric Arteries Before Endovascular Treatment of Aortoiliac Aneurysms

The endovascular treatment using bifurcated stent grafts of an aortoiliac aneurysm which does not have a distal neck on the primitive iliac artery must firstly be preceded by the occlusion of the hypogastric arteries, in order to avoid retrograde injection which can bring about a type II endoleak.

So as to avoid ischemic complications, this exclusion must be carried out at least 1 week before the aortoiliac aneurysm treatment.

Key Points

- Iliac aneurysm: theoretically 1.5 times the diameter of the healthy artery; obvious above 25 mm.
- Iliac aneurysms of more than 3 cm must be treated.
- Often asymptomatic; prognosis of rupture: severe.
- Associated with 20 % of infrarenal AAA.
- Endovascular treatment (embolization using coils, stent graft) is the first-line treatment; the choice of the technique depends on the vascular anatomical configuration.
- Post-embolization buttock claudication is not rare, more commonly seen in the cases of distal embolization of the hypogastric artery and its branches, and in the case of bilateral embolization, if a bilateral exclusion is needed, it is better to do it in two steps.
- Exclusion of the hypogastric arteries before the endovascular treatment of iliac aneurysms should be performed if possible 8 days beforehand, thus avoiding ischemic complications.

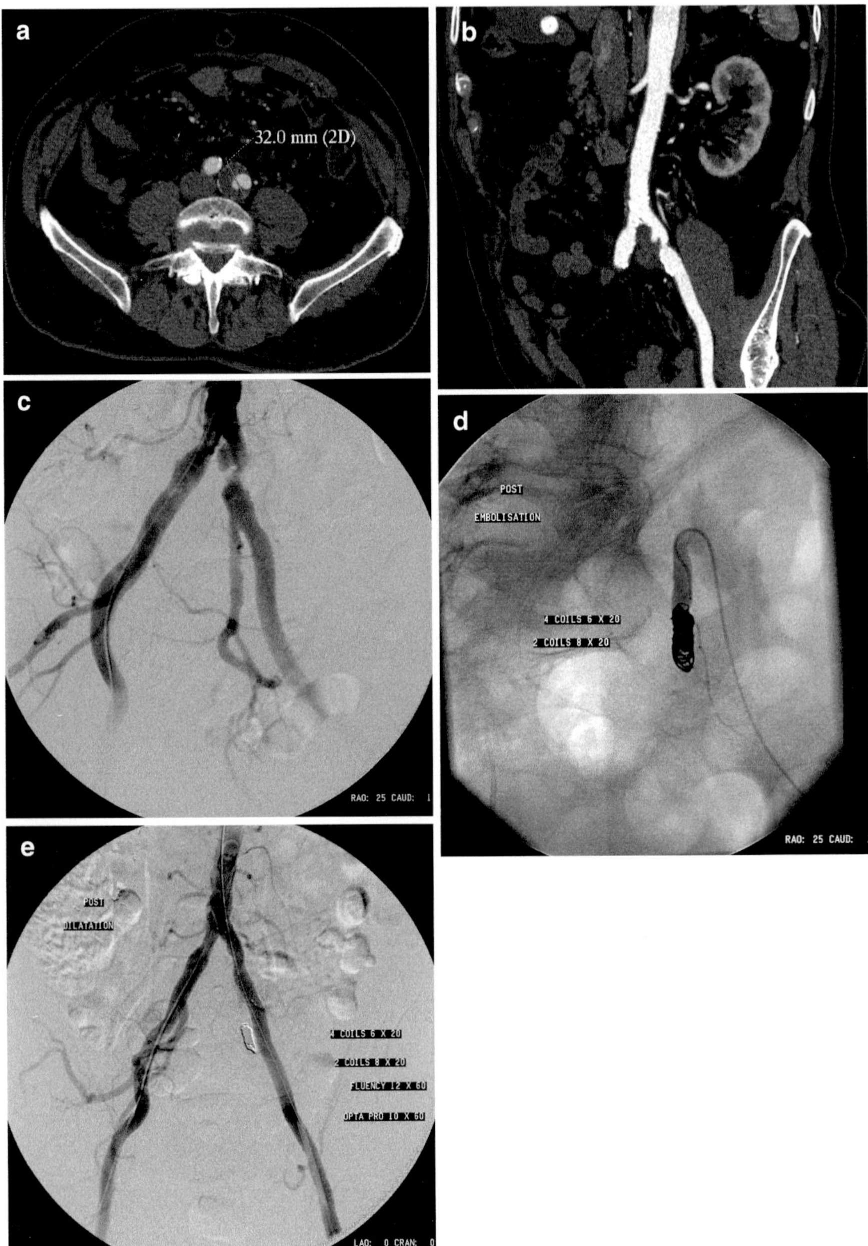

Fig. 12.1 (**a**, **b**) Axial transverse CT (**a**) and MPR reconstruction (*curved*) (**b**): partially thrombosed left common iliac artery aneurysm. With the growth in size (up to 32 mm), appeared an intermittent claudication related to the partial thrombosis of the left common iliac artery: the exclusion of the aneurysm with an iliac stent graft was planned, which involved first the occlusion of the ipsilateral hypogastric artery by coils, to avoid a later reinjection. (**c**) Aortography (25° RAO): short stenosis downstream of a proximally enlarged left common iliac artery. (**d**) Occlusion of the end of the hypogastric trunk by coils, via a distal ipsilateral femoral access. (**e**) Control aortography after deployment of a stent graft excluding the aneurysm and also treating the stenosis

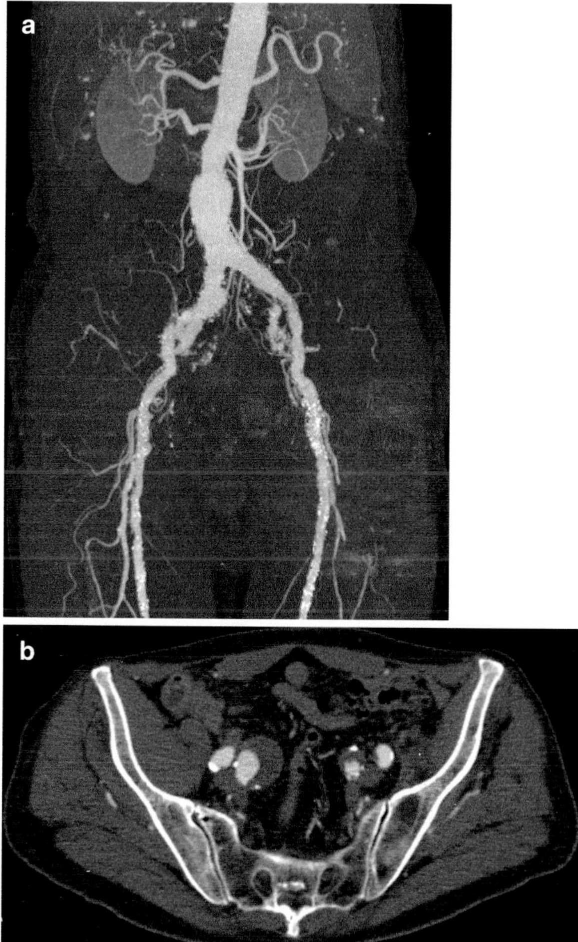

Fig. 12.2 Infrarenal aortic aneurysm extended to common iliac and hypogastric arteries. Embolization before bifurcated aortoiliac stent grafting (EVAR). (**a**) MIP reconstruction with calcified structures substraction showing the flowing lumen: infrarenal aortic aneurysm, respecting an infrarenal proximal neck, extended to the common iliac arteries; partially thrombosed internal iliac aneurysm. (**b**) Axial transverse CT scan through the origin of the two hypogastric arteries: partially thrombosed right hypogastric aneurysm, smaller left hypogastric aneurysm, partially flowing. (**c**) Aortography. (**d**) Right hypogastric aneurysm treatment: from a left femoral artery puncture, cross over to the right common iliac artery, and selective catheterization of the right hypogastric artery (Cobra catheter). (**e–g**) Hyperselective catheterization of the right gluteal artery (downstream of the aneurysm) (**e**), to be first excluded by coils + plug, to avoid any reinjection after the coverage of the common iliac aneurysm by a stent graft (**f**, **g**). (**h**) Control aortography via a right femoral access 3 weeks later: correct exclusion of the right hypogastric artery. (**i**) Selective catheterization of the left hypogastric artery from a right femoral access: after crossing over the aortoiliac bifurcation, injection before truncal plug exclusion, to avoid any reinjection after implantation of an aortoiliac stent graft. (**j**) Final aortographic control: exclusion of both hypogastric arteries, allowing the aorto-bi-iliac stent grafting (EVAR). (**k–m**) CT scan 1 month after the EVAR: axial scan (**k**), volume rendering, and MIP reconstruction (**l**, **m**): decrease in size of the internal iliac aneurysms, which are not enhanced. Right iliac limb of the stent graft: *white arrow*; coils at the end of the right hypogastric trunk and in the right gluteal artery (*black arrow*)

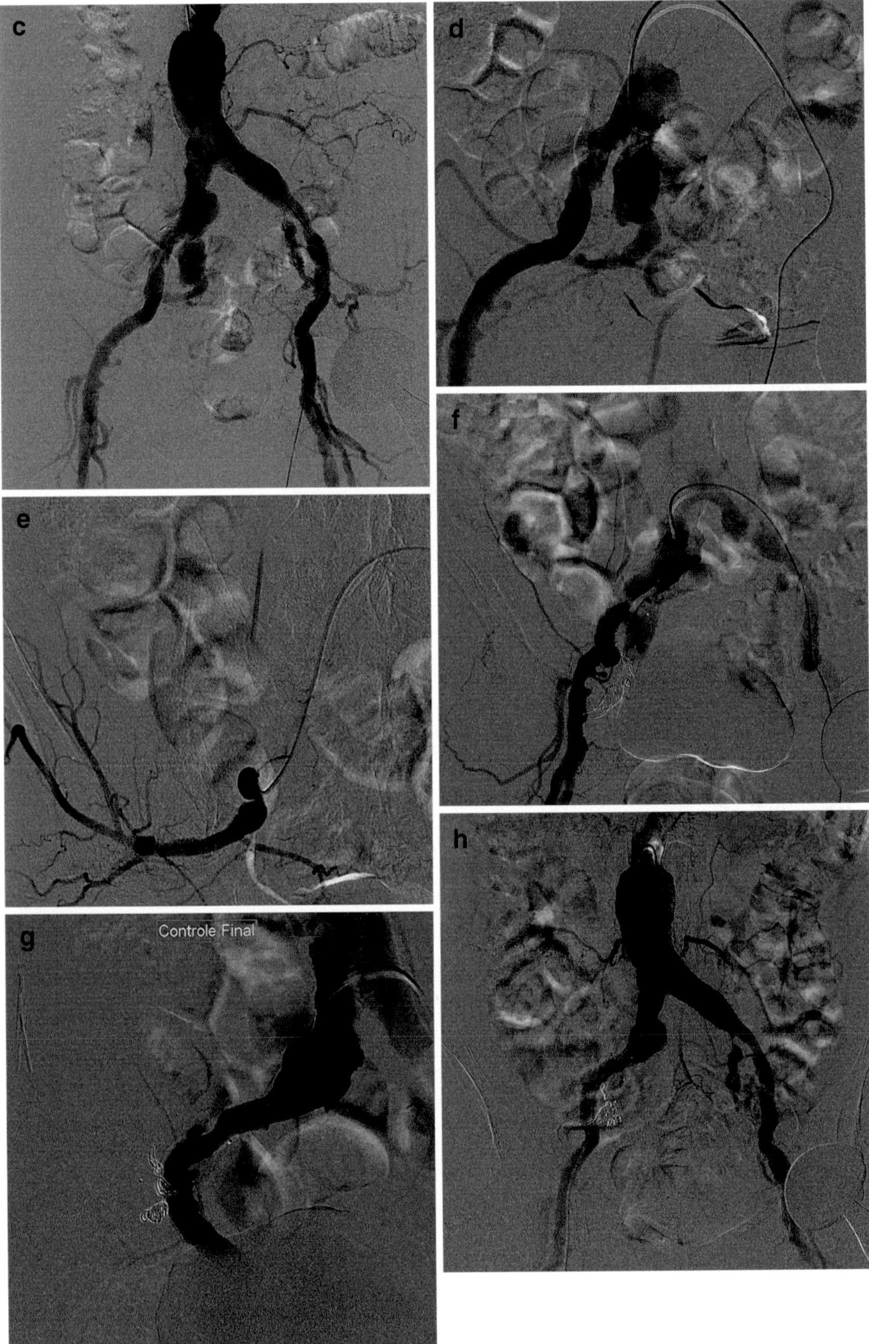

Fig. 12.2 (continued)

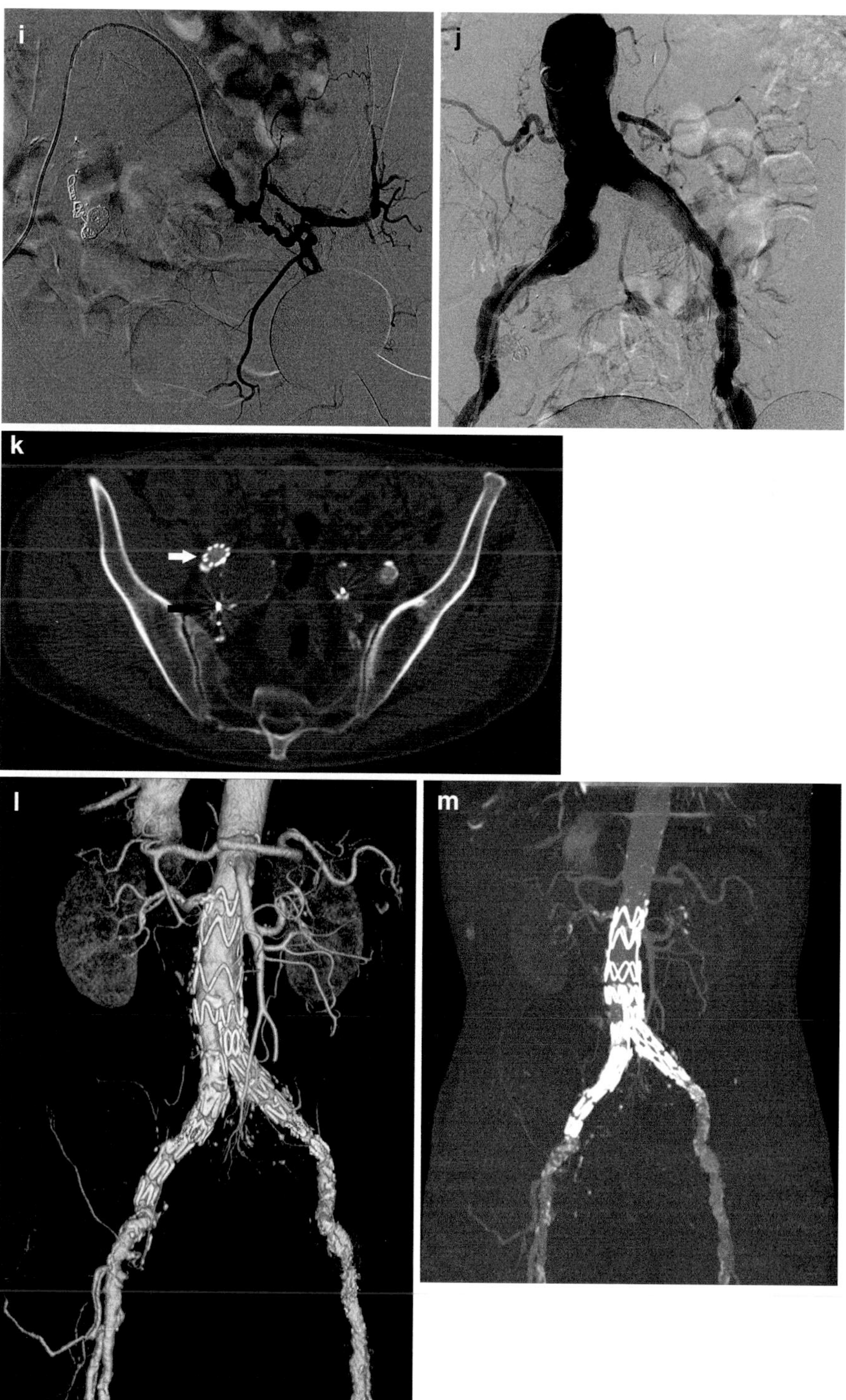

Fig. 12.2 (continued)

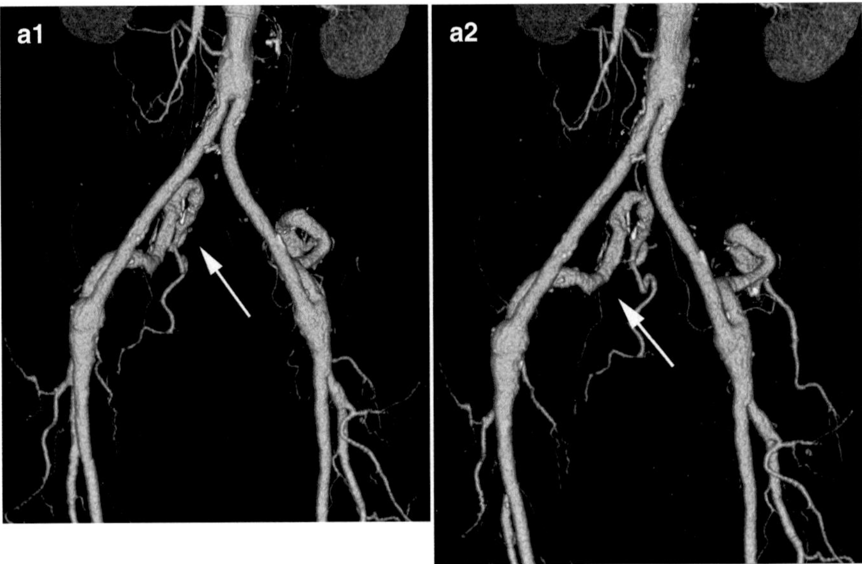

Fig. 12.3 Patient operated 10 years ago: an aortobifemoral bypass was performed to treat an occlusive aortoiliac disease. The native external iliac arteries were left in charge to ensure a retrograde perfusion of the hypogastric artery territories, with end-to-side low iliofemoral anastomosis. A 5 cm aneurysm of the left hypogastric artery has been discovered during the follow-up, meaning the risk of rupture. (**a1–a6**) CT: (MPR/volume rendering) showing the retro-reinjection, from the low anastomosis, of the external iliac and hypogastric native arteries (*arrows*). (**b**) Large left gluteal artery (*thick arrow*), in communication with the left hypogastric aneurysm (*thin arrow*). (**c**) Transverse CT scan 2 cm higher than the previous (b) figure, showing the right and left iliac branches of the aortobifemoral bypass (*thick arrows*), the native external iliac arteries retrogradely injected (*arrow*), and the left iliac aneurysm (*black arrow*). (**d**) Three centimeters above CT scan showing the native iliac bifurcation: large left internal iliac aneurysm, partially flowing. (**e**) Puncture of the left common femoral artery, downstream of the aortobifemoral bypass anastomosis, and retrograde catheterization of the native left external iliac artery limited dimensions of the flowing lumen of the hypogastric aneurysm. (**f**) Final control after the occlusion with coils of the efferent collateral branches of the hypogastric aneurysm

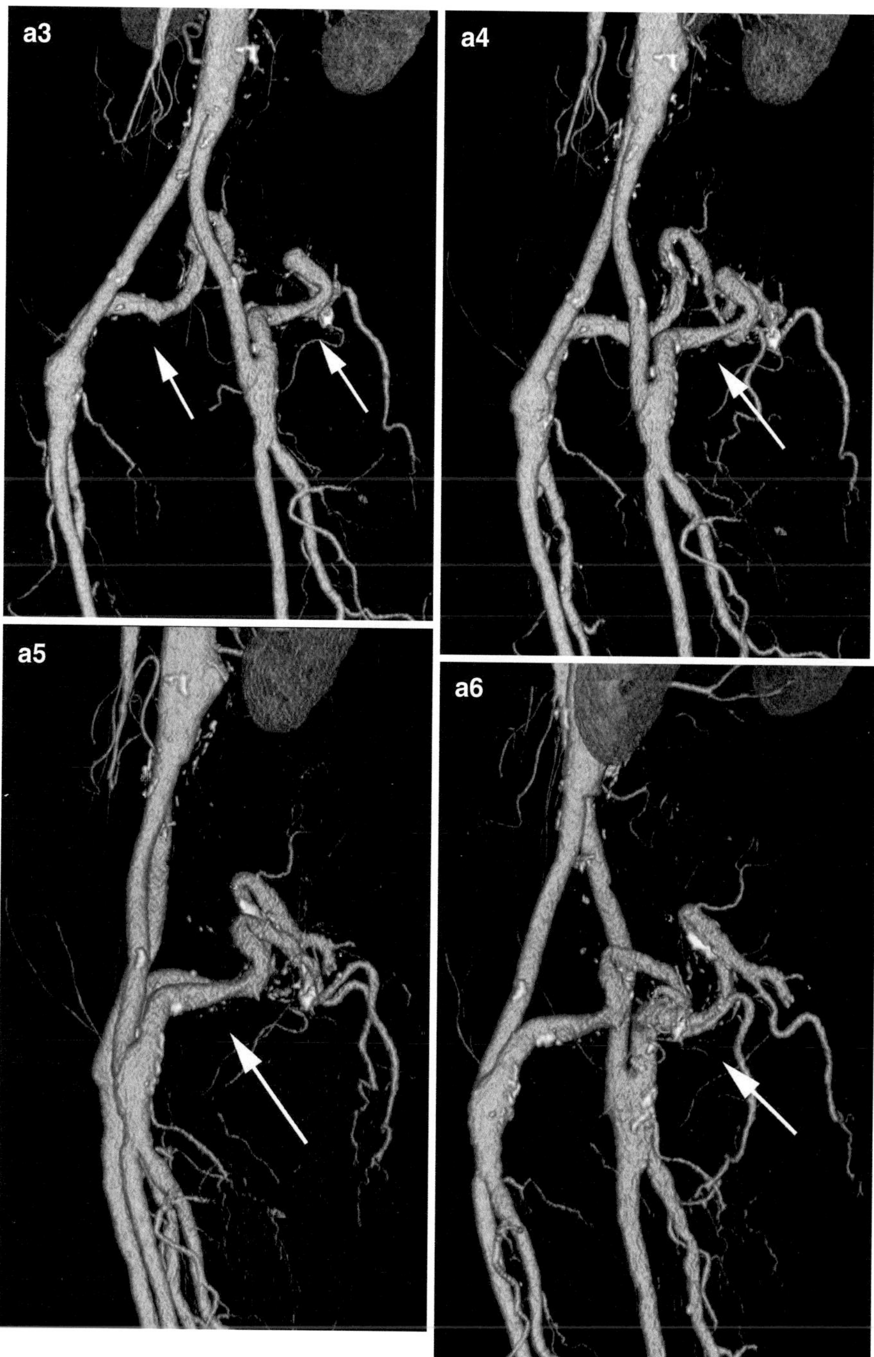

Fig. 12.3 (continued)

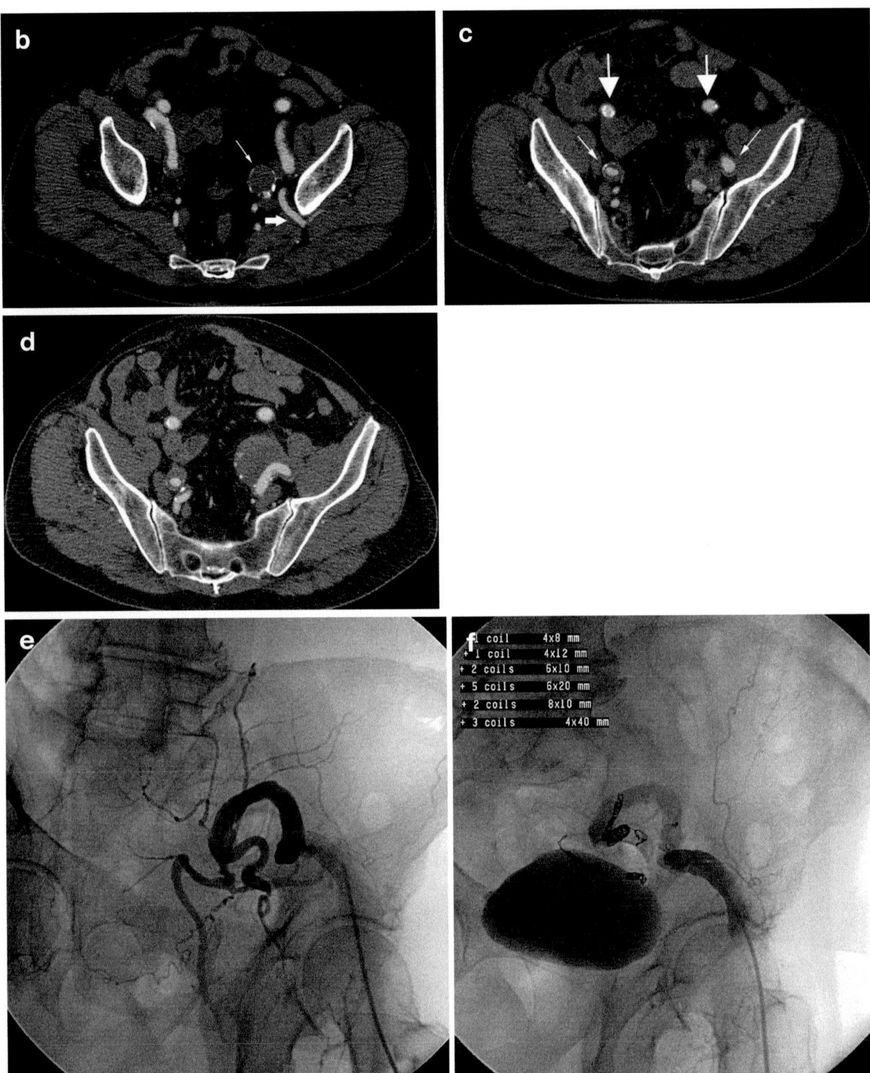

Fig. 12.3 (continued)

Suggested Reading

Pellerin O, Caruba T, Kandounakis Y, et al. Embolization of the internal iliac artery: cost-effectiveness of two different techniques. Cardiovasc Intervent Radiol. 2008;31:1088–93.

Stroumpouli E, Nassef A, Loosemore T, et al. The endovascular management of iliac artery aneurysms. Cardiovasc Intervent Radiol. 2007;30:1099–104.

Uberoi R, Tsetis D, Shrivastava V, Morgan R, Belli AM. Standard of practice for the interventional management of isolated iliac artery aneurysms. Cardiovasc Intervent Radiol. 2011;34:3–13.

Part VI
Situations and Strategies: Kidney, Retroperitoneum, and Male Pelvis

Chapter 13
Renal Arterial Embolizations

Louis Boyer, Laurent Guy, Anne Ravel, Lucie Cassagnes, Rami Chemali, and Pascal Chabrot

13.1 Background

Renal embolization can be indicated in parenchymal or vascular diseases such as cancer, trauma, iatrogenic injury, hypertension, or end-stage renal failure, as a planned procedure or taking place in emergency situation.

These procedures do not expose to major risk, providing that the radiological team is well informed on patient's clinical and laboratory workup and ensures post-procedure management with an emphasize on pain control, as well as follow-up.

13.2 Relevant Radiological Anatomy

The left and right renal arteries generally arise from the abdominal aorta, at the level of the L1–L2 intervertebral disk or the body L2 vertebrae. The left renal artery emerges from the posterolateral part of the aorta, with a direction with an oblique, posterior, and lateral course. The right renal artery, which is longer, frequently originates from a slightly higher position, ventrally and/or laterally, with a curvilinear posterior course: so the depiction of the renal arteries ostia is optimally generally obtained on a left anterior oblique view with an angle of 15–20°.

L. Boyer, MD, PhD (✉) • A. Ravel, MD • L. Cassagnes, MD • P. Chabrot, MD, PhD
Department of Radiology, University Hospital of Clermont-Ferrand, Clermont-Ferrand, France
e-mail: lboyer@chu-clermontferrand.fr; pchabrot@chu-clermontferrand.fr

L. Guy, MD, PhD
Department of Urology, University Hospital of Clermont-Ferrand, Clermont-Ferrand, France

R. Chemali, MD
Department of Radiology, Saint Georges Hospital, Beyrouth, Lebanon

P. Chabrot, L. Boyer (eds.), *Embolization*,
DOI 10.1007/978-1-4471-5182-1_13, © Springer-Verlag London 2014

The renal artery trunk is musculoelastic with a diameter of 4–7 mm which can be reduced by stress-induced vasoconstriction and which is also autoregulated by the renin-angiotensin-aldosterone system, thus ensuring an adequate flow in the event of obstructive lesion.

The renal artery branches off in a lower capsular collateral (exo-renal circle, adrenal), and four terminal branches: a spindly one (superior polar) and three larger ones: prepyelic, retro-pyelic (classically with a curvilinear course and external convexity on a frontal 2D projection), and inferior polar (which beforehand crosses in front of the ureter in 80 % of the cases). Beyond, the intrarenal arterial tree is terminal.

The variations are numerous and frequent:

- Early division of the renal artery into branches supplying the kidney
- Variable arising of the terminal inferior polar artery: from the trunk of the renal artery, both with the prepyelic and the retro-pyelic arteries; from the prepyelic artery only; or from the retro-pyelic artery only
- Multiple renal arteries: unilateral: 15–18 % or bilateral: 10 %, up to four arteries on each side, which can sometimes originate, for the most caudal one, at the level of the common iliac artery. The parenchymal territory of the supernumerary arteries is variable, and sometimes considerable, meaning potential ischemic disease after their exclusion by embolization or coverage by stent graft

13.3 Techniques

Before the procedure, it is necessary to ensure the sterility of the urine.

For permanent exclusion of the renal parenchyma, a prophylactic antibiotic treatment is advocated by some (see Chap. 2). We do not administer systematic antibiotherapy.

An EKG and blood pressure monitoring must be carried out during the procedure and beyond during 24 h.

Parenchymal embolizations are painful and should be realized in collaboration with an anesthesiologist who administers analgesics on demand, according to the degree of pain and to the importance of infarcted area. They can be administered with an automatic syringe pump or even better self-administered by the patient himself (PCA: patient controlled analgesia).

- Ipsilateral puncture site to the treated kidney optimizes the harmonious curve approach of small-caliber catheters. We nevertheless prefer a contralateral access that usually enables a more stable catheterization. In patients with atheroma or sinuous arteries, the procedure is facilitated by using a long introducer sheath (25–40 cm), whose tip is placed just below the renal arteries' ostia.
- A preliminary arterial tree mapping includes the study of abdominal aorta and its branches and the analysis of the kidney. One will take into account a possible early venous flow and arteriovenous shunts, an associated vascularization by the

exo-renal circle in case of tumor. In the conservative indications, the arterial supply to the adrenal glands, gonads, ureters, and healthy renal parenchyma will be identified and spared.

- Embolization agents: the choice depends on the indication. Proximal agents allow the occlusion of renal artery. If the goal is to destroy parenchyma, then intraparenchymatous branches must be occluded by distal agents, with a possible additional proximal occlusion, and the first 2 or 3 cm of the trunk must be spared to facilitate surgical arterial ligation in case of nephrectomy or to make a second procedure possible should embolization be incomplete or should tumor reoccur.
- During the procedure, having a stable catheter position is an important prerequisite in order to avoid out of target embolization. The distribution of the embolization agent as well as the residual flow in the embolized territory must be carefully monitored: the slowing down of the flow is a sign of progressive downstream occlusion that should lead to the reduction of the injection speed.

Post-procedure control injection must be carried out far from of the embolized area, with a perfectly clean catheter, to avoid reflux and out of target embolization agent migration.

13.4 Technical Results

Global morbidity and mortality rates are respectively estimated at 8 and 2.5 %.

The side effects largely depend upon the infarcted volume:

- Pain generally occurs during the embolization and can last from 1 to 5 days. It must be prevented and managed by appropriate premedication and sedation.
- Post-embolization syndrome almost systematically occurs as soon as there is a consequent tissue necrosis. It includes nauseas, vomiting, fever, and abdominal pain. A paralytic ileus is often associated. Leukocytosis and an increased LDH level are observed. These symptoms resolve generally after a symptomatic treatment for a few days.
- Hypertension: a transitory increase of the blood pressure is usually observed during a few hours and up to 24 h. A permanent hypertension, consequence of renal ischemia, can develop.
- Renal failure depends on the importance of the parenchymal necrosis, the precautions taken with the use of iodinated contrast agents, and can be prevented with a correct pre- and post-procedure patient hydration.
- Hematuria: a moderate hematuria may occur following the embolization, in relation with a hemorrhagic infarction, and usually disappears within 24–48 h.
- Infection: the risk of outbreak of a latent infection can be minimized by a perfect knowledge of the medical file (history of lithiasis or infection?). A cytobacteriological examination of the urines must be systematically carried out before the procedure: an ongoing untreated urinary infection is a temporary contraindication

for the embolization. Small air bubbles on CT, 3–16 days after a renal embolization, do not always mean an abscess; they can also be due to a normal aseptic infarction.
- Accidental out of target embolization.

13.5 Indications

Acute coagulation disorders or infectious syndromes are contraindications which must always be ruled out before procedure.

13.5.1 Malignant Tumors

13.5.1.1 Preoperative Embolization of Adenocarcinoma

In patients who are candidates for radical surgery, embolization facilitates tumor excision and reduces blood loss. It is indicated in highly vascularized large-sized lesions (in our group the threshold is 7 cm).

Embolization must be complete in these cases, with distal obstruction of the vessels, in order to devascularize, as completely as possible, the segment that will be secondarily excised.

Ethanol associated or not with Lipiodol®, glue, and gelatine sponge have been used. Today we generally use microparticles, in the absence of intratumoral arteriovenous shunts. If coils are set up in the renal arterial trunk, they must be released within a few centimeters of the ostium, so as not to hinder its ligature.

Similarly, embolization has been advocated before radiofrequency ablation of adenocarcinomas.

13.5.1.2 Palliative Embolization

In patients for which a nephrectomy is not possible because of their advanced age and/or disease stage, embolization can be carried out as a symptomatic treatment to improve the quality of life and treat some complications: persistent macroscopic hematuria with anemia due to blood loss, lumbar pain unresponsive to medical treatment, cardiac insufficiency due to arteriovenous shunts and hyper-flow, hypertension, hypercalcemia, and polycythemia.

We use microparticles and/or coils and always preserve a vascular access should ulterior catheterization be necessary.

A complete embolization is not always necessary in these cases: it must be limited to resolving the symptoms while avoiding the complications of massive parenchymal necrosis [1].

The combination of embolization and radiofrequency ablation can be an interesting therapeutic alternative among incurable patients or poor candidates for surgery; it can give more complete results than embolization alone [2].

13.5.2 Angiomyolipoma (AML) [3]

13.5.2.1 As a Curative Treatment

The embolization is the method of choice to treat a hemorrhagic syndrome, allowing bleeding control and in many cases complete devascularization of the AML. Surgery is then not always necessary.

Bleeding is the most serious complication related to AMLs.

The diagnosis of AML must be considered in the event of spontaneous hemorrhage around the kidney, all the more so in young or average-aged woman; CT is the key test.

Arteriography and embolization must then be considered.

Microcatheters and microparticles (100–300 μ) enable ideal and elective devascularization of AML. In case of rupture of an arterial aneurysm, coils are more appropriate.

Embolization is effective to rapidly stop the bleeding. The complete exclusion of the tumor might necessitate a second embolization session or additional conservative surgery.

13.5.2.2 Preventive Embolization

When the AML is larger than 4 cm in diameter, the risk of hemorrhage is about 20 % per year. It depends on its size, multifocality, and the presence and size of intralesional aneurysms. Pregnancy increases the risk of growth and bleeding.

- A noninvasive imaging follow-up is recommended for the AML of less than 4 cm.
- For the AMLs of more than 4 cm, preventive embolization can be performed as an alternative to the surgery or can precede surgical resection which can then be limited. For diffuse lesions, especially when the masses are large and bilateral, embolization helps to preserve a maximum of renal parenchyma.

Symptomatic AMLs of more than 4 cm must be treated.

The treatment of asymptomatic AMLs of more than 4 cm remains controversial: multiplicity of the lesions, a context of tuberous sclerosis (Bourneville's disease), patient's way of life, and desire of pregnancy lead some authors [4] to carry out embolization rather than surgery. Others [5] consider that in case of Bourneville's disease a yearly noninvasive imaging follow-up is sufficient to keep an eye on the low-growth-rate lesions and the patients older than 30.

Today, inert particles are the most used. In some cases, glue is used. It is necessary to be cautious with proximal micro-coiling as it exposes to a risk of revascularization.

The reduction in size but also the reduction of the vascular component on CT or MRI are the radiological criteria of embolization's effectiveness.

Post-embolization syndrome, frequent after preventive embolization of AML, is generally not observed after an emergency embolization.

13.5.3 Renal Hemorrhages Related to Anticoagulants

Anticoagulant-related hemorrhagic complications occur more readily in the abdomen and the pelvis and concern the soft tissues (see Chap. 14), the GI, and urinary tracts.

The bleeding can be extracapsular, subcapsular, intraparenchymal, in the renal sinus, submucosal, or in the wall of the upper urinary tract.

CT contributes to a precise location of the bleeding and can show an underlying cause (often a renal tumor). A contrast extravasation is not a sign of severity: it corresponds to capillary bleeding.

Correction of homeostasis disorders is mandatory. Embolization is rarely needed in emergency and should be discussed only in case of poor hemodynamic tolerance.

13.5.4 Traumatic or Iatrogenic Lesions

Lumbar trauma, especially caused by stabbing weapons, biopsies, and percutaneous procedures of the kidney, can cause vascular lesions which all are indications for embolization. For a long time, Chatelain's classification [6] was the standard reference. Today we usually refer to the classification of the American Association for Surgery of Trauma (AAST) [7] (Appendix 13.1).

13.5.4.1 Acute Phase

An emergency embolization can be required for serious trauma involving large parenchymal fractures and voluminous perirenal hematomas: active bleedings are identified on CT as a contrast blush during the arterial phase. They are related to a wound or a rupture of the renal artery itself or its branches.

The higher the AAST grade is, the more severe are the vascular lesions and bigger is the risk of post-embolization parenchymal loss. Therefore, embolization and homeostasis nephrectomy benefits/risk ratios must always be compared. A massive embolization of the kidney (main branches, even trunk of the renal artery) can however be indicated in case of severe trauma, thus allowing to postpone nephrectomy until a phase of clinical stability.

Some renal parenchyma traumas spontaneously stop bleeding within a few hours because of the relative inextensibility of the perirenal space. A careful monitoring is thus essential. In a very large majority of the cases, hemodynamically stable patients with a CT evaluation can be monitored. AAST grade IV and V lesions, although often requiring a surgical exploration, can also be managed without a surgical intervention if they are well evaluated, selected, and monitored [8].

In the hours following the injury, clinical or biological worsening can lead to a new CT evaluation and to an arteriography with embolization.

- Embolization is indicated if an active bleeding is seen on CT in hemodynamically stable patients or in case of a controlled shock.
- Embolization has also been proposed in patients with uncontrolled shock, but this indication must not compromise vital prognosis, and surgery must be discussed.

The treatment of AAST grades I to III is generally a conservative approach; embolization can be indicated for active bleeding. For the AAST grade IV, the treatment is if possible conservative, with embolization in case of active bleeding. For the AAST grade V, the treatment can be conservative if the patient is stable; embolization may be required if the patient is unstable.

Depending to the morphology of the lesions, coils, particles, and/or absorbable agents will be used.

- It must also be noted that in some cases an endoprosthesis can restore the lumen of a traumatic renal artery trunk
- A CT scan monitoring during the hospitalization is recommended for all grades, with a systematic reevaluation between the fifth and the seventh day after the trauma.

For severe traumas, a scintigraphy or an MRI must be planned 6 months later, in order to evaluate the residual renal function of the traumatic kidney.

On the follow-up imaging, renal infarction is often more limited than one would expect.

13.5.4.2 Secondary Period

- Persistent hematuria due to an induced arterio-ureteral fistula is very common after a renal biopsy; it usually spontaneously clogs up after a few days. If it persists beyond 1 week, the occlusion of the responsible vessel, which is usually a peripheral artery, will be performed using inert particles or microcoils.
- Around the tenth day, an obstructive thrombus can break off and lead to a sudden and potentially severe bleeding. The patient is not always under medical surveillance at that moment. As in the acute phase, an emergency embolization is a good option in this case.

13.5.4.3 Late Complications

False aneurysms and arteriovenous fistulas are not exceptional. Their rate increases with the number of percutaneous procedures and renal biopsies. After a renal biopsy puncture, nearly 15 % arteriovenous fistulas occur, of which only 4 % would persist after a few months; most of them spontaneously occlude. A rupture of these false aneurysms and traumatic AVFs lead to delayed hemorrhages; embolization using coils allows conservative management. These same complications can be observed after partial surgery.

Proximal arteriovenous fistula can also be seen after a nephrectomy, especially if a unique and common arterial and venous ligation of the vascular pedicle was performed.

13.5.4.4 Bis: Malformative Arteriovenous Fistulas

Much more rare, may be discussed here because they are treated the same way. The decision to treat depends on the flow rate of the fistula (cardiac insufficiency, hypertension), to the risk of rupture for large-size false aneurysms, and to repeated hematuria.

Occlusion should preferably concern the communication zone between the artery and the vein or the false aneurysm if it exists. Larguable balloons and coils can be used, with glue (cyanoacrylate) in some cases; in our group, we prefer using Amplatzer occluders.

Today, noncommunicating false aneurysms are more readily occluded with coils. A covered stent can also be deployed. Generally, it is possible to preserve the downstream vascular bed and almost all of the renal parenchyma.

Embolization is currently the technique of choice to treat all these lesions: its results are superior to those of the surgery.

13.5.5 Other Intrarenal Communications: Cirsoid Arteriovenous Malformations

These AVM (involving a nidus, which is interposed between artery and vein instead of a capillary bed) include multiple small tortuous arterial afferences and a venous drainage of the same sort; they are often called "cirsoid" in the literature. Symptoms include a hematuria which can be exceptionally serious, a hypertension, a lumbar murmur, or even a heart failure.

Their detection is based on the color Doppler ultrasound (shunts with perivascular artifacts, increase in circulatory speeds in the afferent branches, reduction in the resistance index, arterialization of venous flow). They can also be recognized on CT.

Embolization is the first-line treatment to occlude the shunt while preserving a maximal functional renal parenchyma. The use of a microcatheter is mandatory in order to reach the afferent pedicles. Liquid agents (glues, alcohol) are usually used.

13.5.6 Renal Arterial Aneurysms (See Also Chap. 5)

Pedicular aneurysms can have a congenital origin and are then often associated to elastic tissue diseases (Ehlers-Danlos syndrome, Recklinghausen's disease). These aneurysms are not rare in renal artery fibromuscular dysplasia. They can also be of inflammatory or infectious origin (false aneurysms). Polyarteritis nodosa involves very frequently microaneurysms, which are typically very peripheral. Traumatic false aneurysms can be the consequence of a direct wound or a tear of the media due to a deceleration shock. Lastly, atheromatous aneurysms are often associated with stenosing lesions.

Most are asymptomatic. The risk of spontaneous peripheral embolism and infarction depends on the circulatory turbulences and to the sacciform aspect of the aneurysm. Renovascular hypertension, renal artery thrombosis, hematuria, and constitution of arteriovenous fistula make up the other complications, among which the most serious is the rupture.

Endovascular treatment can be indicated to treat a rupture depending on the configuration of lesions, the experience, and the availability of the operators. A temporary preliminary upstream balloon occlusion limits blood loss before obtaining the exclusion of the ruptured aneurysm.

Apart from the emergency situations, the therapeutic indications must be carefully discussed, ideally in a multidisciplinary medical discussion, and then the different therapeutic alternatives must have been explained to the patient.

All false aneurysms must be treated.

The risk of rupture of the true aneurysms depends on their size. Symptomatic aneurysms should be treated. According to the recommendations of the AHA [9], the preventive standard treatment for ruptures concerns aneurysms of 2 cm or more in women who are of child-bearing age (class I, level of evidence B) (and it must then be carried out outside of pregnancy). The treatment of aneurysms of more than 2 cm in older women and in men is, according to the same recommendations, "probably indicated" (class IIa, level of evidence B).

The low morbid-mortality rate of endovascular treatment has led some authors to lower the cutoff value for treatment to less than 2 cm and consider as aneurismal an arterial diameter twice or more than that of the parent artery diameter.

Aneurysms of 20 mm or less can thereby be treated, especially in young patients: in women in child-bearing age desiring to become pregnant; when they are symptomatic, responsible of renal ischemia and hypertension; when they are associated to a significant renal artery stenosis; in the case of a dissecting aneurysm or with distal embolization; and in the case of an obvious increase in size as shown on successive imaging controls.

Planned surgery is a highly reliable technique.

But in case of a narrow-neck aneurysm or in case of favorable anatomical configuration, an endovascular treatment can be considered as the first-line treatment. It should ideally preserve the downstream vascular bed and the arterial lumen. The aneurysm's occlusion can be achieved by coiling the aneurysmal sac. An occlusion balloon can be temporarily inflated upstream, slowing the flow and thus securing the procedure. When the neck is wide, it is possible either to release the coils while having inflated a balloon at the level of the neck (remodeling technique) or to initially implement a bare stent to bridge the affected segment, then to release coils through the mesh of the stent. The use of liquid agents (Onyx…) has been recently reported: it implies an excellent technical mastery. Covered endoprosthesis and multilayered stent are other options. Finally, a surgical bypass may precede embolization.

Rundback et al. [10] proposed an angiographic classification helpful in discussing therapeutic indications : type I lesions are truncal or segmental branches saccular aneurysms that can be excluded using stent graft; type II lesions are fusiform aneurysms or close to a bifurcation, and they are generally surgically treated: some of these aneurysms can nevertheless be treated by embolization (coils, Onyx) with protection technique (remodeling) or even by covered or multilayer ("flow diverter") stents; type III lesions concern small segmental branches, feeding a limited fraction of renal parenchyma, which could be occluded by embolization. Each case must be carefully analyzed (configuration of lesions, state of the carrier vessel, etc.) taking into account the complexity of the surgical procedures. Even though arteriography remains the standard reference test for establishing therapeutic indications, it however depicts arterial lumen only and must always be preceded by a CT (which for the moment is our preference) or an MRI scan.

If therapeutic abstention is decided (small lesions), an imaging follow-up (US, CT, MRI) is essential. In the absence of precise recommendation, we propose a yearly cross-sectional imaging follow-up.

13.5.7 Functional Exclusions

In end-stage renal disease associated to a hypertension which is poorly controlled by medical treatment, or to a massive proteinuria responsible for a nephrotic syndrome, or in case of endless urinary fistula or of a hydronephrosis unresponsive to usual treatments, an exclusion of the renal parenchyma may be discussed. Elsewhere, it can be a urinary ascites or imperious urges on a neobladder.

In patients suffering from end-stage renal disease, the kidneys preserve three important functions: metabolism of vitamin D, erythropoiesis, and sometimes elimination of a certain quantity of water; the loss of these functions must be balanced with the expected gain of a functional exclusion.

Surgery in these fragile patients has a non-negligible morbidity rate (20 %), and the mortality rate can reach 5 %. Embolization ensures with few complications a total infarction of the kidney (there must not remain any viable parenchyma which might compromise the result, particularly in case of hypertension). Pure ethanol could be used in these cases. The injection is ideally slowly carried out downstream an occlusive balloon, to avoid reflux in other abdominal arteries. Microparticles and glues can be also used.

Another indication is the embolization using particles ± coils of polycystic kidneys, as an alternative to nephrectomy before renal transplantation [11], when these native polycystic kidneys are too voluminous.

Key Points

- For planned indications: sterile urines.
- Systematic analgesia during and after embolization, to deal with the pain induced by infarction; ideally: PCA pump.
- Complete prior angiographic assessment (arterial cartography, angioarchitecture, venous return).
- Overall morbidity and mortality: 8 and 2.5 %.
- Post-embolization syndrome (nausea-vomiting, fever, pain, possible ileus) almost constant for a few days.
- Monitoring of the BP: regular disturbances during approximately 24 h. a hypertension can then develop.
- Preoperative embolization of the adenocarcinomas (our threshold = 7 cm) minimizes blood loss and facilitates the oncologic surgery.
- Palliative embolization for inoperable symptomatic kidney tumors (hematuria, anemia, polycythemia, hypertension, hypercalcemia, pain, heart failure).
- Embolization = treatment of choice for hemorrhagic AML; = alternative to surgery for the preventive treatment of AML which are larger than 4 cm, whether they are symptomatic or not.
- Renal hematoma related to anticoagulants: embolization is only performed in case of bad hemodynamic tolerance.
- Traumatic or iatrogenic lesions: hemostasis embolization in acute phase, in case of an active bleeding shown on CT; treatment of secondary arterio-urinary fistula (tenth day hematuria); exclusion of false aneurysms or late AVF.
- Embolization is very interesting to treat some malformative AVF, AVM, and some renal artery aneurysms exceeding 20 mm in diameter (AHA recommendations) or even less if they are observed in women of child-bearing age, if their size increases, or if they are associated to a downstream ischemia with hypertension, to an RA stenosis, or to a dissection with distal embolization.
- Stent grafts = alternative to exclusion for some traumatic lesions, AVF, and aneurysms.
- Embolization for functional exclusion in patients with terminal renal failure and poorly controlled hypertension, massive proteinuria, urinary fistulas, hydronephrosis, etc.

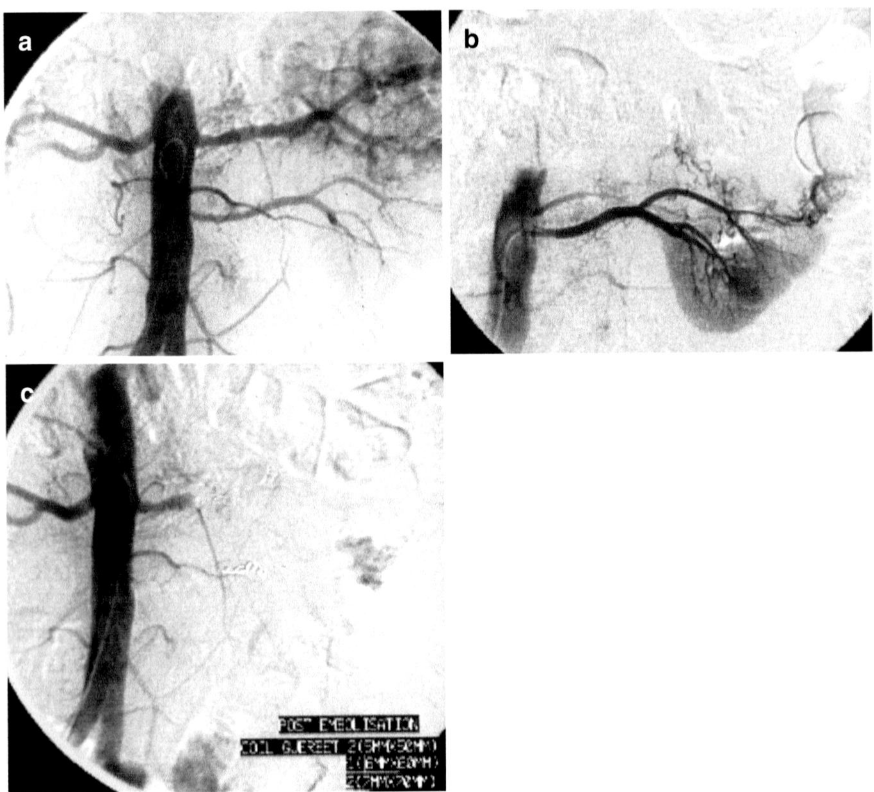

Fig. 13.1 Large adenocarcinoma of the left kidney: preoperative embolization. (**a**) Arteriography: two arteries feed the left kidney, a main renal artery and an inferior accessory artery. (**b**) Selective injection of the inferior accessory artery, which clearly reveals that it also participates to the perfusion of the tumor. (**c**) Truncal embolization by coils, relatively distal to allow surgical ligation while accessing the pedicle

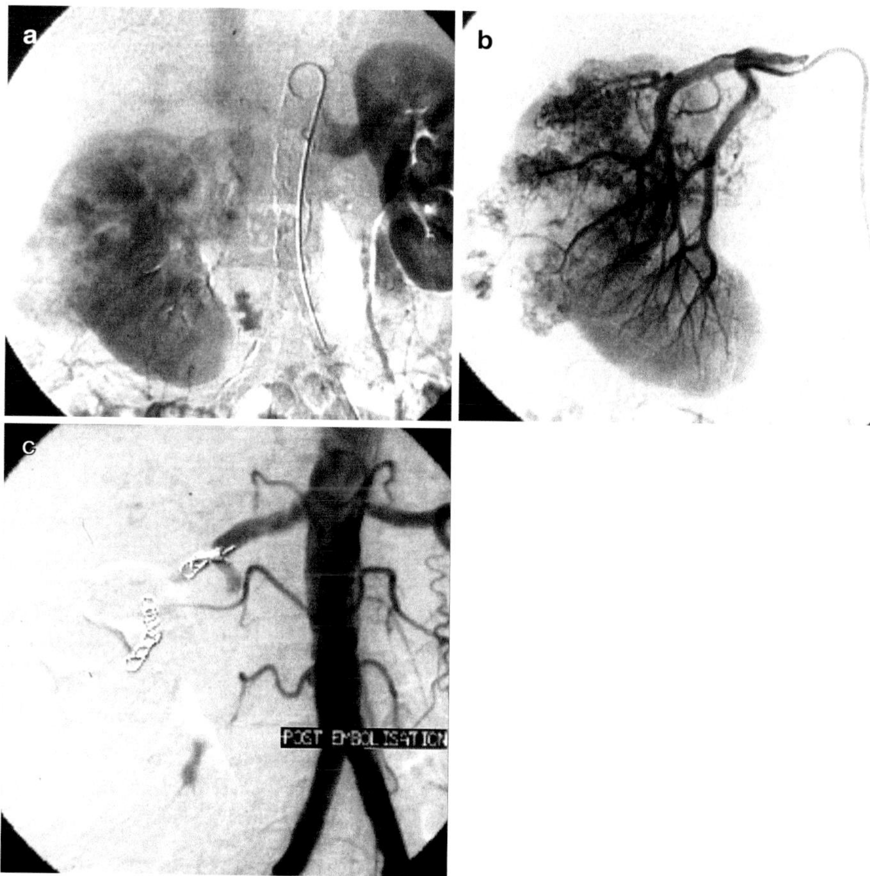

Fig. 13.2 Large adenocarcinoma of the right kidney: preoperative embolization, the morning before surgery. (**a**) Late phase of arterial opacification: patent renal vein, without abnormal arteriovenous communication, allowing the use of microparticles. (**b**) Selective catheterization to embolize with particles the branches feeding the tumor, followed by a proximal truncal occlusion. (**c**) Final aortographic control, sparing of few centimeters of the trunk of the patent right renal artery, in order to simplify surgical ligation during nephrectomy

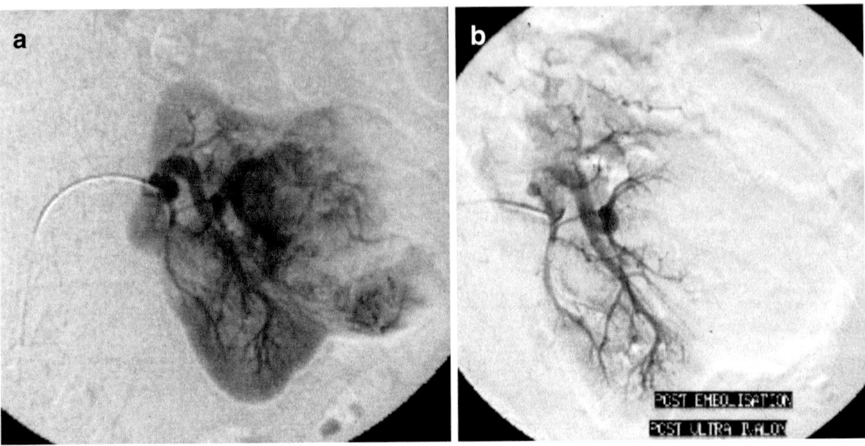

Fig. 13.3 87 years old, large adenocarcinoma of the left kidney judged as inoperable. Back pain+hematuria. A palliative embolization was planned. (**a**) Selective injection at the nephrographic phase: the tumor spars the lower pole of the kidney. A hyperselective embolization with particles was decided. (**b**) Arteriographic control after palliative tumoral exclusion by particles

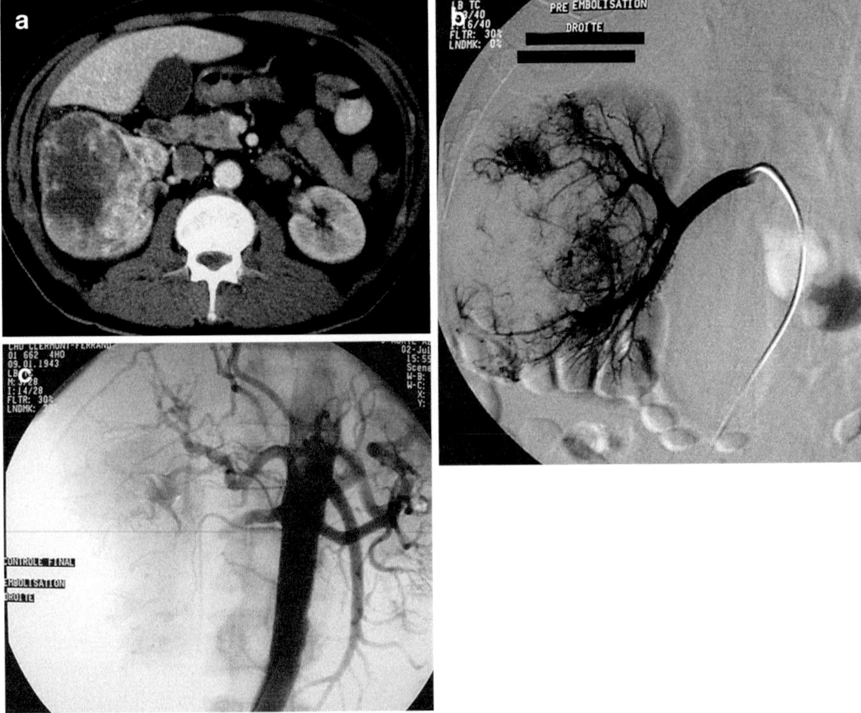

Fig. 13.4 Very large adenocarcinoma of the kidney with extension to the inferior vena cava and lung metastases, causing a severe deterioration of the general condition with fever, back pain, and hematuria. The patient was considered as inoperable. Palliative embolization was decided, in order to decrease the hematuria and the paraneoplastic syndrome. (**a**) CT: massive tumor involving the entire kidney with venous invasion. The left kidney is normal. (**b**) Selective injection of the right renal artery: almost all of the right kidney was involved, and a complete exclusion of this kidney was then performed (normal left kidney). (**c**) Control after exclusion with particles (microparticles of 500–700 and 900–1,200 μm)

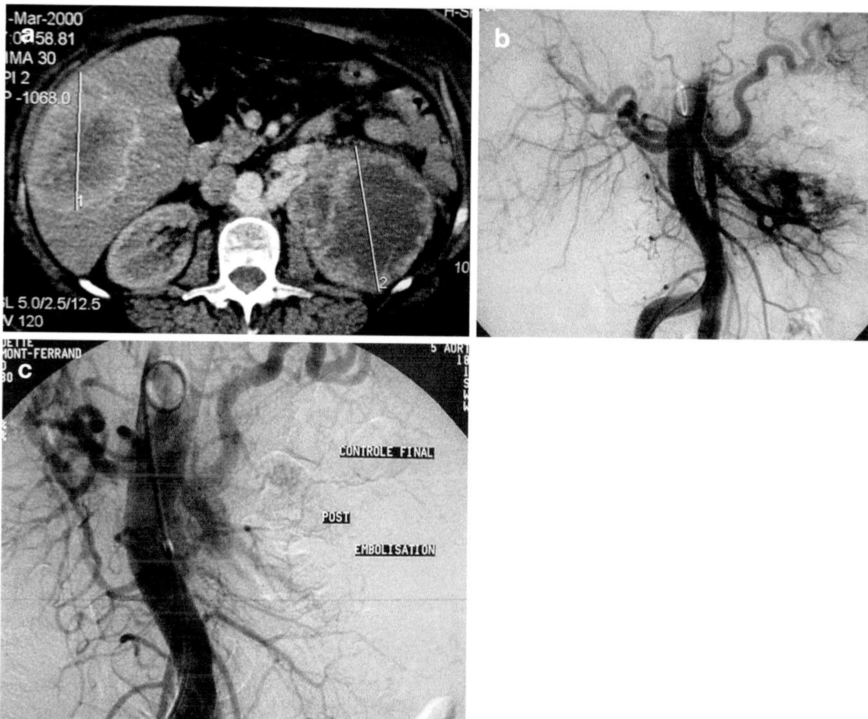

Fig. 13.5 Very large left renal tumor with liver metastases in a 75-year-old W with hematuria and polycythemia. (**a**) CT: renal tumor and liver metastasis; note a retroaortic patent left renal vein. (**b**) Aortography. (**c**) Control aortography after exclusion by microparticles

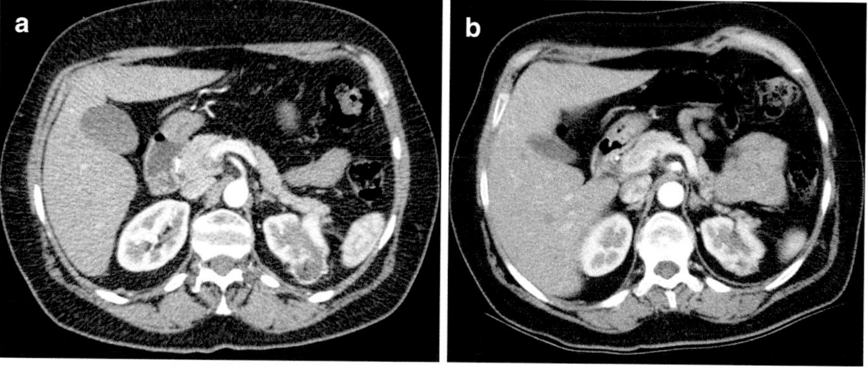

Fig. 13.6 Preventive embolization of an angiomyolipoma. (**a**) Asymptomatic 35 mm angiomyolipoma, discovered on a CT scan indicated for back pain in a 57-year-old M. Taking into account its size, imaging follow-up of this kidney was initially decided. (**b–d**) CT scan 1 year later: the exorenal angiomyolipoma, measuring now 55 mm, is fed (coronal reconstruction) by a large arterial pedicle designated to the upper pole. Given this growth in size, an embolization was decided to prevent bleeding complication. (**e**) Selective arteriography: the vascularization of the angiomyolipoma was provided by upper pole branches that have been hyperselectively catheterized to exclude the tumoral territory by microparticles (100–300 and 300–500 μm in diameter). (**f**) CT scan 2 years later: note the retraction of the external cortex (*arrow*) and a small residual tumor (less than 15 mm in size), warranting further follow-up

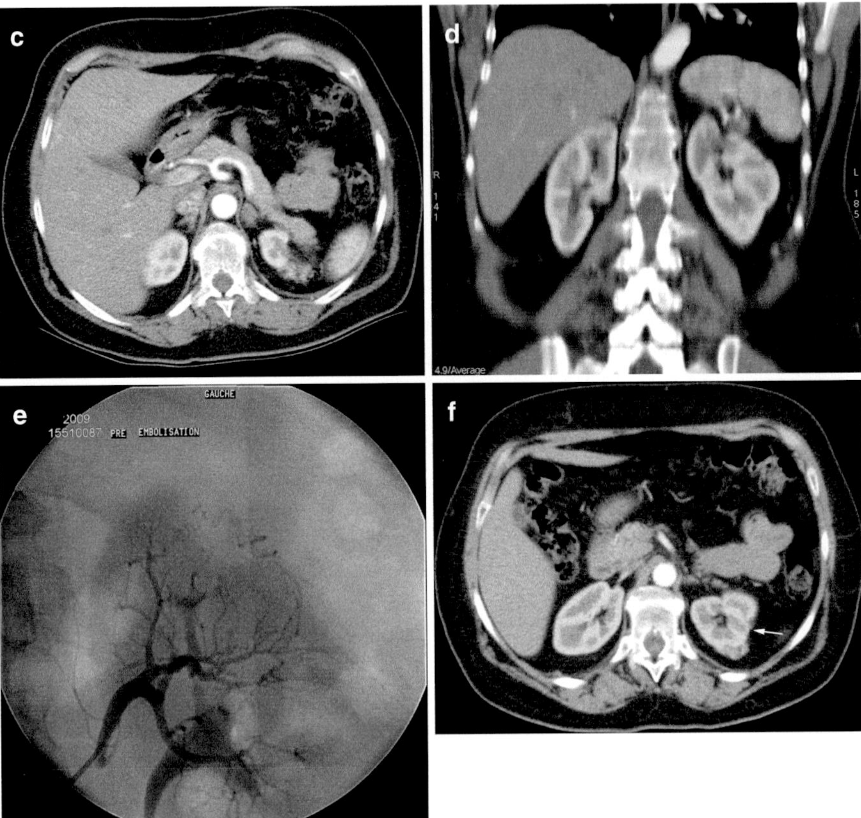

Fig. 13.6 (continued)

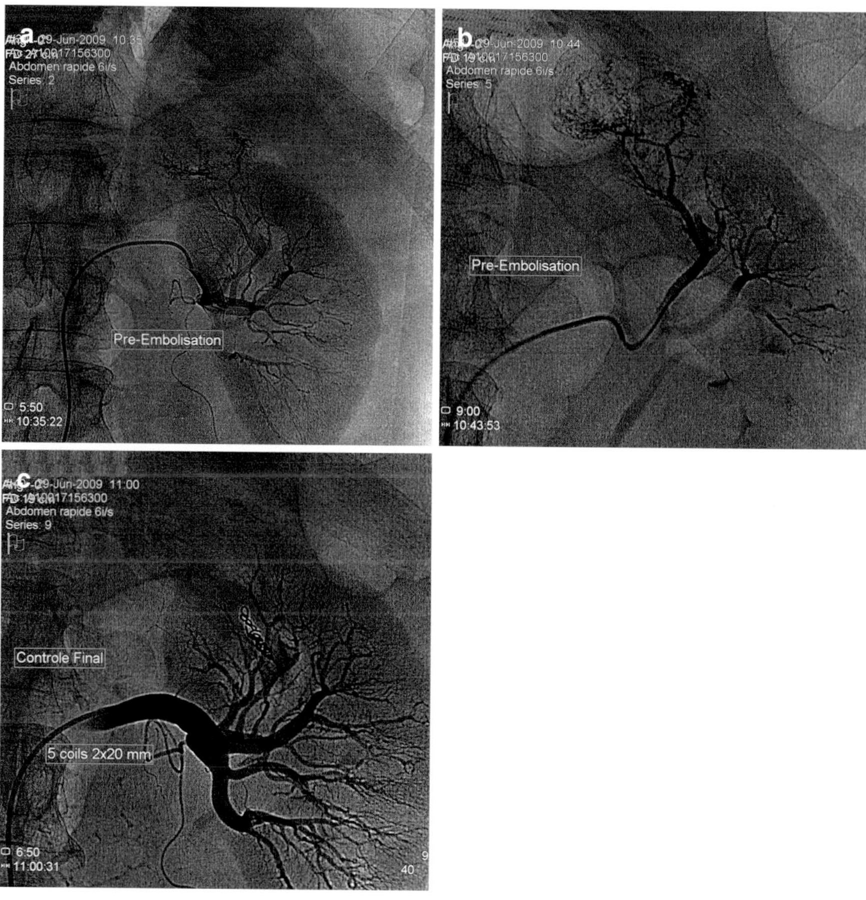

Fig. 13.7 Growth in size of an angiomyolipoma, measuring now 7 cm in a 65-year-old M: a preventive exclusion was decided. (**a**) Selective catheterization: tumoral hypervascularization with exo-renal development from the left upper pole. (**b**) Hyperselective injection. (**c**) Arteriographic control after selective exclusion with particles + coils

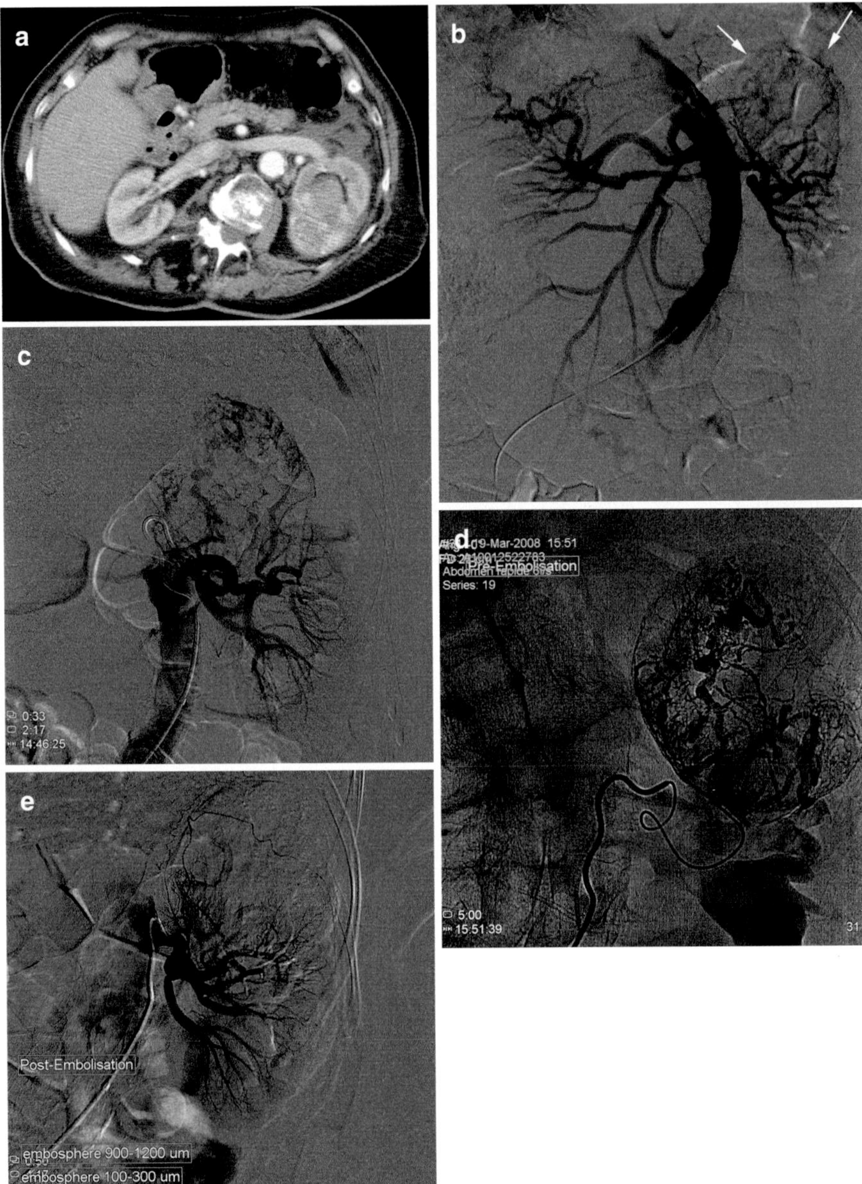

Fig. 13.8 Anticoagulation treatment for 6 months for thromboembolic disease; hospital admission for severe hematuria and left back pain. The assessment of hemostasis showed a PT = 27 %. (**a**) CT: large expansive process in which fat density was individualized: a hemorrhagic complication of an angiomyolipoma was suggested. (**b**) Aortography: the aorta and renal arteries are tortuous; hypervascular expansive process of the upper pole of the left kidney (*arrow*). (**c**) Selective renal artery injection. (**d**) Hyperselective catheterization using a microcatheter. (**e**) Selective renal arteriographic control after exclusion of the tumor by microparticles

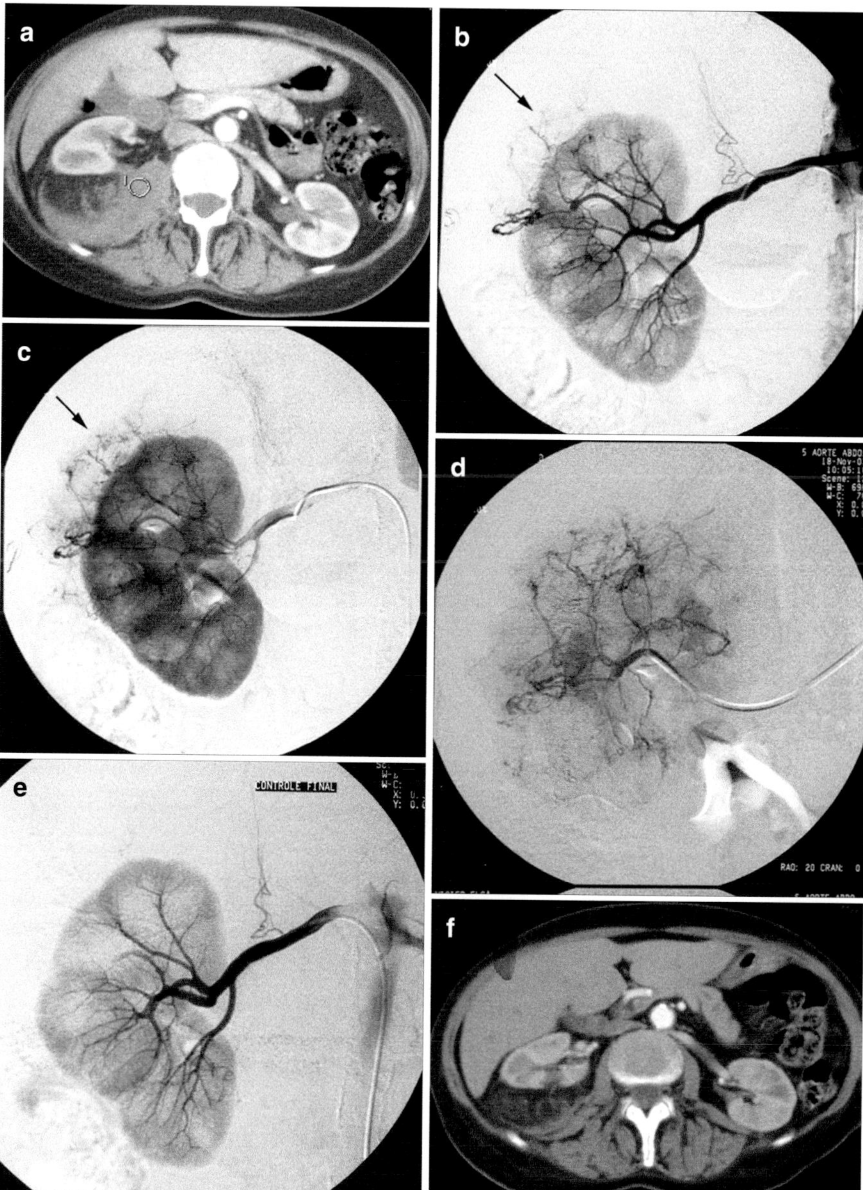

Fig. 13.9 Severe back pain and hemodynamic collapsus in a 57-year-old W. (**a**) Large kidney, associated with an important hematoma (hematoma HU densities in the circle) in the surrounding fat, suggesting a ruptured angiomyolipoma. (**b**, **c**) Selective catheterization of the right renal artery: normal intrarenal vascularization; abnormal vessels providing blood supply to an angiomyolipoma developed from the external face of the upper pole (*arrow*) (arteriographic phase: **b**, then nephrographic phase: **c**). (**d**) Selective catheterization of the vascular pedicle feeding the angiomyolipoma. (**e**) Selective arteriographic control after tumoral devascularization. (**f**) CT scan 1 month later: resorption of perirenal hematoma

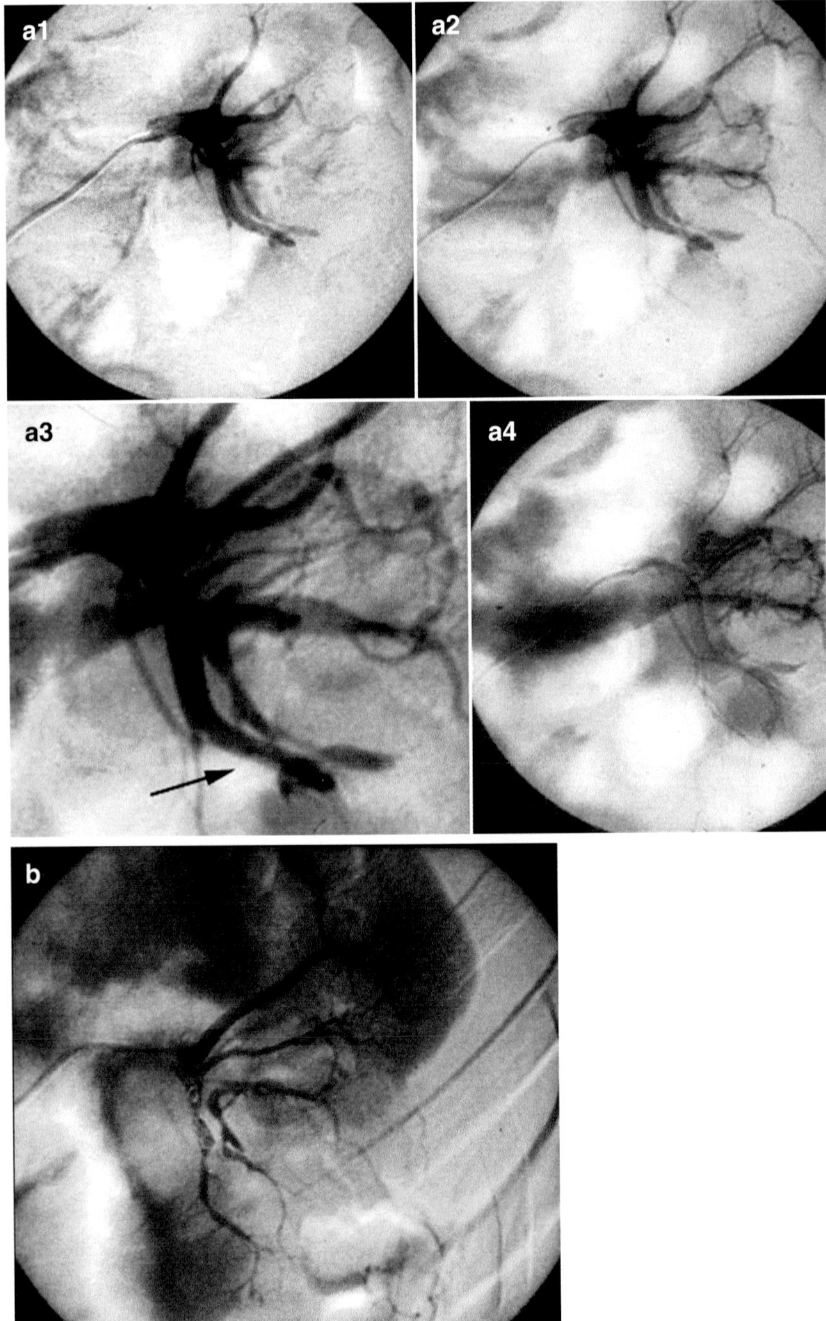

Fig. 13.10 Arteriography performed 4 h after renal biopsy because of the association of back pain, collapsus, and perirenal hematoma on ultrasound. (**a1**–**a4**) Selective injection of the artery feeding the left kidney that was biopsied: a massive venous return was noted from the first second, corresponding to a traumatic arteriovenous fistula in the lower part of the sinus (*arrow*). (**b**) Control after distal occlusion by coils of the artery supplying the fistula

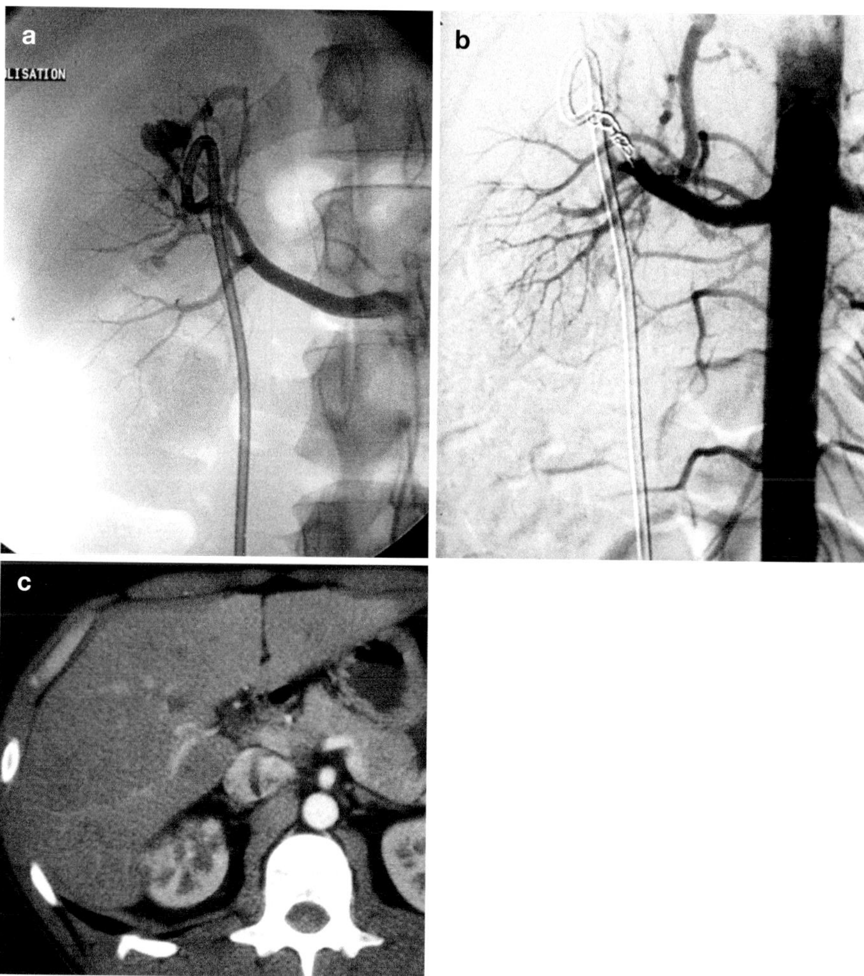

Fig. 13.11 Hematuria 10 days after a traumatic injury of the kidney. (**a**) Selective arterial injection of the right renal artery: arteriovenous fistula and a very likely arterio-calyceal fistula (note the proximity of the traumatic arteriovenous fistula and the upper end of the double J catheter). (**b**) Coils exclusion of the artery supplying the lesion. (**c**) Control CT of the upper pole 6 months later

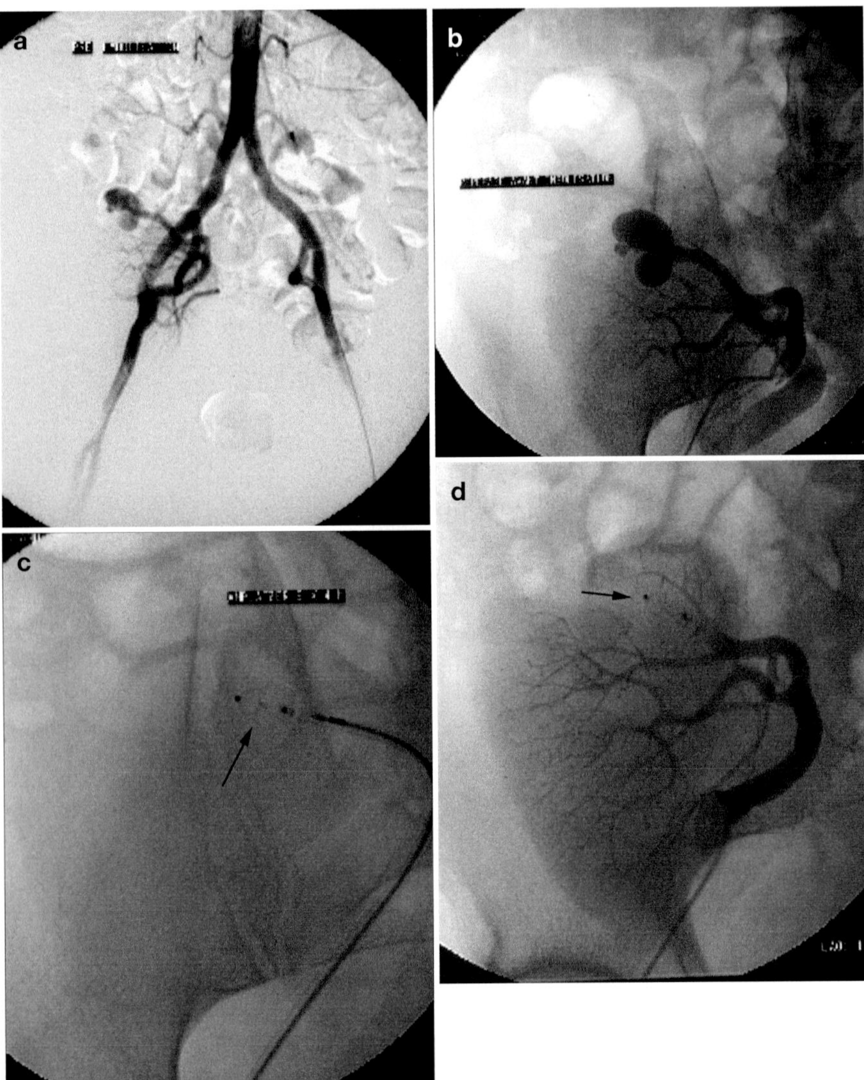

Fig. 13.12 Transplanted kidney in the right iliac fossa, 6 weeks after a renal biopsy, severe deterioration of renal function: the duplex Doppler suggested a hilar arteriovenous fistula. (**a**) Aortography conducted by a left femoral access: arterial additional image to the hilum of the transplant, with early venous return. Endovascular occlusion was decided, to which an ipsilateral access was finally chosen. (**b**) Selective injection of the artery of the transplanted kidney via the right femoral access: bilobed additional large hilar image, very mild parenchymography, while the iliac vein and vena cava are early and heavily opacified. (**c**) Amplatzer occluder (*arrow*) was brought close to the arteriovenous communication. Its position could be checked before release. (**d**) Arteriographic control after releasing of the plug (*arrow*): exclusion of the fistula, the renal parenchyma now appears properly enhanced with the treatment of this steal syndrome, allowing significant restoration of renal function

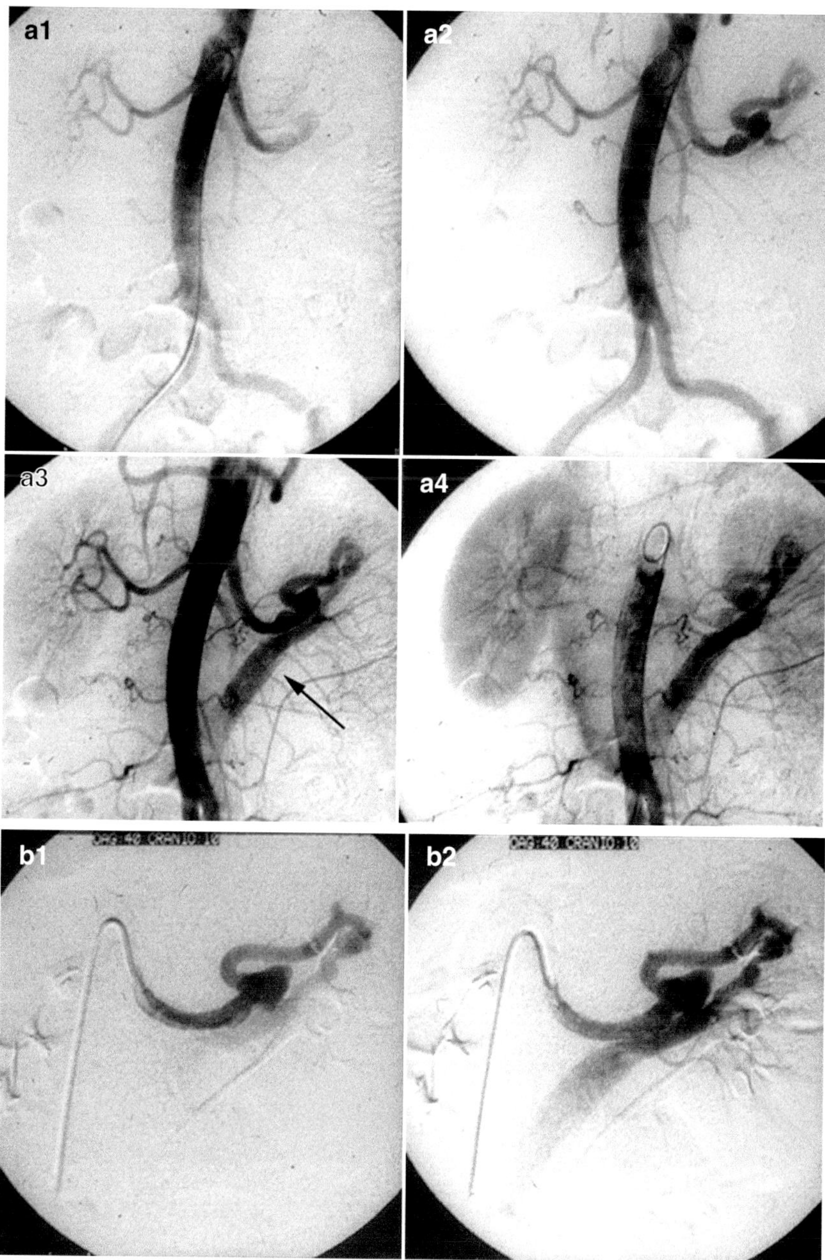

Fig. 13.13 Hypertension, important vascular murmur in the lumbar fossa, and suspicion on Doppler of an arteriovenous communication. (**a1–a4**) Dynamic sequences show massive opacification of an arteriovenous communication and an early venous return from the left renal artery. Note the light nephrography on this side and the descending path of the renal vein (*arrow*) (which should evoke typically a retroaortic renal vein). (**b1–b4**) Selective injection: wide arteriovenous communication from the trunk of the left renal artery. (**c**) Exclusion by a larguable balloon: arteriographic control before releasing the balloon. (**d**) Arteriographic control 6 months later

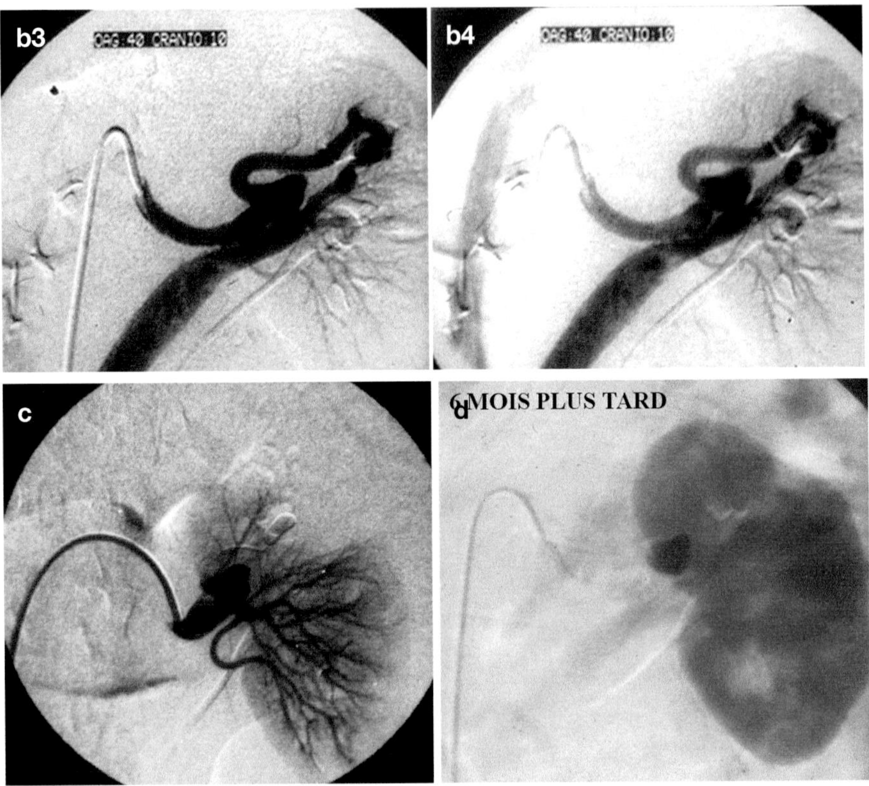

Fig. 13.13 (continued)

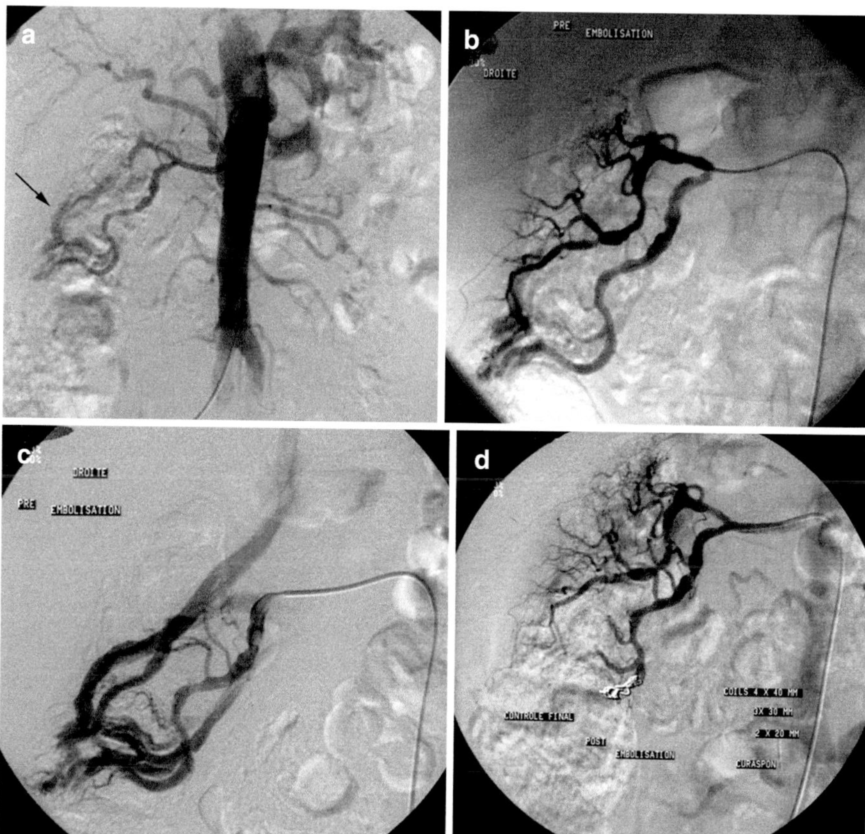

Fig. 13.14 Intermittent recurrent hematuria for 18 months in a 76-year-old W. The assessment showed no anomaly, except an important vascular network in the renal hilum and in the inferior part of the kidney on CT scan. Arteriography was decided to complete the workup. (**a**) Arteriography: large pre-pelvic arterial branch with early venous return (*arrow*). (**b**, **c**) Selective injection: cirsoid arteriovenous malformation. (**d**) Arteriographic control after exclusion by coils

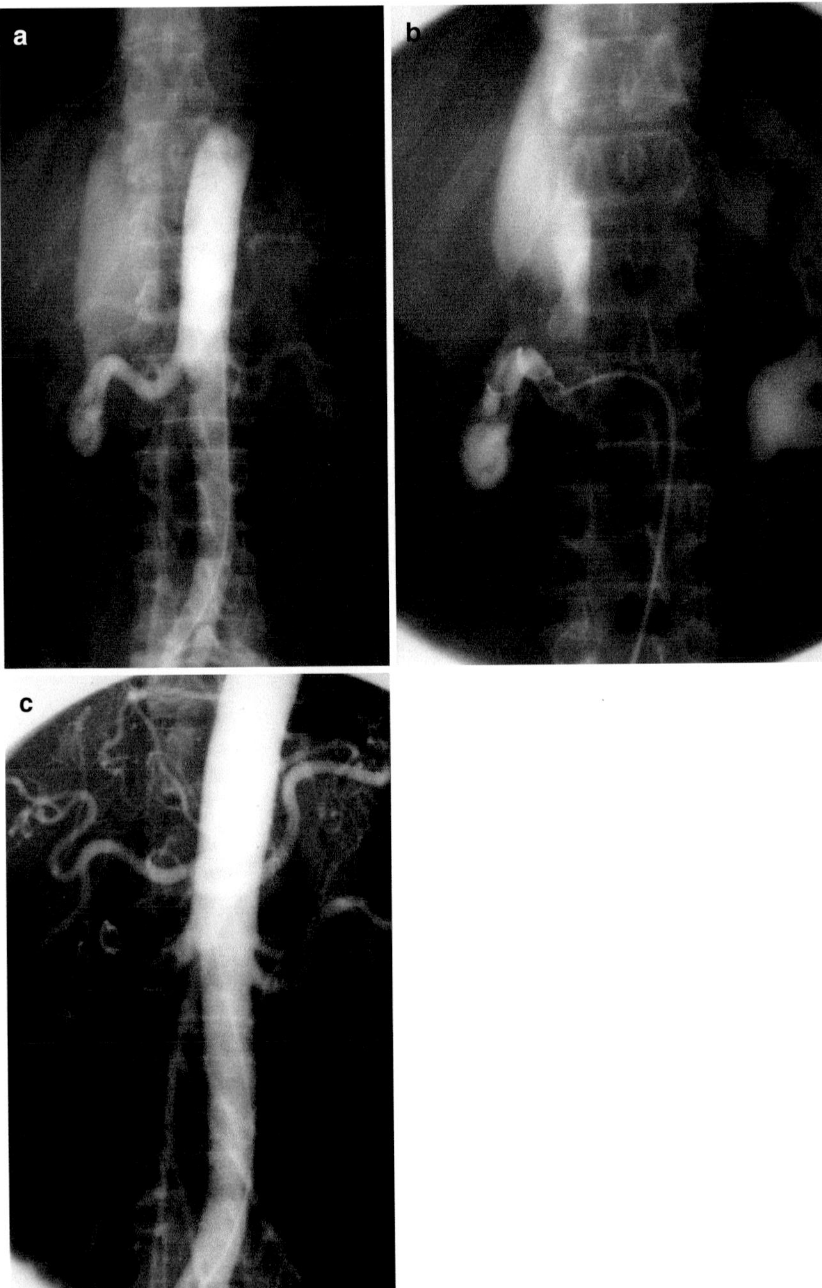

Fig. 13.15 A 75-year-old W with a progressive heart failure for which a high flow was suggested. Ultrasound suggested an abdominal arteriovenous fistula. The main antecedent of the patient was a right nephrectomy at the age of 25 to treat a urogenital tuberculosis. (**a**) Aortography: large arteriovenous fistula developed from the remaining segment of the right renal artery, suggesting a mass ligation (artery + vein) of the pedicle. (**b**) Selective injection: fully channeled massive arteriovenous fistula. (**c**) Aortographic control after exclusion by macro-coils of Gianturco

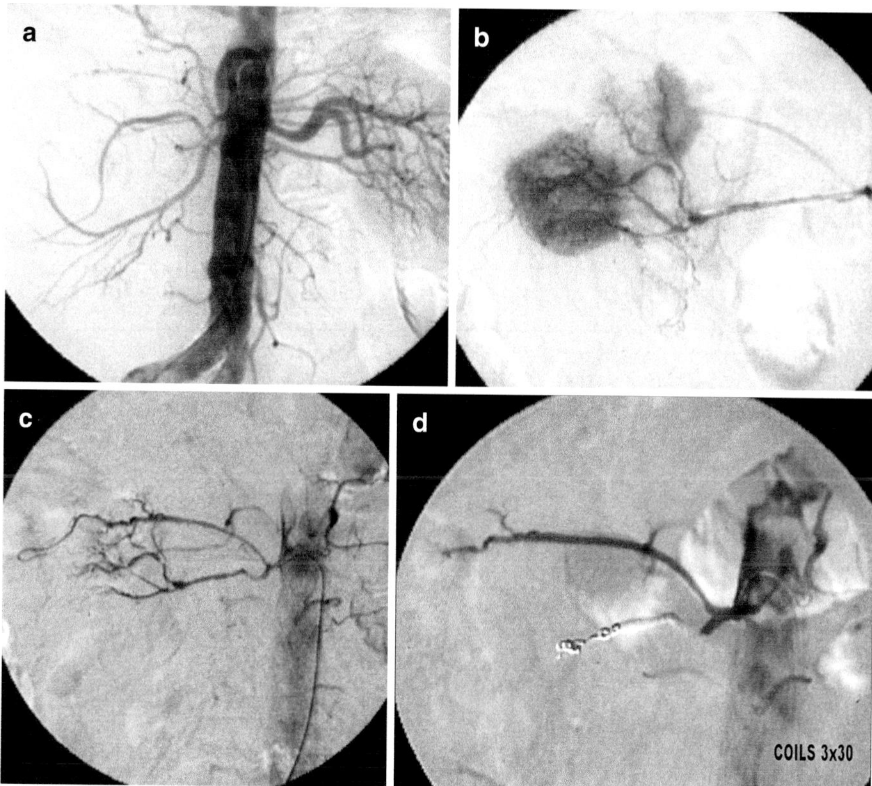

Fig. 13.16 Refractory hypertension in a 78-year-old patient with a history of severe left recurrent pyelonephritis. The assessment of this severe hypertension showed a secondary hyperaldosteronism. An isotopic nephrogram noted that the left kidney provides 95 % of the function. (**a**) Aortography: normal left renal artery feeding a normal kidney; on the right side: disharmonious, small atrophic kidney, fed by a very thin artery. (**b**, **c**) Selective injection of the right renal artery. Note the early division and the predominant participation of the superior branch to the exo-renal circle. The lower branch, which terminal branches are subject to advanced nephroangiosclerosis, vascularizes a very small nephronic volume. (**d**) Exclusion of the first-order lower branch by particles + coils, which will lead to a better control of hypertension, at the price of a moderate 48 h post-embolization syndrome. The exo-renal and parietal branches were spared

Appendix: AAST Classification (Kidney) [7]

Grade[a]	Injury type	Description of injury	AIS
I	Contusion	Microscopic or gross hematuria, urologic studies normal	2
	Hematoma	Subcapsular, nonexpanding, without parenchymal laceration	2
II	Hematoma	Nonexpanding perirenal hematoma confirmed to renal retroperitoneum	2
	Laceration	<1 cm parenchymal depth of renal cortex, without urinary extravasation	2
III	Laceration	>1 cm parenchymal depth of renal cortex, without collecting system rupture or urinary extravasation	3
IV	Laceration	Parenchymal laceration extending through renal cortex, medulla, and collecting system	4
	Vascular	Main renal artery or vein injury with contained hemorrhage	4
V	Laceration	Completely shattered kidney	5
	Vascular	Avulsion of renal hilum that devascularizes kidney	5

AIS Abbreviated Injury Scale
[a]Advance one grade for bilateral injuries up to grade III

Chatelain's classification of kidney injuries [6]	
Type 1	Simple contusion: benign lesion, capsular integrity
Type 2	Ruptured capsule, with parenchymal lesions, possibly involving the urinary tract
Type 3	Serious contusion, large gap between fragments, urohematoma, ischemia
Type 4	Pedicle vascular lesions

References

1. Guy L, Alfidja AT, Chabrot P, et al. Catheter transarterial embolization of renal tumors in 20 patients. Int Urol Nephrol. 2007;39(1):47–50.
2. Mondshine RT, Owens S, Mondshein JI. Combination embolization and radiofrequency. J Vasc Interv Radiol. 2008;19:616–20.
3. Dabbeche C, Chaker M, Chemali R, et al. Rôle de l'embolisation dans les angiomyolipomes du rein. J Radiol. 2006;87:1859.
4. Nelson CP, Sauda MG. Contemporary diagnosis and management of renal angiomyolipoma. J Urol. 2002;168:1315–25.
5. Harbayashi T, Shinohara N, Katano H, et al. Management of renal angiomyolipoma associated with tuberous sclerosis complex. J Urol. 2004;171:102–6.
6. Chatelain C. Essai de classification des lésions et proposition d'une tactique dans les traumatismes fermés récents du rein. Ann Urol. 1981;15:210–4.
7. Tinkoff G, Esposito TJ, Reed J, et al. American Association for the Surgery of Trauma Organ Injury Scale 1: spleen, liver and kidney, validation based on the national trauma data bank. J Am Coll Surg. 2008;207:646–55.

8. Santucci RA, McAninch JW. Diagnosis and management of renal trauma: past, present, and future. J Am Coll Surg. 2000;191(4):443–51.
9. Hirsch AT, et al. ACC/AHA guidelines for the management of patients with peripheral arterial disease (lower extremity, renal, mesenteric, and abdominal aortic). J Vasc Interv Radiol. 2006;17:1383–98.
10. Rundback JH, Rizvi A, Rozenblit GN. Percutaneous stent graft management of renal artery aneurism. J Vasc Interv Radiol. 2000;11:1189–93.
11. Cornelis F, Couzi L, Le Bras Y, et al. Embolization of polycystic kidneys as an alternative to nephrectomy before renal transplantation: a pilot study. Am J Transplant. 2010;10:2363–9.

Chapter 14
Anticoagulant-Related Hematomas

Louis Boyer, Lucie Cassagnes, Agaïcha Alfidja Lankoande, and Pascal Chabrot

14.1 Background

Anticoagulants, such as heparin, low-molecular-weight heparins and warfarin, and presumably the newer classes, are responsible for hemorrhagic complications in up to 4 % of the patients, which can potentially be life-threatening.

The soft tissues, retroperitoneum, psoas muscles, and rectus sheath, are the commonest sites of these nontraumatic hematomas, followed by the gastrointestinal and urinary tracts (renal anticoagulant-related hemorrhages are discussed in Chap. 13).

The risk factors for anticoagulant-related hematomas include patients' age, specific comorbidities (severe heart disease, liver dysfunction, renal insufficiency, hypertension, cerebrovascular diseases, and long-term hemodialysis), association to other drugs with a potentiating effect (nonsteroidal anti-inflammatory agents and diuretics), duration of the treatment, as well as intensity of the anticoagulant effect.

The clinical presentation is often not specific.

Ultrasound can detect hematoma, but CT is nowadays the gold standard, due to its performance in the detection, quantification, and delimitation of hematoma in the retroperitoneum, the psoas and/or iliac muscles, and/or the rectus sheath. Type III rectus sheath hematoma as defined by Bernat spreads into Retzius prevesical space and can diffuse into the peritoneum. It can contain up to 2 l of fluid without any palpable mass. A GI tract parietal hematoma (small bowel generally) can also be

L. Boyer, MD, PhD (✉) • L. Cassagnes, MD • A. Alfidja Lankoande, MD
P. Chabrot, MD, PhD
Department of Radiology,
University Hospital of Clermont-Ferrand,
Clermont-Ferrand, France
e-mail: lboyer@chu-clermontferrand.fr; pchabrot@chu-clermontferrand.fr

P. Chabrot, L. Boyer (eds.), *Embolization*,
DOI 10.1007/978-1-4471-5182-1_14, © Springer-Verlag London 2014

detected. After injection of contrast medium, CT can detect an active bleeding by depicting a vascular blush.

Similar situations are:

- Rare spontaneous hematomas caused by contractions or extreme muscle stretching induced by coughing, vomiting, exercising, and/or vascular and muscular fragility caused by arteriosclerosis, inflammatory diseases, pregnancy, delivery, obesity, age…
- Posttraumatic and/or iatrogenic hematomas (especially after percutaneous punctures and/or biopsies)

14.2 Relevant Radiological Anatomy

14.2.1 Retroperitoneum and Psoas

The posterior abdominal wall is mainly vascularized by the lumbar arteries which participate in an anastomotic network with the subcostal (12th intercostal) and the deep circumflex iliac arteries.

The psoas muscles regularly receive arteries branching off the lumbar arteries but also from the iliolumbar, obturator (branches of the internal iliac artery), external iliac, and common femoral arteries. There is sometimes a unique voluminous branch issuing from the external iliac artery (main artery of the psoas muscle).

14.2.2 Rectus Sheath

A vertical epigastric arterial axis proceeds along the deep face of the rectus sheath: the lower epigastric artery, which originates from the external iliac artery, joins the upper epigastric artery (branch of the internal mammary artery), at the upper third level of the rectus sheath. A full communication between these arteries is found in only 20 % of the cases; more frequently the arteries end in small branches. This arterial axis receives transversal branches from the subcostal, lumbar, and deep circumflex iliac arteries.

14.3 Technique

Catheterization is usually carried out after a femoral access using the Seldinger technique.

In the case of retroperitoneal hematoma, the lumbar arteries are usually involved.

When hematoma is localized in the psoas, the third and the fourth lumbar arteries are concerned; if necessary, the hypogastric arteries will also be catheterized.

In the case of a hematoma of the rectus sheath, the epigastric artery is generally responsible. But other arteries can also be involved: intercostals, external circumflex iliac, abdominal subcutaneous, iliolumbar, superior gluteal arteries, and other branches of the hypogastric arteries.

The use of microcatheters can simplify the navigation.

Before embolization of the lumbar arteries, a selective opacification must be carried out in order to eliminate all aberrant branches vascularizing the spinal cord.

Various embolization agents are used: gelatin sponge, PVA particles, microparticles, and glues. Like many teams, we prefer using microcoils which are ideally placed both proximally and distally to the bleeding site of the artery; if the catheterization is too difficult, we perform proximal occlusion.

When angiography does not confirm the extravasation depicted by angio CT, we perform empiric embolization of the third and the fourth lumbar arteries ipsilateral to the hematoma of the psoas and of the ipsilateral epigastric artery in the case of rectus sheath hematoma, using gelatin sponge.

14.4 Results

To our knowledge, case reports have mainly been published; in his review of the literature, Zissin pooled 26 cases in addition to four personal observations.

Technical success was the rule.

Endovascular treatment has a lower morbi-mortality than surgery. Several patients died after the procedure due to critical clinical status and morbidities, but no embolization-related complication has yet been reported such as infection, cutaneous, and neurologic ischemia.

Gradual resorption of the hematoma can be easily be monitored by ultrasound. The regression of nerve damages consecutive to psoas hematoma has also been observed.

14.5 Indications

A conservative approach was classically advocated to deal with anticoagulant-related hematomas: discontinuation and if necessary reversal of anticoagulants with warfarin or heparin antidotes, fluid resuscitation, as well as blood transfusion. These treatments remain mandatory in all cases.

- A conservative treatment with careful medical supervision (“wait and see”) is usually sufficient for small hematomas; it is also the first-line treatment for hemodynamically stable patients.
- The indications of surgical or percutaneous decompression/drainage of hematoma remain limited.

- If the embolization of posttraumatic or iatrogenic retroperitoneal hematoma is a proven effective and safe treatment option (see Chap. 13), it had been considered for a long time that spontaneous anticoagulant-related hematomas were not indications for catheterization. But it has now been proven that in the case of life-threatening hematomas or in the case of lumbar plexus nerve suffering (psoas hematoma with active bleeding), an embolization has to be preferred to surgery which has a higher morbidity rate.

Arteriography to embolize is also indicated in patients with a vascular blush on CT scan that remain hemodynamically unstable despite fluid resuscitation, blood transfusion, and reversal of anticoagulation.

- In the case of an extended rectus sheath hematoma in hemodynamically unstable patient, even in the absence of extravasation on CT and angiography, an ipsilateral epigastric arterial embolization has even been advocated (Zissin).

Key Points

- Anticoagulant-related abdominal parietal hematomas can be life-threatening.
- A hemodynamic shock occurring in anticoagulated patients must be explored by CT; a vascular blush means active bleeding.
- Embolization is indicated in hemodynamically unstable patients with a vascular blush on CT when conservative treatment seems insufficient; embolization must be preferred to surgery.

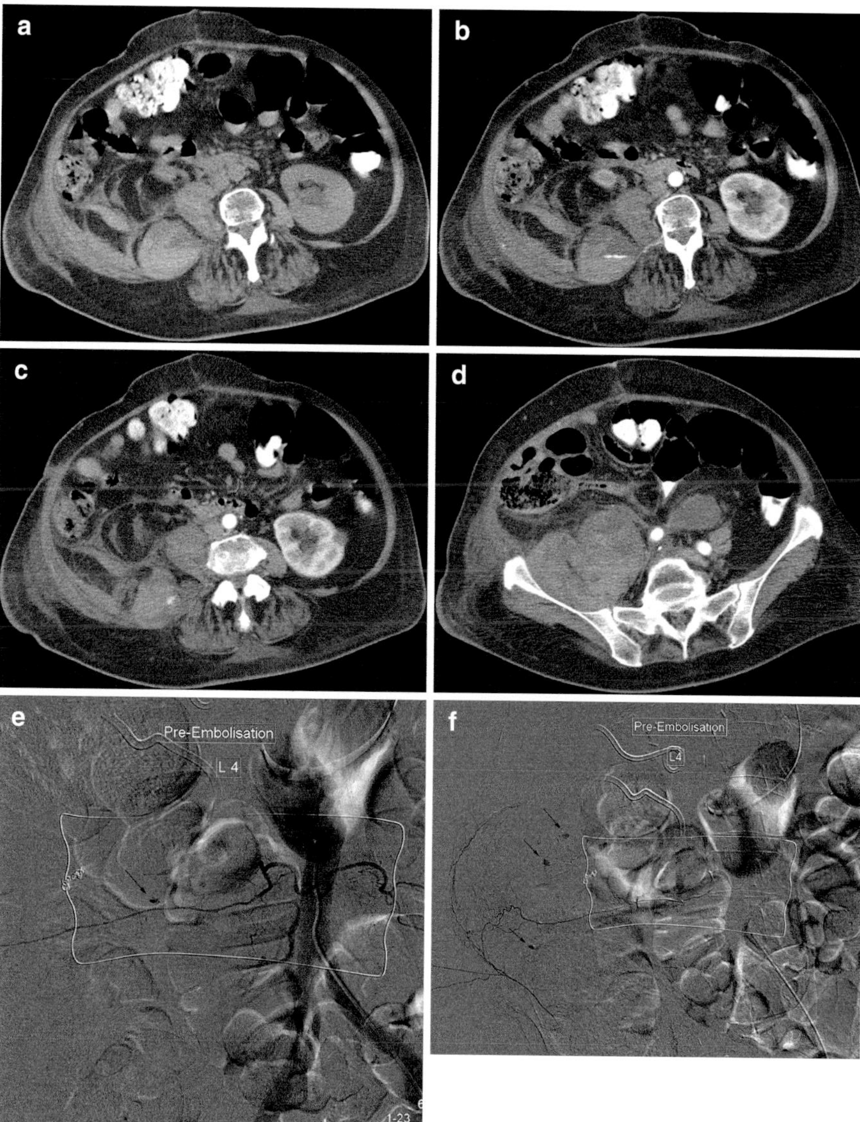

Fig. 14.1 Hemorrhagic shock related to a retroperitoneal hematoma 2 weeks after pelvic surgery, with a discharge right nephrostomy to treat an iatrogenic lesion of the right ureter, while the patient was treated with low-molecular-weight heparin at curative dose because of a postoperative deep venous thrombosis of the lower limbs. (**a**) Non-enhanced CT scan: heterogeneous hypertrophy of the right lumbar psoas: hematoma, associated with an adjacent dense and heterogeneous wall hematoma. (**b**, **c**) Enhanced CT: several foci of blush in the lumbar wall hematoma. (**d**) CT scans few centimeters below: the hematoma involves the abdominal wall, the psoas, and iliac muscles. (**e**, **f**) Two selective lumbar arterial injections: the blush is found in the territory of the fourth right lumbar artery (*arrow*), leading to a hyperselective microcatheterization (**f**), before exclusion by microparticles and gelfoam

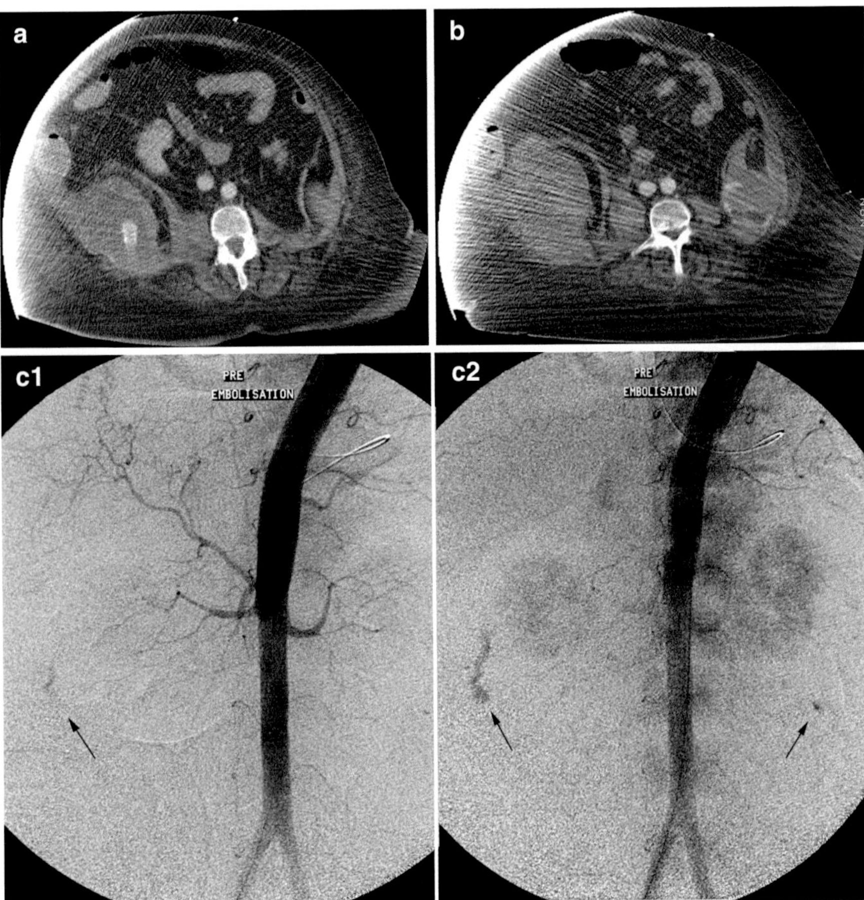

Fig. 14.2 Hemorrhagic shock in an obese patient treated by coumarin because of a rhythmic cardiopathy, in a status of DIC and multiple organ failure. (**a**) CT: right lumbar parietal hematoma, with important blush. (**b**) A few centimeters below: less important left lumbar parietal hematoma but also with important blush. (**c1** and **c2**) Aortography: splanchnic generalized vasoconstriction, massive extravasation in the right lumbar wall, and blush in the left lumbar wall (*arrows*). (**d**) Selective catheterization of the third right lumbar artery supplying the extravasation: exclusion using microparticles. (**e**) Selective catheterization of the fourth left lumbar artery: hypervascularization of the psoas but also of the lumbar wall. The catheterization was very difficult because of an extreme fragility of the vascular wall, leading to an exclusion by coils

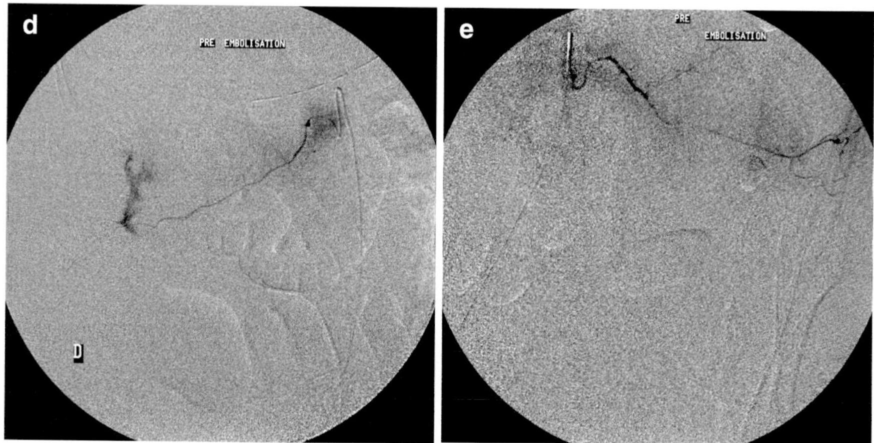

Fig. 14.2 (continued)

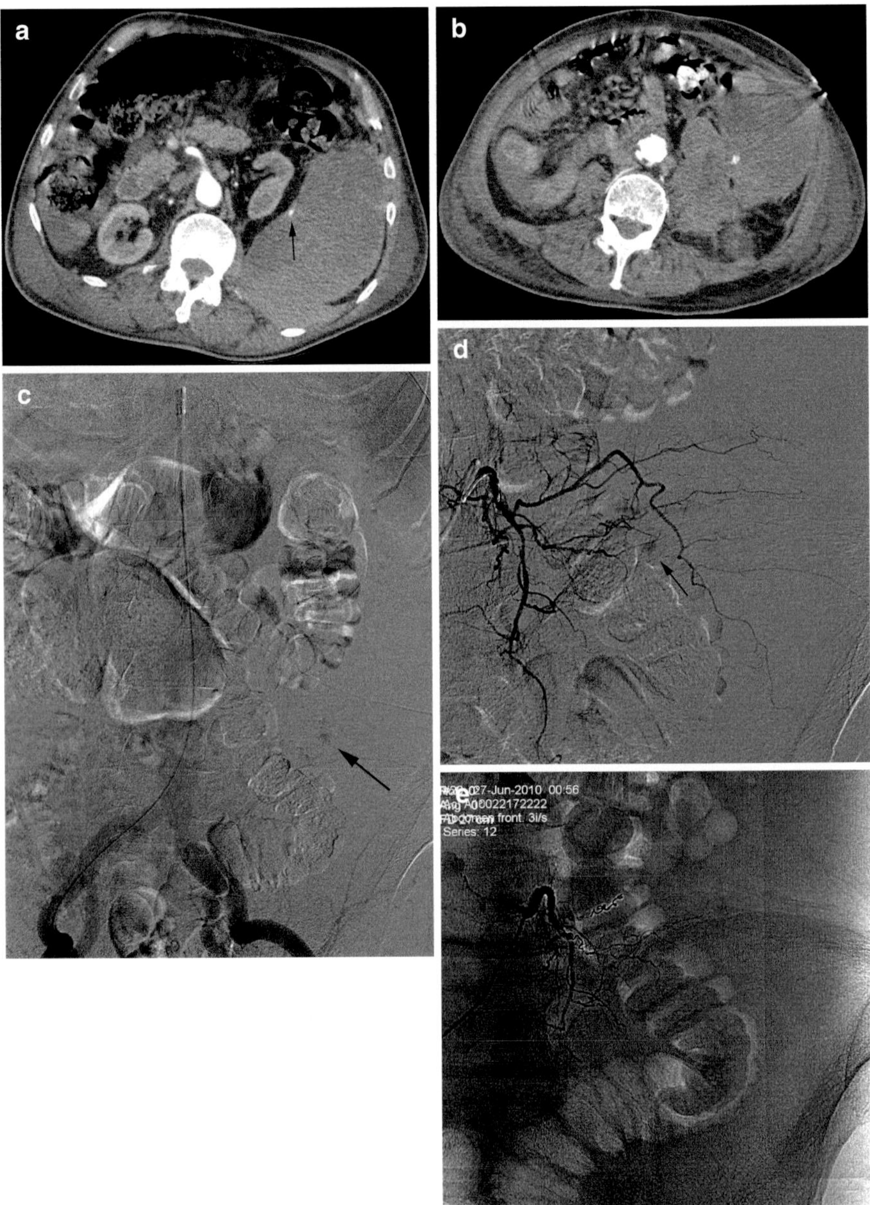

Fig. 14.3 Hemorrhagic shock in a 84-years old male suffering from a non-Hodgkin lymphoma, preventively anticoagulated: severe abdominal pain and deglobulization, leading to a CT. (**a**) CT large lumbar parietal hematoma with blush (*arrow*), anteriorly displacing the left kidney. (**b**) A second blush few centimeters below the hematoma is also extended to the psoas. (**c**) Aortography, late phase: extravasation in a territory presumed dependent of a left lumbar artery (*arrow*). (**d**) Selective injection of the fourth lumbar artery during a difficult and unstable catheterization (agitated patient): parietal blush (*arrow*), embolized by gelfoam and microcoils (**e**)

Suggested Reading

Berna JD, Garcia Medina V, Guirao J, et al. Rectus sheath hematoma classification by CT. Abdom Imaging. 1996;21:62–4.

Zissin R, Gayer G, Kots E, et al. Transcatheter arterial embolization in anticoagulant related hematoma – a current therapeutic option: a report of 4 patients and review of the literature. Int J Clin Pract. 2007;61(8):1321–7.

Chapter 15
Embolization of Varicoceles

Louis Boyer, Anne Ravel, Laurent Guy, Bruno De Fraissinette, Jean-Marc Garcier, Rami Chemali, and Pascal Chabrot

15.1 Background

The abnormal dilatation of the pampiniform venous plexus is not always symptomatic. It is much more frequent on the left side. It can extend from the spermatic vein up to its anastomosis in the renal vein and the inferior vena cava. It is observed in 10–15 % of the adult male population, and it sometimes can be symptomatic: pain, scrotal swelling, or testicular atrophy. It is also found in 20–40 % of the population of infertile men, but it does not necessarily imply male infertility. Various theories have been developed to explain its responsibility, with respect to alterations in the fertilizing qualities of the sperm: scrotal hyperthermia above all, venous refluxes exposing the testis to adrenal or renal metabolites, consequences of venous stasis on testicle, immunological mechanisms, etc.

Various etiological factors have been advocated to explain the varicocele: nutcracker syndrome (renal vein compression between the aorta and superior

L. Boyer, MD, PhD (✉) • A. Ravel, MD • P. Chabrot, MD, PhD
Department of Radiology, University Hospital of Clermont-Ferrand, Clermont-Ferrand, France
e-mail: lboyer@chu-clermontferrand.fr; pchabrot@chu-clermontferrand.fr

L. Guy, MD, PhD
Department of Urology, University Hospital of Clermont-Ferrand, Clermont-Ferrand, France

B. De Fraissinette, MD
Department of Radiology, University Hospital of Clermont-Ferrand, Clermont-Ferrand, France

Department of Radiology, Clinique La Chataigneraie, Beaumont, USA

J.-M. Garcier, MD, PhD
Department of Anatomy and Radiology, University Hospital of Clermont-Ferrand, Clermont-Ferrand, France

R. Chemali, MD
Department of Radiology, Saint Georges Hospital, Beyrouth, Lebanon

P. Chabrot, L. Boyer (eds.), *Embolization*,
DOI 10.1007/978-1-4471-5182-1_15,

mesenteric artery), dysfunction of spermatic vein valves, and high orthostatic hydrostatic venous pressure. Left renal tumors must systematically be ruled out. In the case of a bilateral disease, the left varicocele is certainly the primum movens. In this case the right varicocele and deferential varicose vein are the consequences of an efferent flow via left-right scrotal anastomoses.

15.2 Relevant Radiological Anatomy

The venous drainage of the testis originates from an anterior pedicle, made up of 8–10 anastomosed veins which constitute, around the spermatic vein, the pampiniform plexus. It drains into 3–5 veins in the deep internal ostium of the inguinal canal and then into the spermatic vein which is usually unique. The posterior pedicle, which is made up of much smaller veins, drains into the inferior epigastric vein.

The spermatic vein courses through the spermatic cord into the retroperitoneum. On the left, it joins the left renal vein. On the right, it most often flows into the subrenal inferior vena cava; it can also, but less frequently, feed into the right renal vein or via more complex anastomoses into the vena cava and the right renal vein.

Duplications are frequent in the pelvic and lower lumbar segments, both richly anastomosed on both sides of the spermatic artery. We systematically look for these duplications and anastomoses which can cause recurrences, by performing oblique angiographic views. Retroperitoneal or lumbar vein drainages can be observed in 5 % of the cases, corresponding to complex networks (type II in Bahren classification) [1].

In 15–20 % cases of varicocele, collateral veins that branch off upstream of a well-functioning valve of the spermatic vein can be observed, draining into the renal vein or one of its affluences.

The left "normal" renal vein can coexist with or be replaced by a retroaortic renal vein draining more caudally into the inferior vena cava.

15.3 Technique

- Femoral venous access is usually performed; jugular or brachial approaches are used by a few teams.
- Local anesthesia and if necessary light sedation. No prophylactic antibiotics in our group.
- In our group embolization is carried out during a brief hospitalization (24–36 h) but in some centers it is an outpatient procedure.
- During the procedure, irradiation of the gonads has to be as low as reasonably achievable.

- *Spermatic venography* is the standard diagnostic test before embolization, preceded by the catheterization of the ostium of the spermatic vein:
  - On the left side, a catheter (Cobra C2, spermatic, etc.) is led into the left renal vein; the ostium of the spermatic vein is usually located on its antero-inferior edge. If it is not found, the injection of contrast medium into the left renal vein can be helpful in identifying its termination.
  - On the right side, the ostium of the spermatic vein is infrequently on the renal vein (10 % of the cases). If not found, the antero-right edge of the subrenal inferior vena cava must be explored. The anatomic variations and the very frequent valvulations explain a lower success rate on this side with respect to the other side.

Two injections are then carried out (10 cc of iodine contrast medium, 3–5 cc), to image the lumbar and pelvic segments of the spermatic vein.

Typically it depicts an enlarged venous caliber, a varicose appearance, and/or avalvulation; a retrograde flow in the spermatic vein is only obtained in patients with varicocele. However, if the catheterization is too distal, beyond the valves, it can induce a nonphysiological reflux.

According to Sigmund [2], two types of varicoceles must be distinguished: the "stop" type, where only a reflux exists in the spermatic vein (infraclinical varicoceles would normally correspond to this pattern), and the "shunt" type characterized by a retrograde flow in the spermatic vein, followed by an anterograde flow through the deferential, cremasteric, and external pudendal veins, which are generally anastomosed.

At last, a venography permits the full assessment of anastomoses and collateral venous network.

After diagnostic ICM injections, a selective distal catheterization is carried out, up to the pelvic segment. Accessory veins must systematically be looked for by performing oblique views before the embolization, as these vicarious vessels can hypertrophy and take over the venous drainage. These accessory veins must therefore be occluded whenever it is possible.

- Various occlusive agents have been used: hot contrast medium, Ivalon, small larguable balloons, biological glues, etc. Sclerosing agents are frequently used (Varicocid, Aetoxisclerol, Trombovar), either alone or associated with metallic coils. By destroying the endothelium, sclerosing agents offer a more durable occlusion, notably in case of collateral drainage network. However, their use exposes the patient to a risk of scrotal backflow and therefore requires, as all liquid agents, a groin compression of the spermatic vein, during and immediately after the injection. Gandini [3] considers that sodium tetradecyl sulfate (STS) mixed with air presents an adequate viscosity in this indication.

We prefer to use coils, whose diameter is defined by [the size of the vein as seen on the venography + 1 mm], deployed in two packs, pelvic and lower lumbar. Amplatzer occluder plugs can also be used.

Taking into account the simplicity of post-procedure follow-up, the patient can often return to work very rapidly; we advise against contact sports for 1 month.

15.4 Results

15.4.1 Technical Results

- Embolization is impossible in 5–15 % of the cases, notably due to an important collateral venous network.
- Complications are rare, and the immediate follow-up is usually very simple.

Pain and an increased scrotal swelling, due to the extension of the inflammatory process or of the thrombosis (0.5–1 %, more frequent with sclerosing agents), can be treated by anti-inflammatory drugs, antibiotics, and testicular uptake.

A 5–30 % recurrence rate has been reported (the variability of the post-procedure follow-up can explain these variations).

The technical results are less interesting when exists, just next to a principal spermatic vein with an intact valve, an avalvulated collateral circulation which cannot be catheterized and which links the spermatic vein to the retroperitoneal or the segmental renal veins.

A high lumbar occlusion of the spermatic vein leads to a greater risk of recurrence, due to the frequency of a collateral network.

According to Gandini [3], it has been observed that the rate of recurrence is lower when using sodium tetradecyl sulfate (3.6 %) than when using coils.

After a recurrence, repeat venography and embolization can be attempted.

15.4.2 Fertility

If the benefits of surgical ligatures are generally admitted, the predictive factors of success have been largely discussed. It appears that the extent of the varicocele has no predictive value, but an early treatment in teenagers or young adults would mean a better prognosis.

The evaluation of the impact on fertility is not well codified (parameters, follow-up, etc.). Nevertheless, embolization results seem interesting and comparable to those of surgery: a significant improvement of sperm density, motility, and morphology and pregnancies occurring 1–3 years after the embolization, in 25–40 % of the cases.

15.5 Indications

A tumor of the left kidney (barrier to the spermatic venous flow?) must always be ruled out.

Embolization of a clinical varicocele can be proposed in case of scrotal discomfort, heaviness or scrotal pain increased when standing up or during physical effort, scrotal swelling, recurrence after a surgical intervention for a varicocele, and infertility.

In case of infertility, it is difficult to establish whether the varicocele is responsible: its presence does not necessary mean male infertility. An oligo-astheno-teratospermia or an azoospermia is argument to treat.

The results of the embolization make it a reliable, reproducible, and safe therapeutic alternative to the surgical ligation; as it is mini invasive, it is advocated by some authors as the first-line treatment. Embolization remains feasible in case of a recurrence after surgical treatment.

For some authors, the varicocele must be treated early in teenagers, in order to avoid infertility, even more so if there is a testicular hypotrophy.

We do not treat infraclinical varicoceles.

Key Points

- Left side +++.
- A varicocele is found in 20–40 % of the infertile men, but its presence does not necessarily imply a male infertility.
- The pathophysiology is not univocal (avalvulation, aorto-mesenteric compression, nutcracker syndrome, etc.); as a rule, a left renal tumor must be ruled out.
- A spermatic venography is mandatory in case of recurrence after surgery.
- Embolization agents: sclerosing agents and/or coils – our preference is coils.
- Embolization is possible in more than 80 % of the cases; post-embolization recurrences in 5–30 % of the cases, even more so if the occlusion was high and if there is an anastomosis between a normally valvulated spermatic vein and an avalvulated collaterality network.
- If there is recurrence, a new attempt for embolization is feasible.
- In 25–40 % of infertile couples, pregnancies have been achieved after embolization.
- Early treatment in teenagers would be predictive of a better fertility.

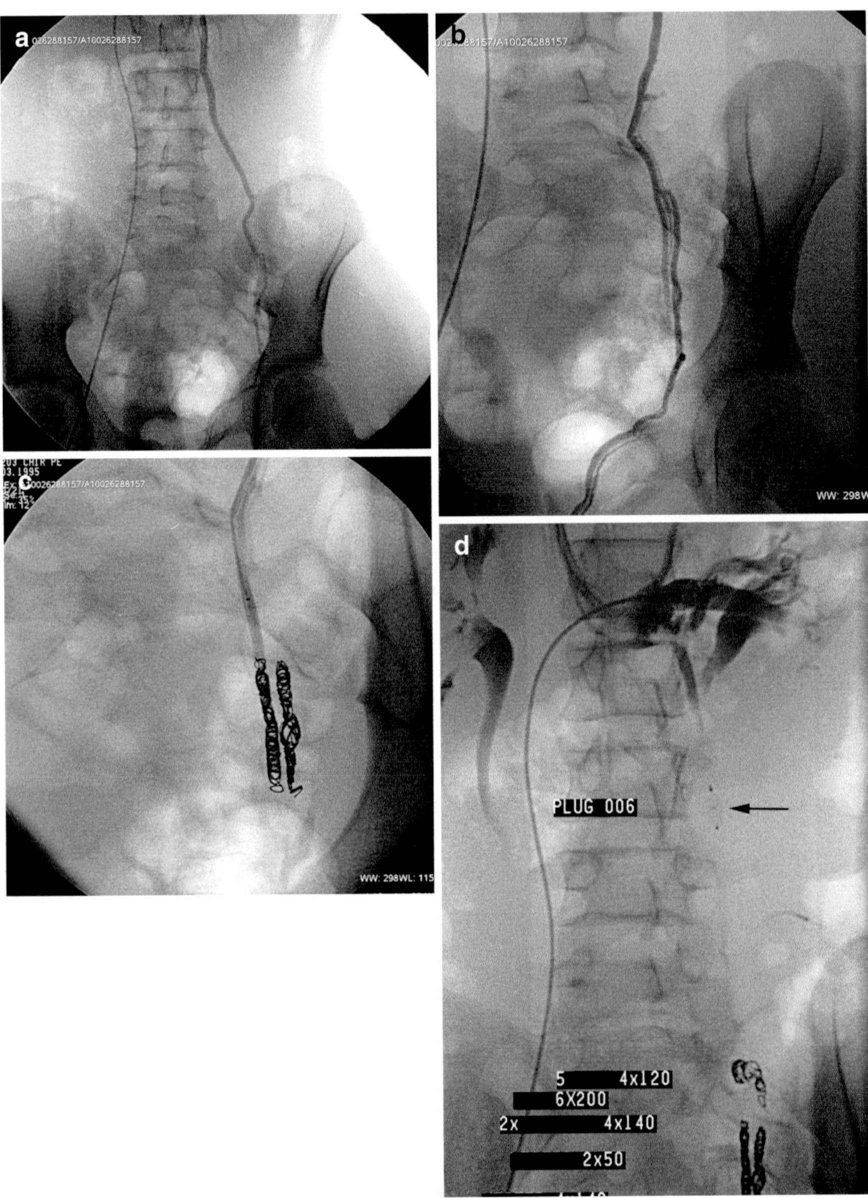

Fig. 15.1 A 16-year-old patient with disabling left varicocele, at rest and with effort, from several months. Renal ultrasound has eliminated any suspicious obstacle to the venous flow. A spermatic venography was requested, in order to perform an embolization if possible. (**a**, **b**) Right femoral vein puncture and catheterization of the left gonadal vein via the left renal vein: no obstacle or valvula was encountered in the path of the guidewire. Injection of 8 cc of ICM (4 cc/s), at the lumbar floor, and then at the pelvic floor. A unique gonadal vein drains into the renal vein, but in the pelvis the gonadal efferent branches are multiple, with two main trunks. (**c**) Control (manual injection by micro-catheter) after occlusion of both main efferent branches by micro-coils in the pelvis. (**d**) Additional lumbar occlusion a few centimeters higher, using an Amplatzer occluder plug (*arrow*). Control injection at the ostium of the gonadal vein, with reflux in the renal vein and the inferior vena cava

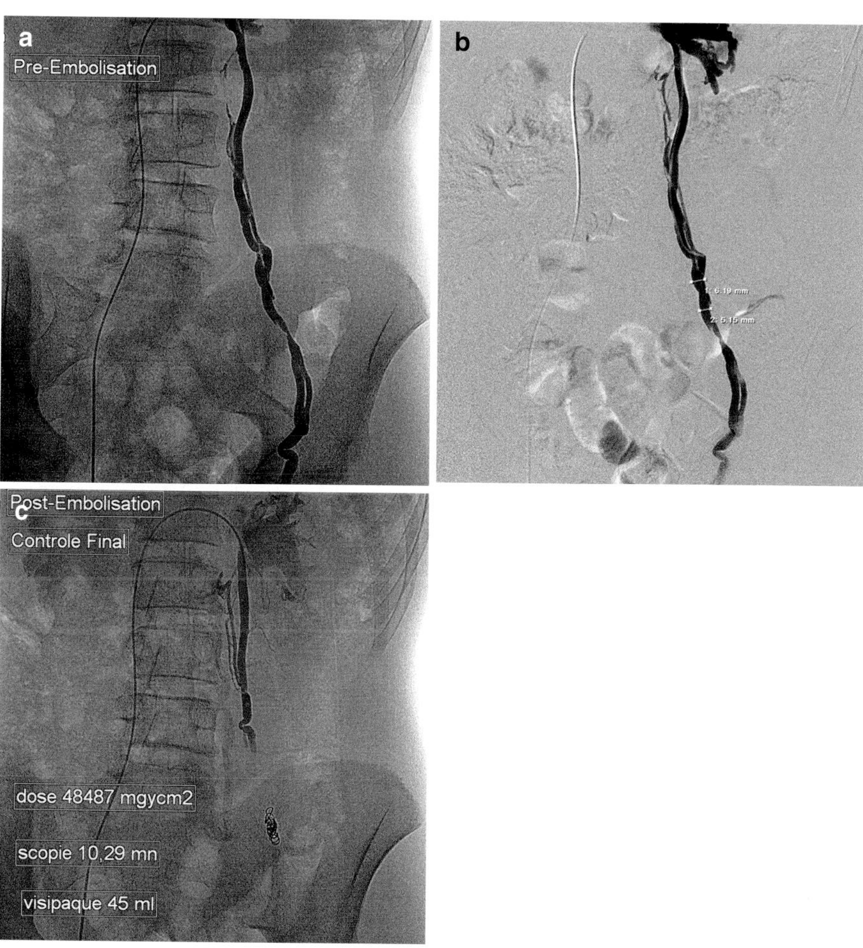

Fig. 15.2 Left varicocele which is very symptomatic on exercise (running) in a young 18-year-old. (**a**) After femoral vein puncture, catheterization of the left renal vein and of the spermatic vein, automatic injection (10 cc at 4 cc/s) in the left genital vein: the gonadal venous drainage is doubled in the pelvic and lumbar floors, but an apparently unique segment was shown in the iliac fossa, at which level we decided to perform the occlusion. (**b**) Sizing of the diameter of the repleted vein downstream of the target segment. To choose the coils, we performed a 10–20 % oversizing: coils of 7 and then 6 and 5 mm diameter were chosen. (**c**) Control after occlusion by coils

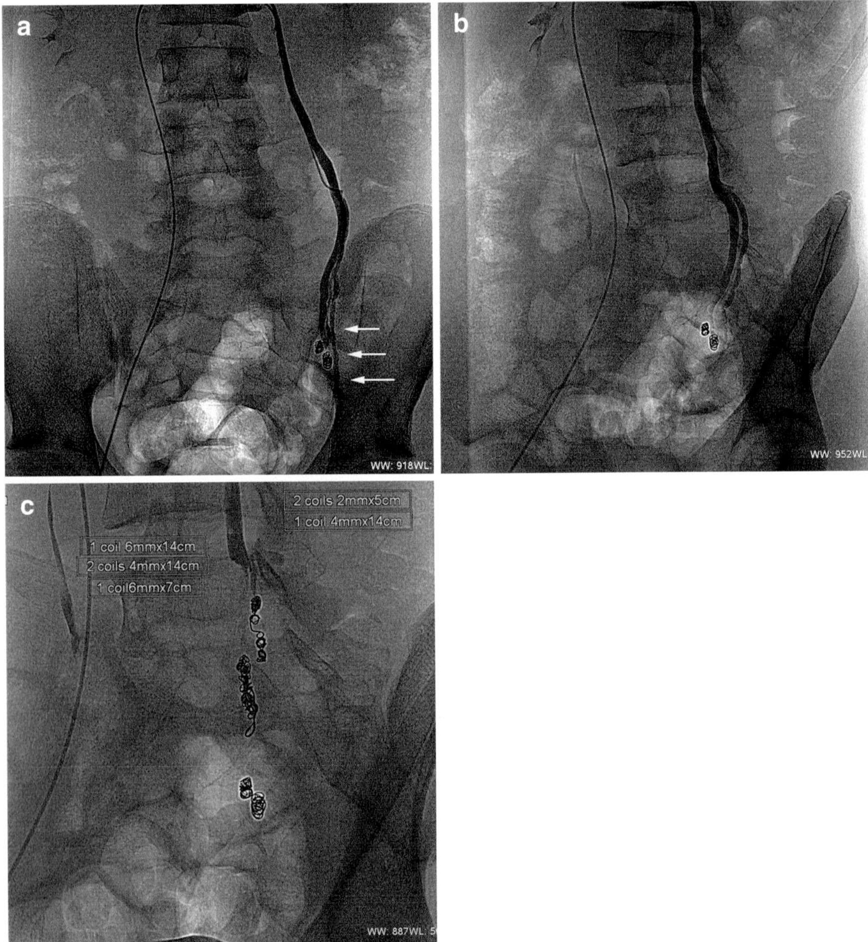

Fig. 15.3 A 18-year-old male; a recurrent symptomatic varicocele has already been surgically operated 3 years earlier; a first embolization has been then performed a few months after this surgery. (**a**, **b**: *frontal and 37° LAO*) Selective catheterization at the ostium of the left gonadal vein. The low pressure (4 cc/s) retrograde opacification showed a patent left gonadal vein (*arrow*), independent of the previously placed coils. This was probably due to the development of vicariances which were not visible on the first angiographic procedure. (**c**) After selective catheterization, the two main efferent branches have been occluded by calibrated coil packs. The manual control injection shows an effective occlusion

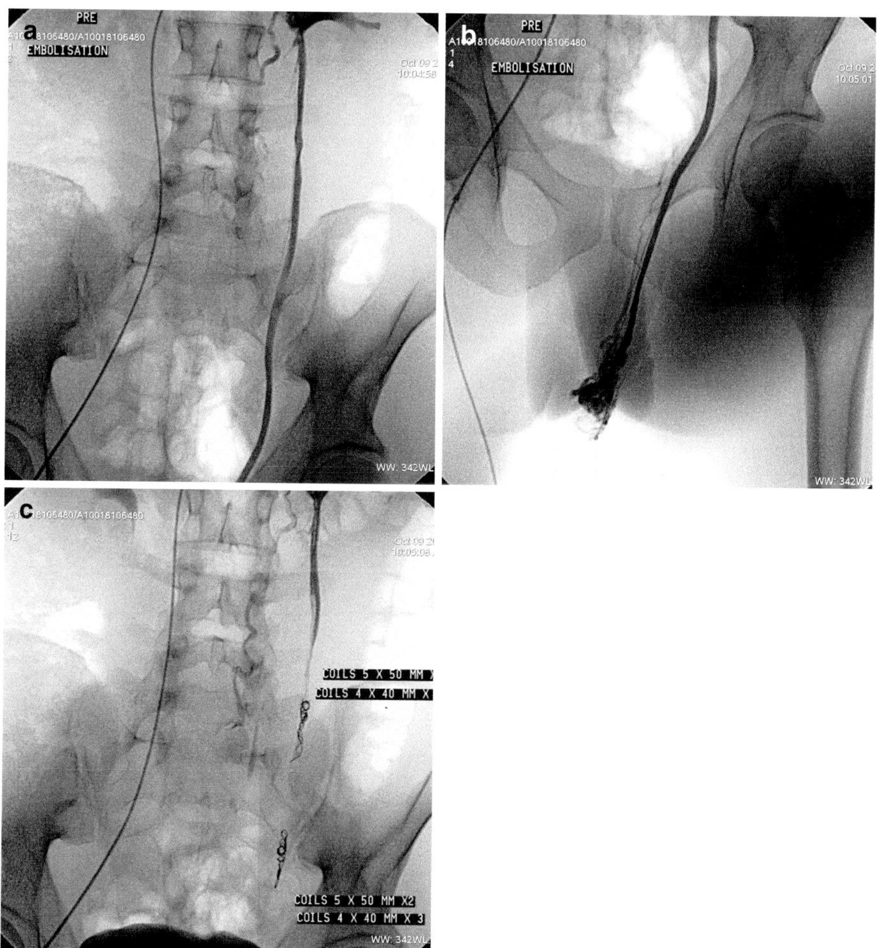

Fig. 15.4 Symptomatic left varicocele in a 29-year-old male, discovered during an infertility work-up (infertility dating at least of 3 years), with oligo-astheno-teratospermia. Left renal ultrasounds eliminated any suspicious lesion which may constitute a mass effect on the left renal vein. (**a**, **b**) Selective injection (low pressure) in the first centimeters of the left gonadal vein (one frame per second, manual travelling making it possible to perform a snapshot at lumbar floor, and another at the pelvis): massive retrograde reflux in a left gonadal vein extending into the scrotum. The efference of the spermatic cord is made of several veins that resolve into one venous axis in the pelvis. (**c**) Final control opacification: two packs of coils were released at the levels of the foot of the sacroiliac joint and of the promontory

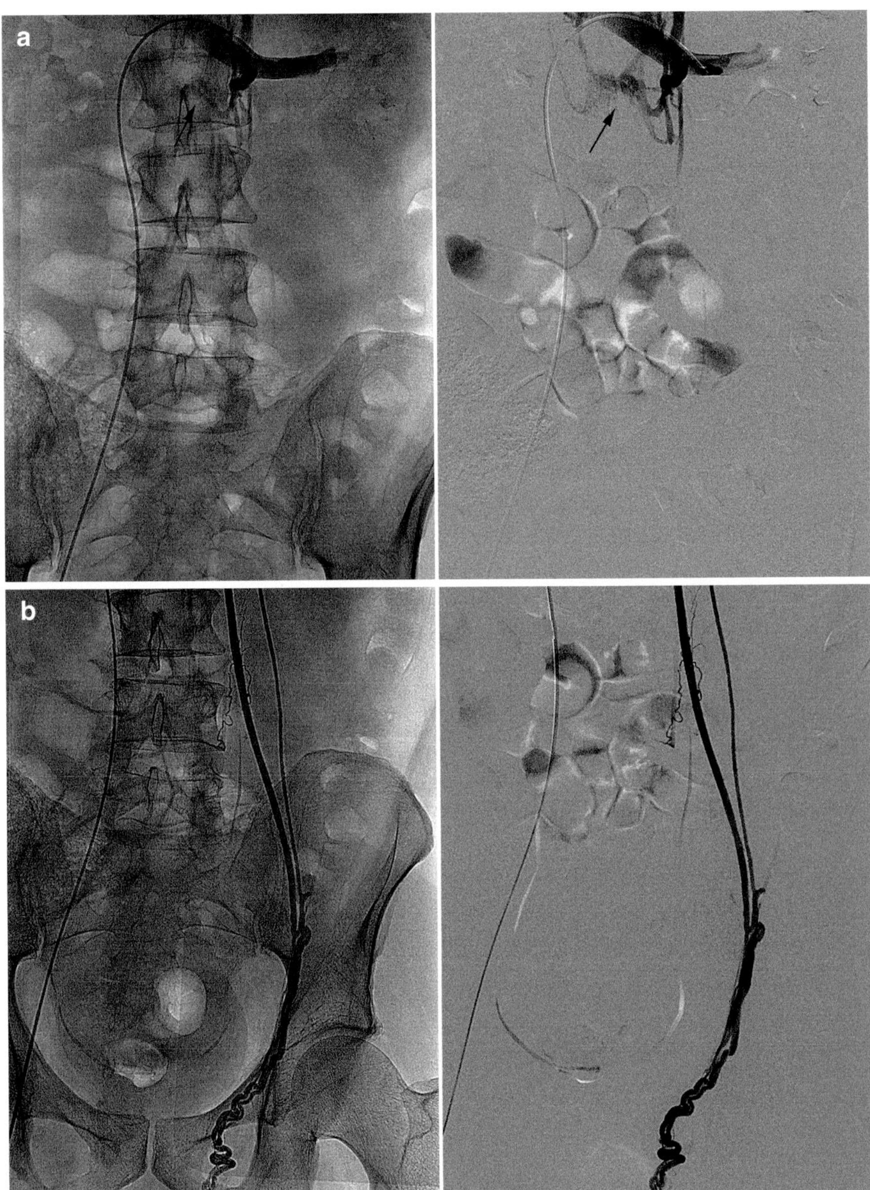

Fig. 15.5 A 52-year-old male suffering from a left scrotal pain related to a known varicocele. A morphological assessment (US + CT) eliminated a retroperitoneal mass. (**a**) Puncture of the right femoral vein, ilio-caval isoflux catheterization, and then left renal vein catheterization (Cobra catheter): several afferent veins, 2–3 cm before the anastomosis to the vena cava, associated with communications with the lumbar venous network (*arrow*), and the affluence of the gonadal vein. (**b**) After selective catheterization (hydrophilic guidewire), an injection was performed 4–5 cm upstream of the end of the gonadal vein (8 cc, 4 ml/s). We observed serpiginous and plexiform efferent gonadal veins, which resolved into two independent pelvic veins, which separately drain in the left renal vein (**c**). (**d**) Ultimate control after exclusion using two packs of coils in the smaller external vein and one pack of coils + one Amplatzer vascular plug in the larger internal vein (*arrow*)

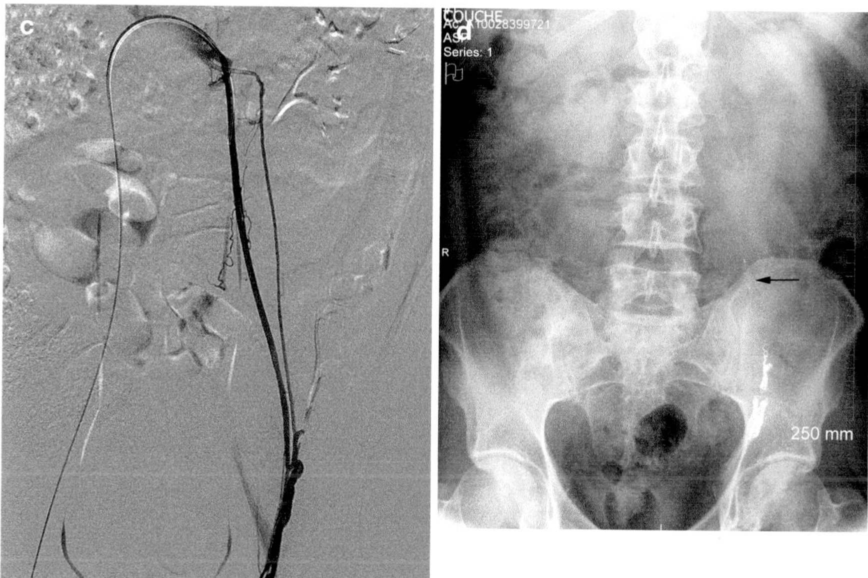

Fig. 15.5 (continued)

References

1. Lenz M, Hof N, Kersting-Sommerhof B, Bautz W. Anatomic variants of the spermatic vein: importance for percutaneous sclerotherapy of idiopathic varicocele. Radiology. 1996;198: 425–31.
2. Sigmund G, Gall H, Bahren W. Stop-type and shunt-type varicoceles: venographic findings. Radiology. 1987;163:105–10.
3. Gandini R, Konda D, Reale CA, et al. Male varicocele: transcatheter foam sclerotherapy with sodium tetradecyl sulfate outcome in 244 patients. Radiology. 2008;246(2):612–8.

Suggested Reading

Demas BE, Hricak H, Mc Clure RD. Varicoceles. Radiologic diagnosis and treatment. Radiol Clin North Am. 1991;29(3):619–27.

Ferguson JM, Gillespie IN, Chalmers N, Elton RA, Hargreave TB. Percutaneous varicocele embolization in the treatment of infertility. Br J Radiol. 1995;68:700–3.

Greiner M, Le Pennec V. Embolisation des varicocèles testiculaires. In: « recommandations de bonnes pratiques en radiologie vasculaire interventionnelle 2007 », Sous la direction de H. Vernhet, SFICV Ed 2007

Marsman JWP. The aberrantly fed varicoceles: frequency, venographic appearance and results of transcatheter embolization. Am J Roentgenol. 1995;164:649–57.

Nieschlag E, Behre HM, Schlingheider A, et al. Surgical ligation vs angiographic embolization of the vena spermatica: a prospective randomized study for the treatment of varicocele related infertility. Andrologia. 1993;25:233–7.

Chapter 16
Embolization of the Internal Pudendal Arteries for High-Flow Priapism

Louis Boyer, Anne Ravel, Laurent Guy, Romain Bellini, Jean-Marc Garcier, and Pascal Chabrot

16.1 Background

Low-flow priapism is due to the obstruction of the venous return, which can be of hematologic, iatrogenic origin or secondary to a spinal cord injury. It is painful and constitutes a urologic emergency, because it exposes the patient to cavernous ischemia. In comparison, high-flow priapism, which is linked to a prolonged, unregulated increase in the arterial flow, is a lot less frequent. It is not painful and does not evolve towards an ischemia and is generally secondary to a perineal or direct-penile trauma. Symptoms are often well tolerated (hence explaining the sometimes prolonged delay before reference); they include a non-painful penis that is not as rigid as in the venoocclusive priapisms, as well as signs of "perineal compression": partial or total detumescence at perineal digital pressure. A puncture with washing out of the corpus cavernosum classically permitted to distinguish low-flow from

L. Boyer, MD, PhD (✉) • A. Ravel, MD • P. Chabrot, MD, PhD
Department of Radiology,
University Hospital of Clermont-Ferrand,
Clermont-Ferrand, France
e-mail: lboyer@chu-clermontferrand.fr;
pchabrot@chu-clermontferrand.fr

L. Guy, MD, PhD
Department of Urology,
University Hospital of Clermont-Ferrand,
Clermont-Ferrand, France

R. Bellini, MD
Department of Radiology, Jean Perrin Cancer Centre,
Clermont-Ferrand, France

J.-M. Garcier, MD, PhD
Department of Anatomy and Radiology,
University Hospital of Clermont-Ferrand,
Clermont-Ferrand, France

P. Chabrot, L. Boyer (eds.), *Embolization*,
DOI 10.1007/978-1-4471-5182-1_16, © Springer-Verlag London 2014

high-flow priapisms with in the latter case bright red blood and arterial oxygen level; it is today only necessary when the diagnosis of high-flow priapism is dubious (absence of obvious traumatic etiology, painful erection, recurrence of symptoms, risk factors for a venoocclusive priapism). Duplex Doppler ultrasound can also confirm a high-flow priapism and sometimes permits the location of some fistulas.

16.2 Relevant Radiological Anatomy

The penis is principally made up of erectile tissues: corpus spongiosum caped at its extremity by the glans and the two corpus cavernosa.

- The corpus spongiosum contains the perineal and penile urethra (anterior urethra); it is enveloped by the bulbo-spongy muscles. Its swollen posterior end (bulb) is located in front of the central tendon of the perineum. The corpus cavernosa are attached to the ischiopubic branches, enveloped by ischiocavernous muscles.
- The glans seems to extend the corpus spongiosum but keeps a structural independence.
- Erectile tissues join together under the pubic symphysis, firmly fixed at the anterior part of the pelvic skeleton.

The arteries of the erectile tissues of the penis arise from the internal pudendal arteries; their origin varies with respect to the division model of the internal iliac artery. The internal pudendal artery is classically the terminal branch of its anterior trunk, but it can arise very high or very distally (small sciatic notch). It sometimes originates from a common trunk with the superior and/or inferior gluteal arteries. An accessory pudendal artery (6–10 %) can arise from the obturator artery, from the ischiatic artery, or directly from the internal iliac artery.

After giving off the artery of the bulb of the penis which courses into the corpus spongiosum and the urethral artery, it gives off the deep artery of the penis which vascularizes the corpus cavernosum and ends in the dorsal artery of the penis which courses along the surface of the corpus cavernosum.

The anastomosis between the left and right network normally occurs in the distal part of the dorsal artery of the penis, at the level of the glans.

This vascularization is not always symmetric; predominance on one side or even the birth of two dorsal arteries of the penis from the same pudendal artery can be observed.

16.3 Technique

- Local anesthesia.
- A cysto-catheter maintains bladder voiding, thus simplifying the selective catheterization when the procedure is prolonged.

- We prefer bilateral punctures of the femoral arteries and access of the hypogastric arteries via a crossover catheterization, from the contralateral puncture site. Vasodilators can be used in case of spasm or, for some authors, as a preventive measure.
- An aortography and selective hypogastric artery injections are performed first, and then a superselective catheterization of the internal pudendal arteries can be carried out. The fistula appears as an extravasation of contrast medium at the level of the penis, from the terminal branches of the internal pudendal artery. The micro-catheter must be positioned as close as possible to the arterio-cavernous fistula.
- Several occlusion agents have been used (autologous clot, absorbable gelatin sponge, biological glues, coils, etc.). According to the AUA recommendations, we prefer absorbable gelatin sponge, easy to handle, even with a micro-catheter, and whose absorption usually after about 3 weeks is very interesting when considering the preservation of the erectile function.

We systematically carry out a contralateral opacification, to detect possible contralateral participation in the feeding of the fistula, and if necessary perform a bilateral embolization using absorbable agents.

16.4 Results

In the review of the AUA, respective rates of technical success and erectile dysfunction of 74 and 5 % are reported after an embolization with absorbable agents, against 78 % success and 39 % erectile dysfunction after an embolization using nonabsorbable agents (coils, PVA particles, glues).

Technical success is confirmed by penile detumescence which is usually observed within hours following the procedure. The evaluation of the erectile function can be made after a few weeks.

Complications related to the procedure are rare (ecchymosis, pain at the injection site, puncture site complications).

16.5 Indications

The aim of treatment is to occlude the fistula and obtain the detumescence, without altering the erectile function.

- Conservative treatment represents a first-line therapeutic option, as a spontaneous resolution of the problem may occur and because of the potential risk of erectile dysfunction after embolization. Furthermore, these priapisms are not painful and do not preclude a normal sexual activity for several. But the long-term effects of high-flow priapism on the erectile tissue have in fact not yet been clearly determined.

- Surgery was the traditional treatment for high-flow priapisms (ligation of the cavernous artery or exploratory corporotomy and in situ micro-ligation of the fistula). The AUA reported a 63 % success rate after surgery, but 50 % erectile dysfunction, and therefore recommends surgery with prior ultrasound guidance as the ultimate alternative, after failure of embolization.
- For the AUA, embolization can be carried out at the patient's request, after informed consent of the procedure risks, of the possibility of a spontaneous resolution of the priapism, and of the absence of significant consequence in the case of a delayed intervention.

Kuefer's review compiled published data of 202 patients: 35 treated surgically with a 20 % success rate and 100 patients having had an embolization with an 89 % success rate (the failures were defined by recurrence of the priapism or erectile function disorder).

In our group the embolization using absorbable gelatin sponge is carried out as the first-line treatment of high-flow traumatic priapisms.

Key Points

- A high-flow priapism is generally the consequence of a perineal trauma.
- Embolization can be carried out as the first-line treatment, after explaining the possibility of spontaneous resolution and of the absence of significant consequences of delayed intervention.
- Embolization is generally immediately effective, with an optimal preservation of the long-term erectile function; its morbidity is very limited.
- Absorbable gelatin sponge gives excellent results.
- Once the fistula is treated by a unilateral embolization, it is necessary to check that the contralateral artery is not also feeding the fistula, justifying in such a case a contralateral embolization.

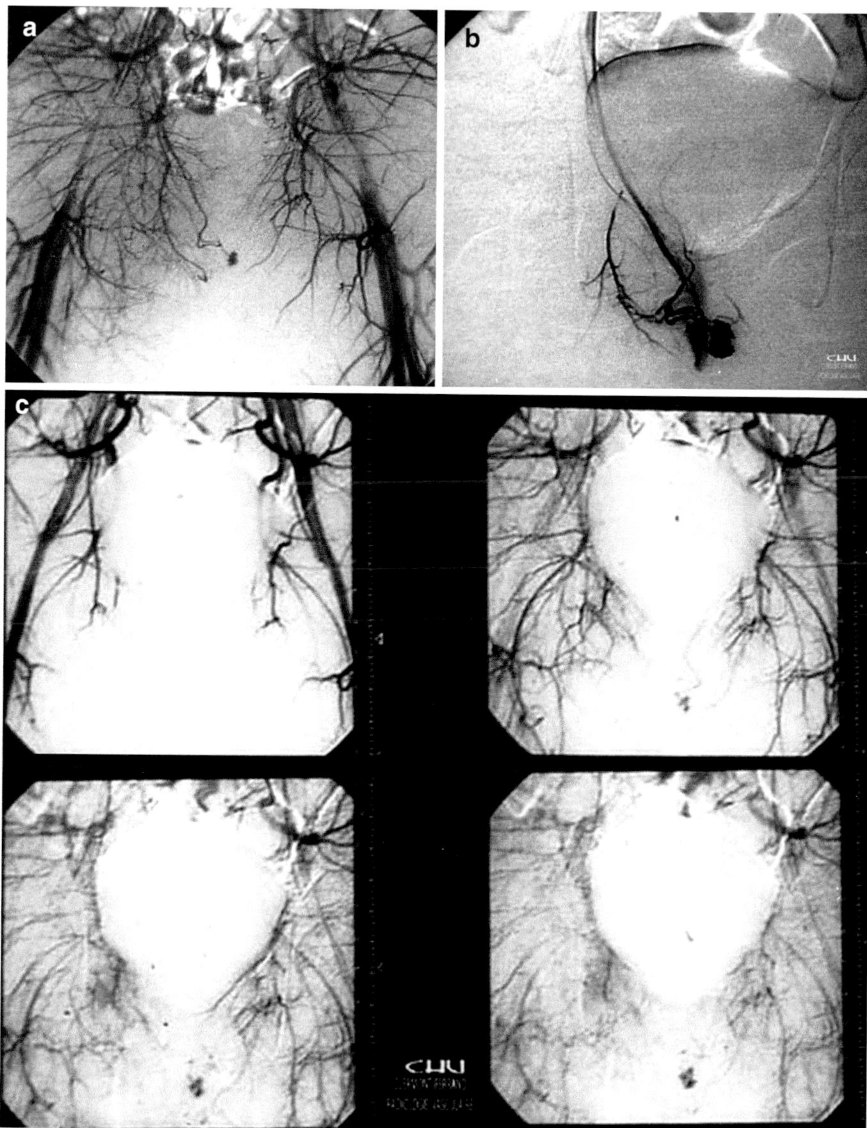

Fig. 16.1 A 12-year-old patient, sustained priapism lasting for 3 days after falling astride on a bar. (**a**) Aortography (injection at the aortoiliac bifurcation): contrast extravasation at the root of the penis. (**b**) Hyperselective catheterization (4 F Cobra catheter): extravasation involving the right internal pudendal artery that was embolized using gelfoam (resorbable gelatin). (**c**) Control aortography: persistent extravasation at the root of the penis. (**d**) Selective catheterization of the left hypogastric artery from a right femoral puncture (crossover), followed by a hyperselective catheterization of the left internal pudendal artery. This artery also contributed to the traumatic cavernous fistula and was also embolized with gelfoam. (**e**) Aortographic final control: exclusion of the fistula

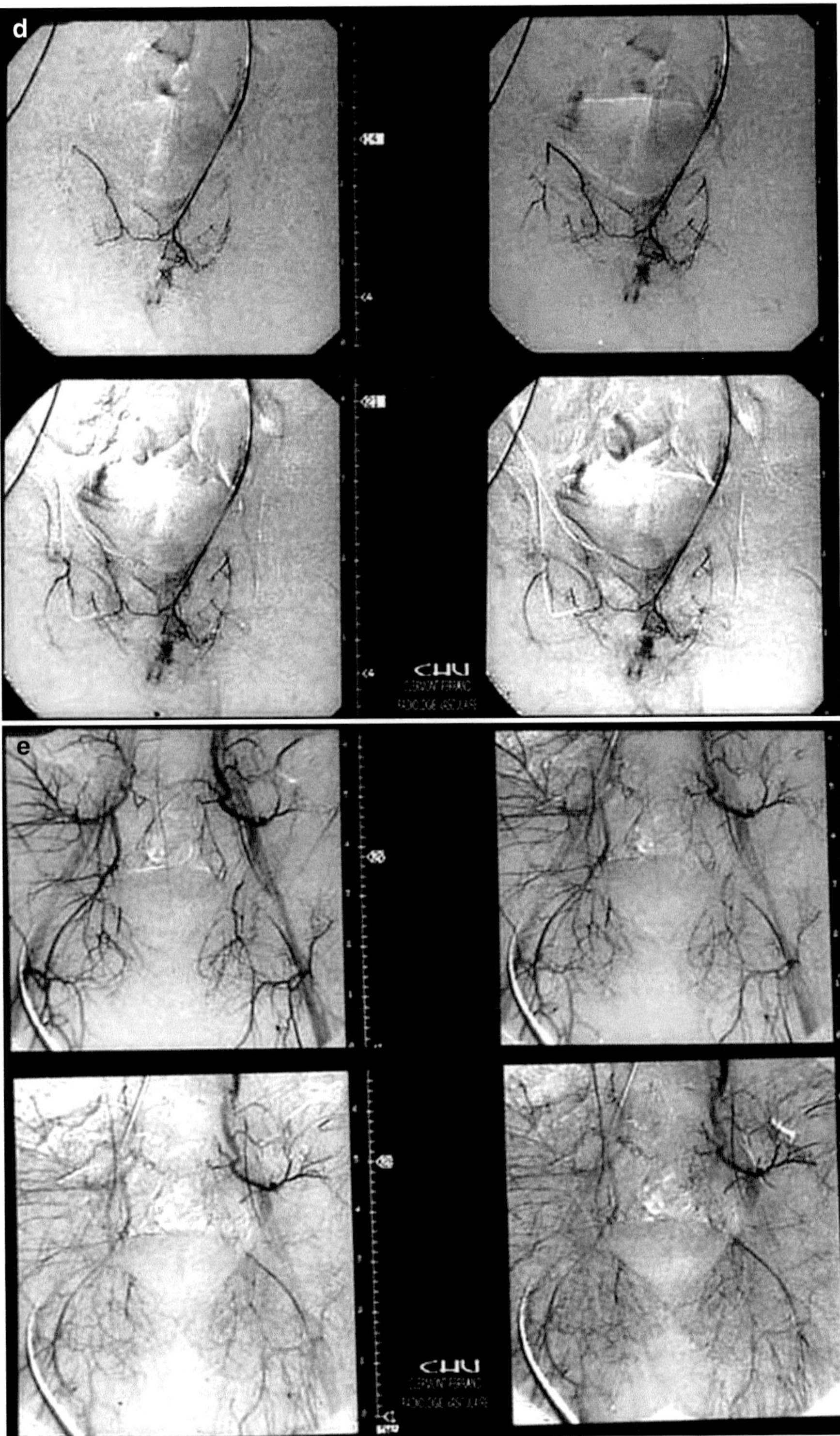

Fig. 16.1 (continued)

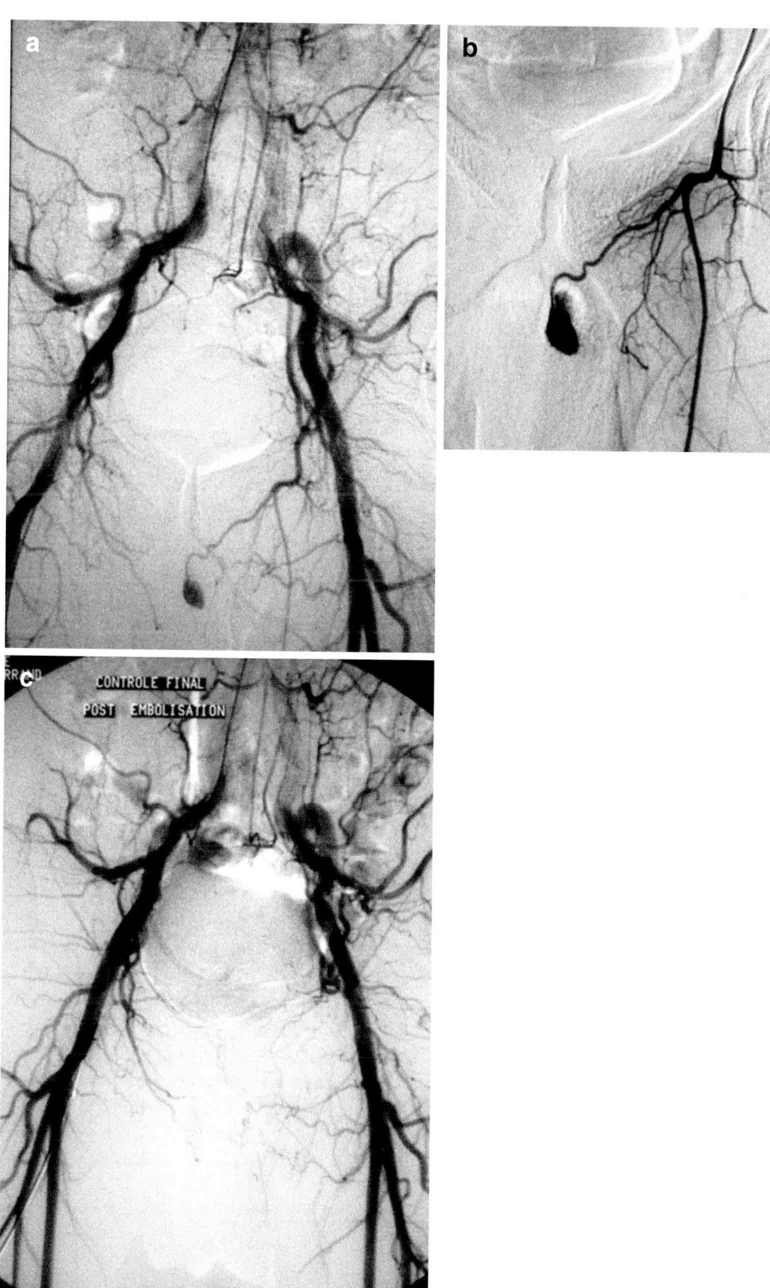

Fig. 16.2 A 25-year-old, highway motorcycle accident: isolated priapism 2 hours later (without any bony traumatic lesion). (**a**) Aortography. Intracavernous extravasation: a left internal pudendal arterial source of the extravasation was suspected. (**b**) From a right femoral artery puncture, a selective catheterization of the left hypogastric artery was performed: it confirmed a significant arterio-cavernous fistula, fed by the left internal pudendal artery. (**c**) Aortographic control (late phase) after embolization of the left internal pudendal artery with resorbable gelatin. Normal erections 1 month later

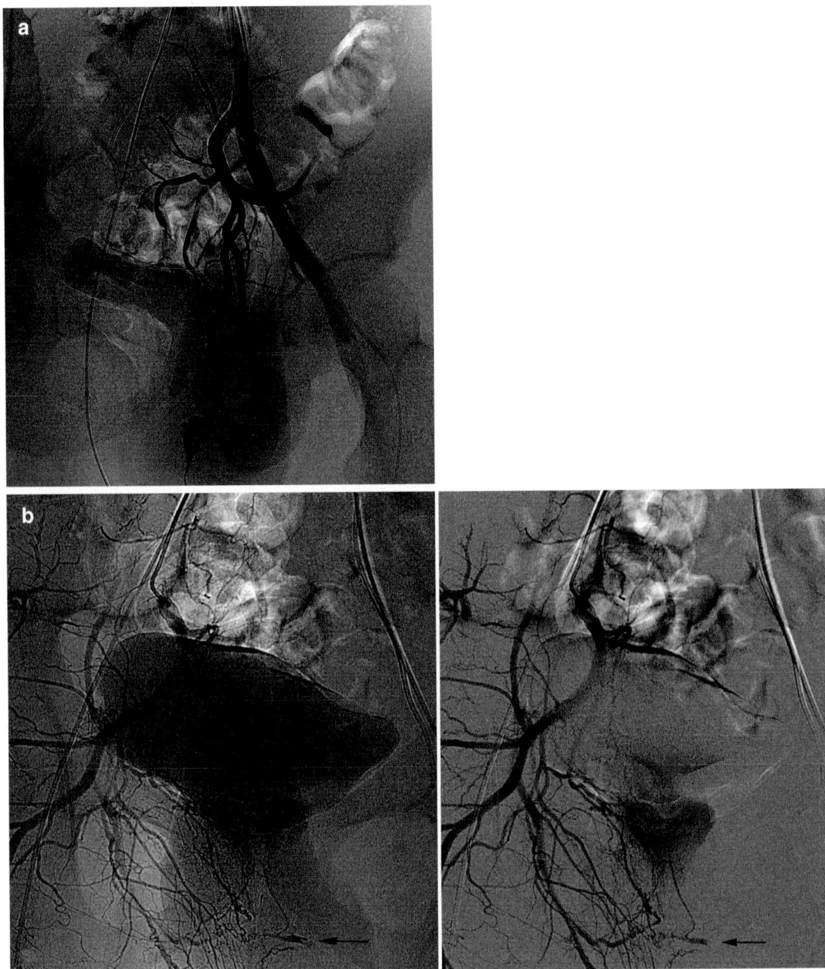

Fig. 16.3 A 23-year-old patient with persistent priapism 10 days after a car accident (driver). No traumatic pelvic bony lesion. (**a**) Selective injection of the left hypogastric artery, from a right femoral puncture: traumatic arterio-cavernous fistula at the root of the penis. Embolization by gelfoam. (**b1**, **b2**) Systematic selective control of the right hypogastric artery: participation of the right internal pudendal artery (*arrow*), leading to an additional hyperselective injection of gelatin

Suggested Reading

American Urological Association. American Urological Association guideline on the management of priapism. J Urol. 2003;170(4 Pt 1):1318–24.

Caumartin Y, Lacoursiere L, Naud A. High-flow priapism an overview of diagnostic and therapeutic concepts. Can J Urol. 2006;13(5):3283–90.

Kim KR, Shin JH, Song HY, et al. Treatment of high-flow priapism with superselective transcatheter embolization in 27 patients : a multicenter study. J Vasc Interv Radiol. 2007;18(10):1222–6.

Kuefer R, Bartsch Jr G, Herkommer K, et al. Changing diagnostic and therapeutic concepts in high-flow priapism. Int J Impot Res. 2005;17(2):109–13.

Montague DK, Jarow J, Broderick GA, et al. Members of the Erectile Dysfunction Guideline Update Panel. J Urol. 1986;135:142–7.

O'Sullivan P, Browne R, McEniff N, Lee MJ. Treatment of "high-flow" priapism with superselective transcatheter embolization : a useful alternative to surgery. Cardiovasc Intervent Radiol. 2006;29(2):198–201.

Chapter 17
Embolization of Endoleaks After Endovascular Abdominal Aortic Aneurysm Repair (EVAR)

Pascal Chabrot, Gérald Gahide, Lucie Cassagnes, Gilles Soulez, Louis Boyer, and Eric Therasse

17.1 Background

A persisting blood flow in the aneurysm sac is one of the main concerns of endovascular treatment of aortic aneurysms. The frequency of these endoleaks after EVAR varies from 15 to 50 % [1, 2]. The persisting blood pressure in the aneurysm sac exposes to the risk of rupture [3].

Depending on their source, location, or mechanism, endoleaks can be classified as follows [4–8]:

- *Type I*: leaks occurring at the proximal neck (IA) or distal (IB) end of the stent graft.
- *Type II*: coming from a branch of the aorta, most often lumbar or inferior mesenteric artery (IMA) with endovascular aortic repair (EVAR), subclavian or intercostal with thoracic endovascular aneurysm repair (TEVAR). Certain authors make a difference between a simple type II, where the entry and the exit take place by the same artery, and the complex type II, where the input and the output are two distinct vessels. This last type would more likely rupture.

P. Chabrot, MD, PhD (✉) • L. Cassagnes, MD • L. Boyer, MD, PhD
Department of Radiology,
University Hospital of Clermont-Ferrand, Clermont-Ferrand, France
e-mail: pchabrot@chu-clermontferrand.fr; lboyer@chu-clermontferrand.fr

G. Gahide, MD, PhD
Department of Radiology, Sherbrooke University Hospital, Sherbrooke, QC, Canada

G. Soulez, MD, MSc
Department of Radiology,
University Hospital Notre Dame, Montréal, QC, Canada

E. Therasse, MD, FRCPC
Department of Radiology, Hôtel-Dieu – University of Montréal, Montréal, QC, Canada
Centre Hospitalier de l'Université de Montréal (CHUM),
3840 Saint-Urbain street, H2W 1T8 Montréal, QC, Canada

P. Chabrot, L. Boyer (eds.), *Embolization*,
DOI 10.1007/978-1-4471-5182-1_17, © Springer-Verlag London 2014

- *Type III*: due to a disconnection of the different components of the stent graft, breaking apart, or to a perforated graft.
- *Type IV*: observed uniquely during implantation and due to a prosthetic porosity.
- *Type V*: type V endoleak, also called endotension, is characterized by a progressive increase of the maximum diameter of the aneurysm, without any leak visible on CT.

Endoleaks can be detected at the end of the implantation procedure on the control arteriography or on follow-up imaging (CT scan or MRI).

The types I and III most often require a rapid treatment.

Initially, the type II endoleaks were considered as being negligible due to the fact that in 50 % of the cases, a spontaneous resolution is observed. However, this type can bring about an aneurysmal rupture. Their treatment thus varies according to the persistence and/or the progression of the diameter of the aneurysm.

Type V endoleaks are surgically treated.

17.2 Relevant Radiological Anatomy

After EVAR, type II endoleaks most often concern the IMA or the lumbar arteries. Even if the leak is clearly depicted on cross-sectional imaging, undertaking an arteriography is most often mandatory to precisely define the anatomy, the hemodynamics of the arterial entries and exits, and the technical feasibility of an embolization.

Mesenteric anastomoses: Accessing the IMA is most frequently done through the Riolan's arch, passing by the left branch of the middle colic artery (issuing from the SMA), towards the ascending branch of the left colic artery, issuing from the IMA. The marginal artery of Drummond is very rarely usable.

Iliolumbar anastomoses: Accessing the lumbar arteries is done through iliolumbar anastomoses coming from the posterior trunk of the internal iliac arteries (IIA), or sometimes from the deep circumflex iliac arteries.

17.3 Techniques

17.3.1 Type I Endoleaks

17.3.1.1 Type IA (Proximal)

The proximal type I endoleaks are more likely to occur if the neck is short, irregular, angular, or conical [9].

If the type IA endoleak is depicted while expanding the stent graft, a compliant balloon angioplasty is the first choice technique to treat it.

However, if this approach is not sufficient and the stent graft mebrane is just under the origin of the renal arteries and if the stent-grafted portion of the aneurysm neck is not too dilated or infiltrated, a balloon-expandable bare stent (Palmaz®) can be used. These stents improve the stiffness and the adhesion to the neck, at the same time respecting the renal artery perfusion.

If there is at least a 5 mm-long segment of infrarenal neck that is not covered by the stent graft mebrane or if distal migration of the stent graft is noted, insertion of a proximal extension cuff having a trans- or suprarenal fixations (Cook, Talent, Endurant) is recommanded [1].

If the infrarenal neck covered by the endovascular graft is too short and/or of bad quality, and if the suprarenal aorta is of good quality, setting up a fenestrated stent graft can be considered.

Surgery stays the last option if the abovementioned endovascular approaches are not possible.

17.3.1.2 Type IB (Distal)

Distal endoleaks are usually accessible to an iliac extension, which can be associated with a prior embolization of the IIA if the extension must be prolonged up to the external iliac artery.

Indications of surgery in case of failure are less frequent than for proximal leaks (IA).

17.3.2 Type II Endoleaks

17.3.2.1 Access

- Endovascular Approach: Catheterization of the Collateral Networks
  - Mesenteric artery catheterization: After a selective opacification of the SMA (4 or 5 French diagnostic catheter: Chuang, Glidecath, Sim, or Cobra), the proximal middle colic artery is catheterized using a micro-catheter. In order to limit a vasospasm, a vasodilator may be injected. A control injection is performed to detail the anastomosis of the ascending left colic artery. The origin of the IMA is progressively catheterized with the micro-catheter. Here the choice of the lengths of both the 4 French catheter and the micro-catheter is very important, the distance to cover being relatively long: for the 4 French cath, a 60 cm catheter allows a sufficiently proximal catheterization to be obtained, at the same time limiting the length of the catheter outside of the patient; for the micro-catheter, a length of at least 135 cm is recommended [1].
  - Lumbar artery catheterization: The IIA is catheterized and then opacified, in order to allow a selective catheter to approach the ostium of the iliolumbar

artery (ILA). Due to its limited length, the ILA is directly cannulated by a micro-catheter after a vasodilator injection, to ensure a prudent progression up to the aneurysmal sac. The collateral vessels reopacifying the lumbar arteries are often tortuous and of small size, thus making navigation up to the aneurysmal sac difficult or impossible: in this case, an embolization at some distance from the sac may turn out to be necessary.

- Transparietal Approach: Direct Puncture of the Sac

In the absence or failure of an endovascular approach, the aneurysmal sac can be accessed by a direct puncture. The percutaneous translumbar approach is carried out under CT, or under C-arm CT, or under fluoroscopic guidance after the procedure was planned on CT (angle, depth of the sac, and distance from spinous processes).

The patient is placed in prone position, and the left paravertebral puncture is performed, may been seen and using a Chiba 20G needle (angle 45–60°).

A pulsating blood reflux confirms the puncture of the aneurysmal sac, which is opacified in order to help positioning the micropuncture device, followed by insertion of a 5 French catheter. A micro-catheter may then be used to navigate into the sac and to possibly cannulate the implicated branches.

Depending of the localization of the leak or of possible in-between structures a right paravertebral approach crossing the inferior vena cava may be performed [10, 11], using the same technique, without reported hemorrhaging complication or arteriovenous fistula.

For these approaches, particular attention must be given to the progression of the needle in the area around the stent by doing several fluoroscopic incidences, in order to avoid puncturing the graft.

17.3.2.2 Embolization Strategy

Embolization of the only afferent or only the efferent artery is marked by an important endoleak recurrence rate: Baum et al. reported an 80 % recurrence rate after an embolization of the origin of the IMA without embolization of the aneurismal sac or others type II endoleak feeders.

In theory, the exclusion of the afferent vessel, the sac, and the efferent vessel ensure an optimal embolization. In practice this goal is rarely realized:

1. It is often difficult to demonstrate all the implicated branches, even when guided by selective injection into the sac.
2. Catheterizing an efferent or afferent branch after crossing the sac is most often very difficult.

When accessing the aneurysm through an endovascular approach, it is important to try to occlude the sac and the vessel which is giving the access to it. With a transparietal approach, the embolization is often limited to the aneurysmal sac.

17.3.2.3 Embolization Agents

- Coils: Initially used for proximal occlusions, coils can be positioned by endovascular or transparietal access into the aneurysmal sac, with favorable results [12]. The aneurysmal sac is filled by using coils of regularly decreasing diameter. However, these coils will limit the sensitivity of subsequent CT scan controls.
- Liquid agents: Most often the flow crossing the leak is slow. A liquid agent is injected into the sac or close to the ostium through an endovascular approach. The liquid agent spreading towards the origin of the patent collateral network causes their exclusion but can also induce downstream ischemic complications (spinal cord, lumbosacral, or colic ischemia) [13].
- Glue: The injection is performed under fluoroscopic control. The dilution is adapted to the flow and to the topography: generally 1:2 ratio is used in case of lumbar injection (0.5 ml of nBCA and 1 ml of lipiodol) and 1:3 ratio in case of mesenteric injection, so as to limit a possible reflux into the IMA.
- Ethylene vinyl alcohol copolymer (Onyx®; eV3, Covidien Vascular Therapies, Mansfield, MA, USA): Onyx is a radio-opaque and progressively gelling agent which is rather simple to use. The results already reported seem promising. The approach is most often translumbar; a progressive injection given under fluoroscopic control generally leads to the exclusion of the aneurysmal sac and of the origin of the concerned vessel [14]. The cost of Onyx limits today its use, especially for voluminous sacs. They are few long-term results concerning the sustainability of the embolization are available. A strong radio-opacity is an important drawback for the CT scan follow-up.
- Thrombin: Its advantages are its cost and the ease of use [13] to treat type II endoleaks. This radiolucent agent is slowly injected after having opacified the sac. The progressive but massive character of the thrombosis makes it difficult to use in a strict endovascular approach because of a major risk of retrograde embolization.

17.4 Results

The reintervention rate after aortic stent graft varies between 10 and 27 %. The initial technical success rate of these secondary interventions, mostly performed through an endovascular approach, varies depending on the type of endoleak: between 50 and 90 % for type I, 57–80 % for type II, and around 75 % for type III [1, 15, 16].

The long-term results are heterogeneous according to the nature of the leak and the different treatment methods. The treatment of endoleaks should be compared to that of arteriovenous malformations: exclsusion of only the afferent artery using coils is insufficient, thus explaining the high failure rates reported in the first series [17] and the favorable results observed after a direct embolization of the sac [18].

In case of type I endoleaks, when possible, treatment with a proximal or distal extension most often gives a durable exclusion.

In case of type II endoleaks, the recurrence rate 1 year after embolization of only the origin of the affected vessel reaches 80 %; on the other hand, an embolization of the sac and its afferent vessels allows a 93 % durable success rate to be achieved in the Baum series [17].

The optimal embolization agent has not yet been determined. The limited number of cases and the variability of the techniques do not allow a comparison of the different agents (coils, thrombin, glue, Onyx). However, a liquid agent allows an easier embolization of the sac and the afferent vessels.

17.5 Indications

- Type I and III endoleaks require treatment because they lead to aneurismal sac pressure equivalent to the systemic blood pressure and, hence, make the SG ineffective to protect the aneurism from rupture.
- For type II endoleaks, the indirect communication via the parietal collateral (iliolumbar, intercostals) or visceral (mesenteric, renal polar) vessels induces a less important pressure into the aneurismal sac. However, the risk of rupture is present if the aneurism increases in size [19]. For most of the authors, endoleaks lasting for more than 6–12 months, associated with a progression of the aneurysmal sac (5 mm or 10 %), are indications for treatment.

Key Points

- Reintervention after EVAR are frequent
- Type I and III endoleaks: major risk of evolution; systematic treatment; according to the characteristics of the neck: bare stent, extension with an endovascular graft (suprarenal or trans-renal fixation), fenestrated stent graft, or surgery
- Type II endoleaks: potential risk of evolution; must be treated if there is growth of the anuerysm (the spontaneous regression rate is about 50 %); ostial occlusion of the IMA is insufficient; transparietal access is required if an endovascular access do not give a satisfactory embolization of the sac or as a second choice in the case of a failure after an endovascular approach.

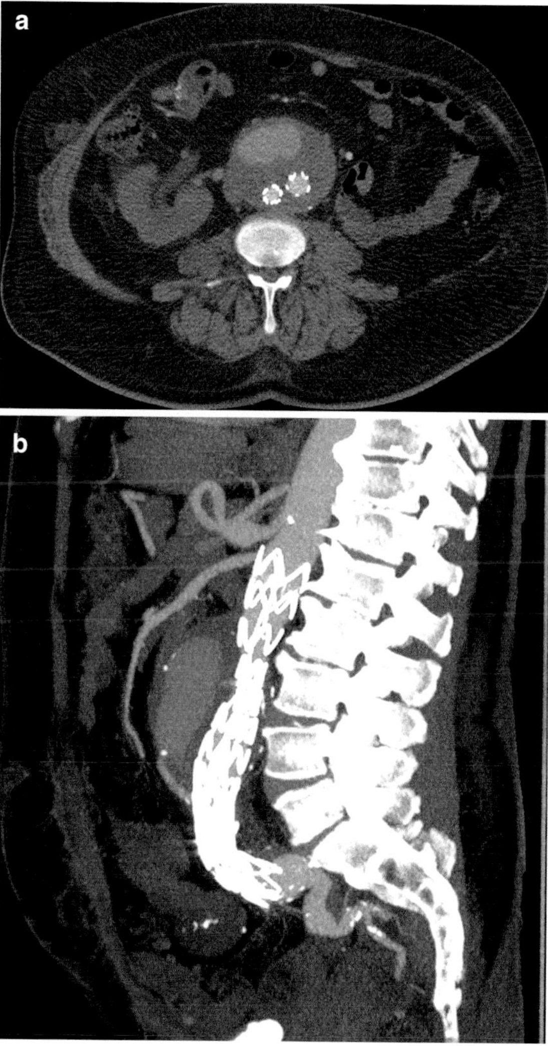

Fig. 17.1 A 69-year-old patient, with end-stage renal failure, under hemodialysis for several years. An infrarenal abdominal aortic aneurysm was treated by stent graft (EVAR) 2 years ago. Due to the oligo-anuric renal failure, it was accepted to cover a right accessory renal artery, originating low in the aorta (L4) follow-up of the aneurysmal sac after EVAR showed an increase in size (10 mm in 6 months). (**a**) Arterial phase CT: extra-prosthetic intra-saccular enhancement. (**b**) MIP reconstruction in the sagittal plane, showing a massive enhancement of the sac, from a type 2 endoleak involving the arcade of Riolan. (**c**) MPR reconstruction. (**d**) Aortography, early phase (from a right femoral catheterization): the arcade of Riolan is very early injected. (**e**) Selective catheterization of the middle colic artery (branch of the SMA) (early phase). (**f**) Selective catheterization, via the arcade of Riolan, of the IMA and of the extra-prosthetic sac and then of the low lumbar right renal artery. (**g**) Control after occlusion by coils of the low lumbar right renal artery. (**h**) Exclusion of the sac by glue embolization (Histoacryl). (**i**) Control after coiling at the origin of the IMA, whose branches stay perfused by the arcade of Riolan

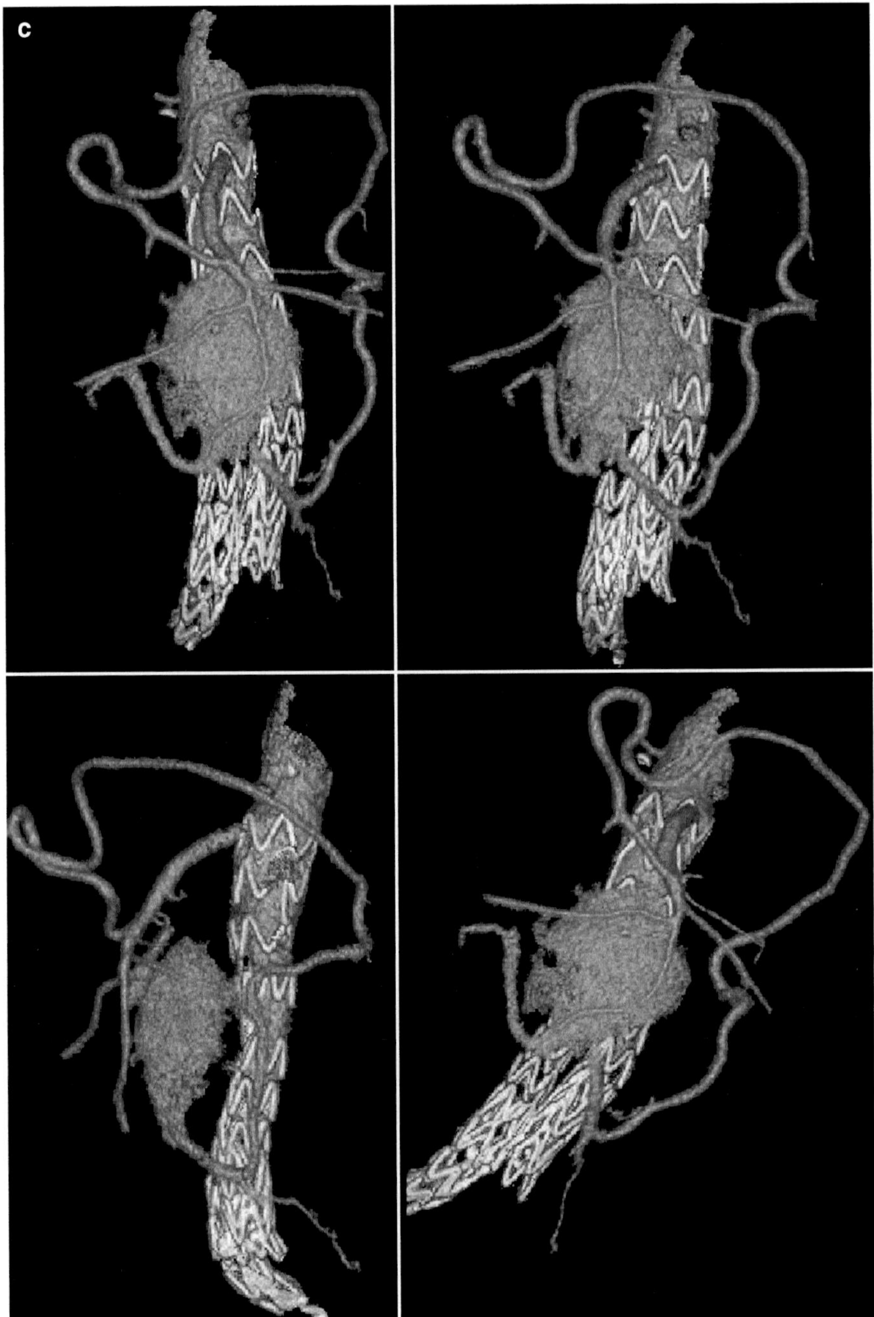

Fig. 17.1 (continued)

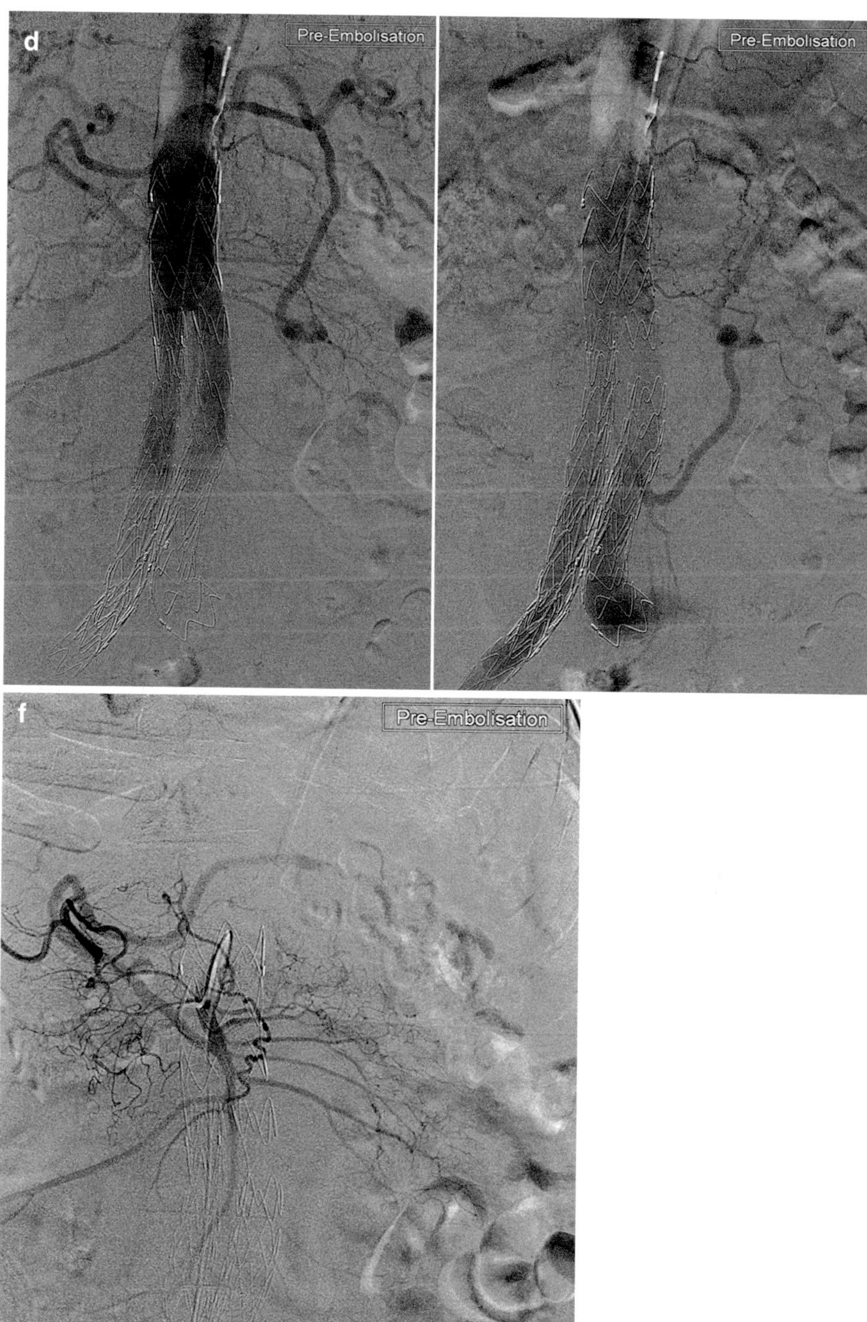

Fig. 17.1 (continued)

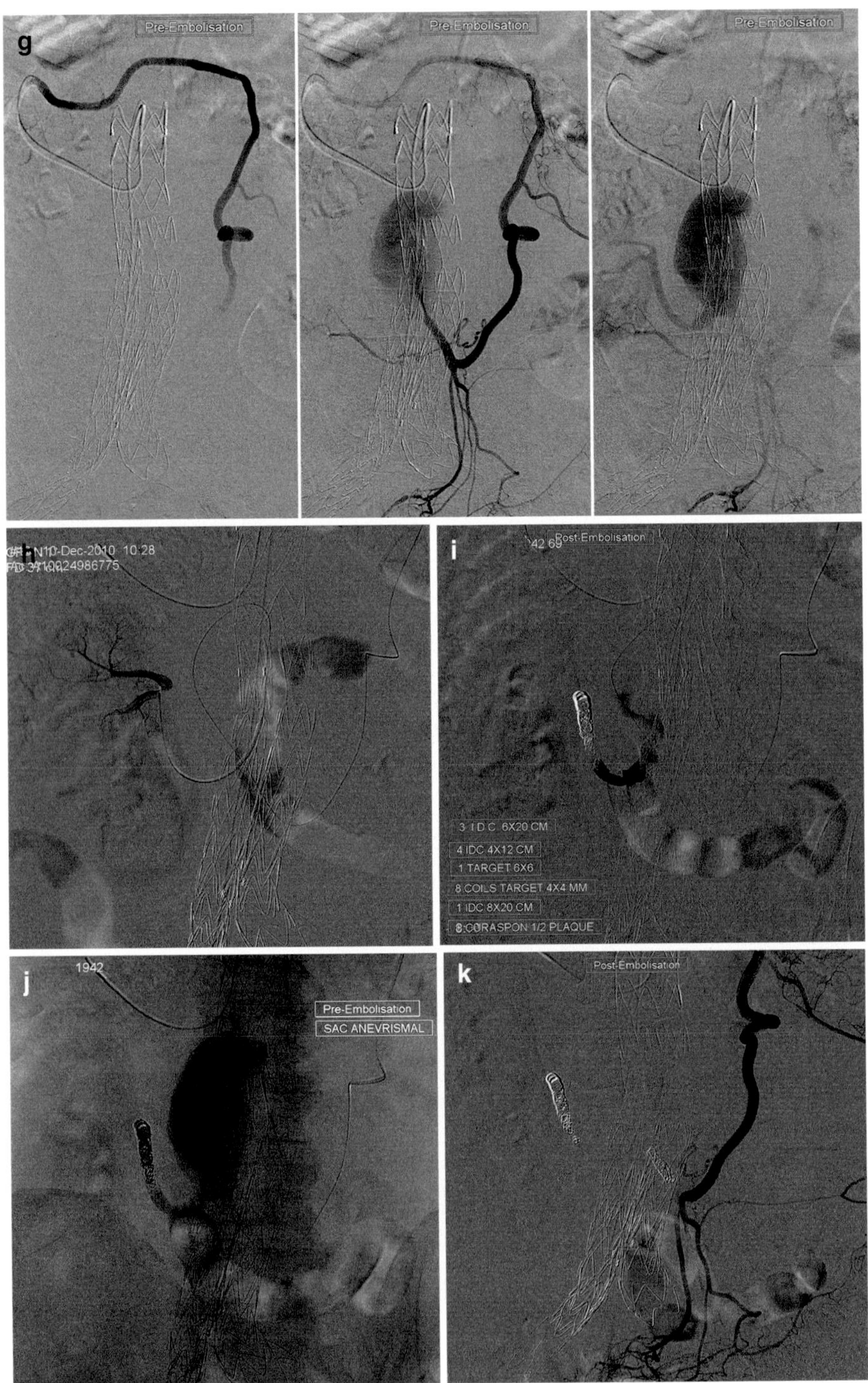

Fig. 17.1 (continued)

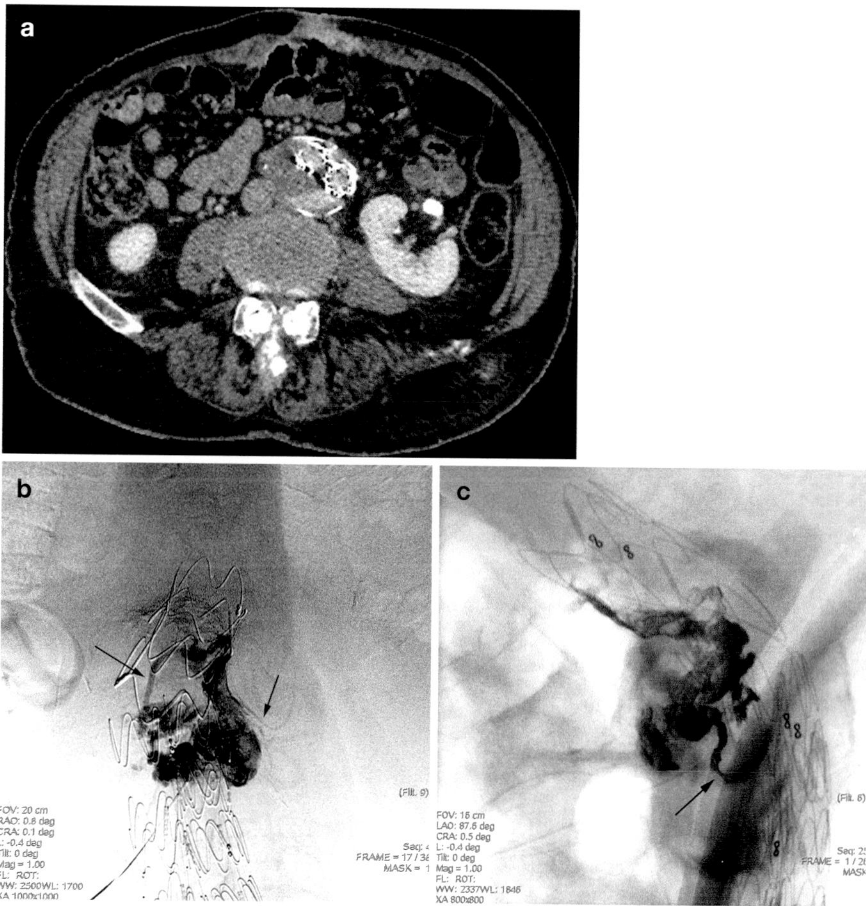

Fig. 17.2 A 67-year-old, with increasing abdominal aortic aneurism diameter 18 months after EVAR (aorto-bi-iliac stent graft). Follow-up CT showed a type II lumbar endoleak, inaccessible to an endovascular treatment. (**a**) CT showing posterior endoleak fed by a lumbar artery. (**b**) (AP) and (**c**) (lateral): Periprosthetic endosaccular access via a CT-guided transparietal puncture: injection of Onyx. Note the opacification of two lumbar arteries (*arrows*)

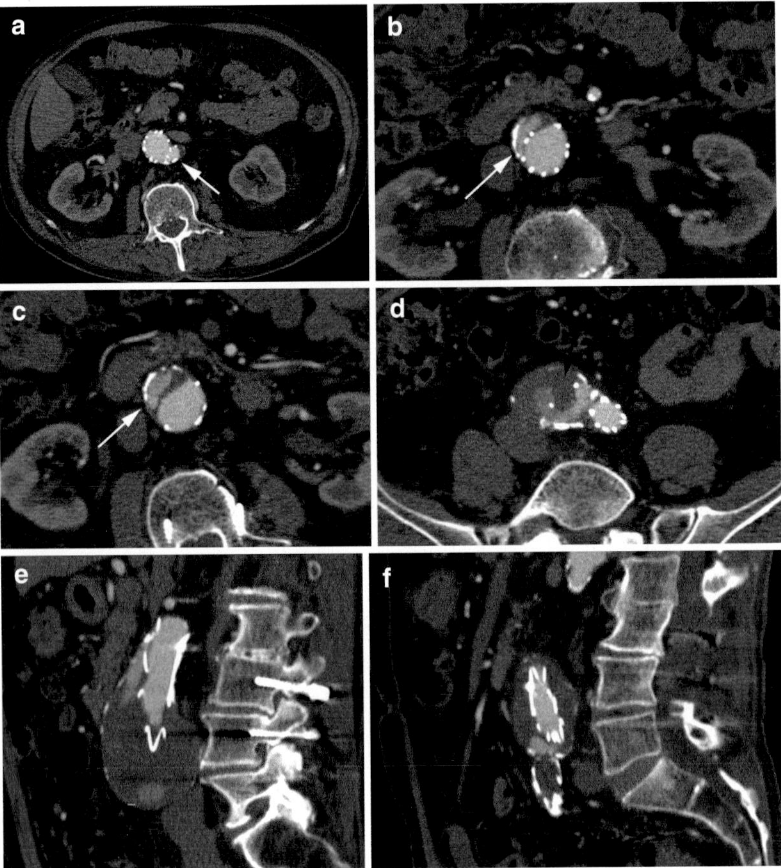

Fig. 17.3 A 83-year-old M, EVAR (aortoiliac stent graft) 3 years ago to treat an infrarenal aortic abdominal aneurysm. An occlusion of the right leg after few weeks had led to a suprapubic left-right cross bypass. Annual CT follow-up has shown an increase in size of the sac. Which was caused by various endoleaks: *type 1*, due to a continuous growth in diameter of aorta above the stentgraft; *type 2*, via lumbar arteries, which seemed contingent; and finally suspected *type 3* endoleak due to the imperfect coaptation between the aortic piece and the left iliac leg of the stent graft. (**a**) CT scan at the upper extremity of the stent graft, at the level of the ostium of the left renal artery (*arrow*). (**b–d**) Scans below the previous: endosaccular extra-prosthetic anterior enhancement (*arrows*), occluded right leg of the endoprosthesis (*black arrow*). (**e**, **f**) Sagittal CT reconstruction: type 1 endoleak; reconstruction passing through the right leg (3–6): type 3 endoleak. (**g**) Aortography conducted via a left humeral access (pigtail), a guidewire was also led via a left femoral access. Late phase (**h**): right endosaccular extra-prosthetic enhancement (*arrow*) (note the presence of a bone screw, from a previous spine surgery). (**i**, **j**) The type 1 endoleak was confirmed by selective catheterization, using a Mikaelsson catheter inserted between the proximal uncovered petals of the stent graft. (**k**) Coils (*arrows*) were positioned in the flowing phase of the endoleak; then a cuff (short cylindrical stent graft) was deployed at the upper neck. On this image, before the release of the cuff, note the ostium of the left renal artery catheterized by a guidewire brought via the humeral access. (**l**) Control after coiling and expansion of the cuff: exclusion of the type 1endoleak. (**m**, **n**) Type 3 endoleak is not clearly shown by the injections at the lower part of the aorta; occlusion of the left prosthetic branch; coils in the right hypogastric artery (that preceded the stent grafting implantation, to avoid reinjection); good patency of the left hypogastric artery, downstream of the stent graft; suprapubic left-right cross bypass. However, a complementary left iliac stent graft was deployed to cover the prosthetic aortoiliac anastomosis. (**o**, **p**) Final control opacification

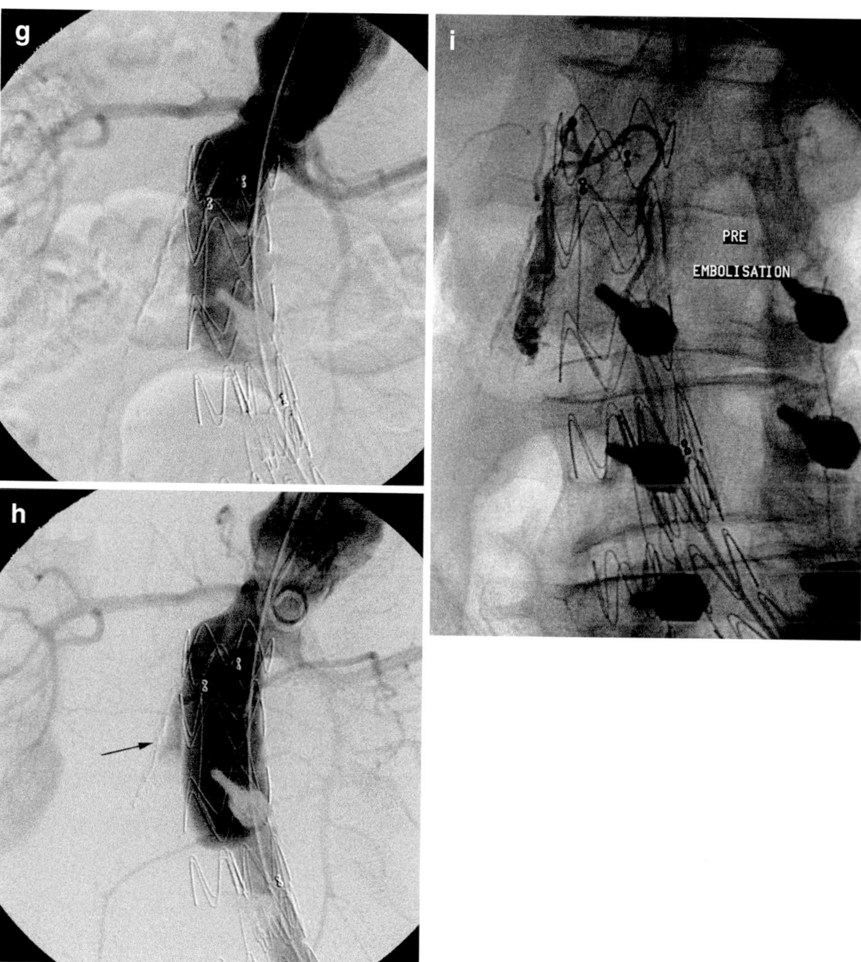

Fig. 17.3 (continued)

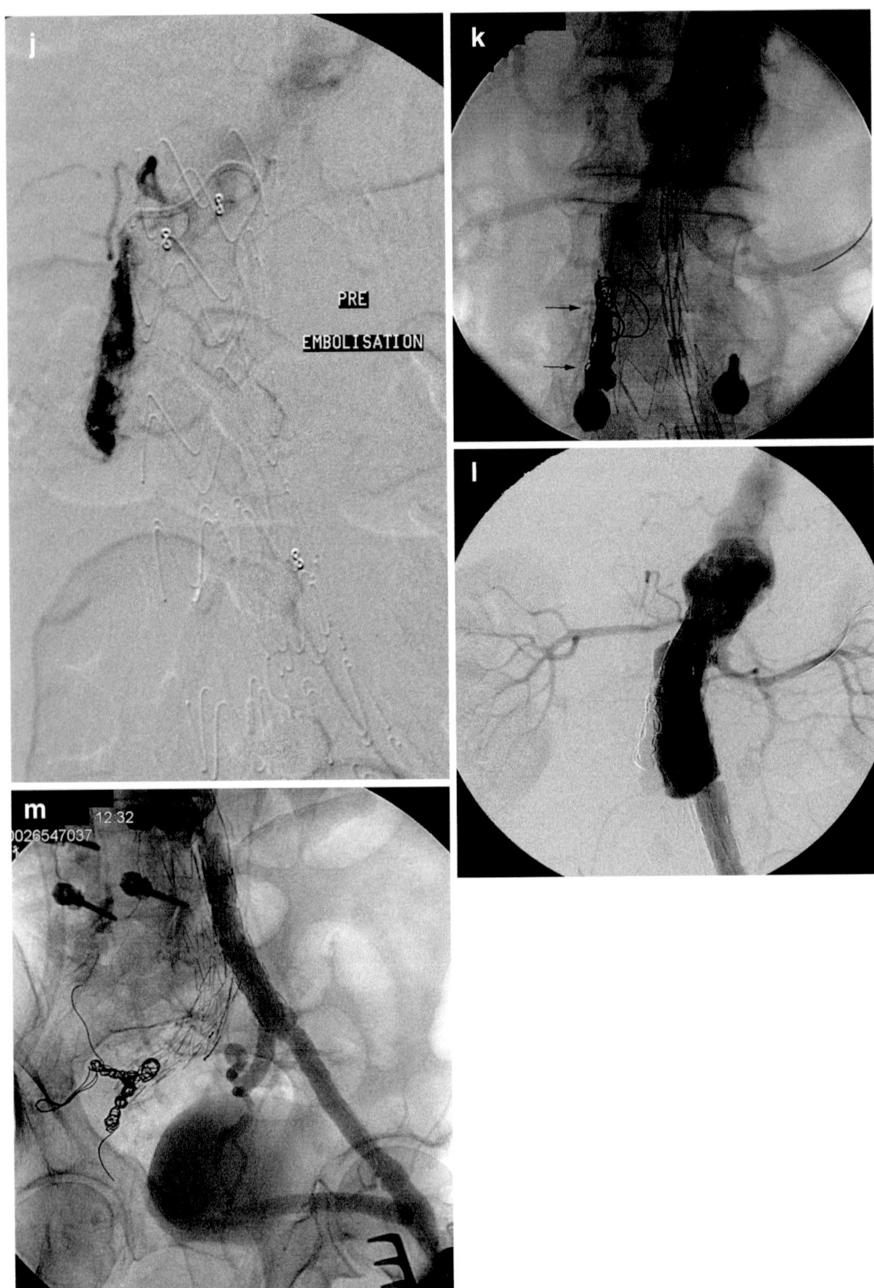

Fig. 17.3 (continued)

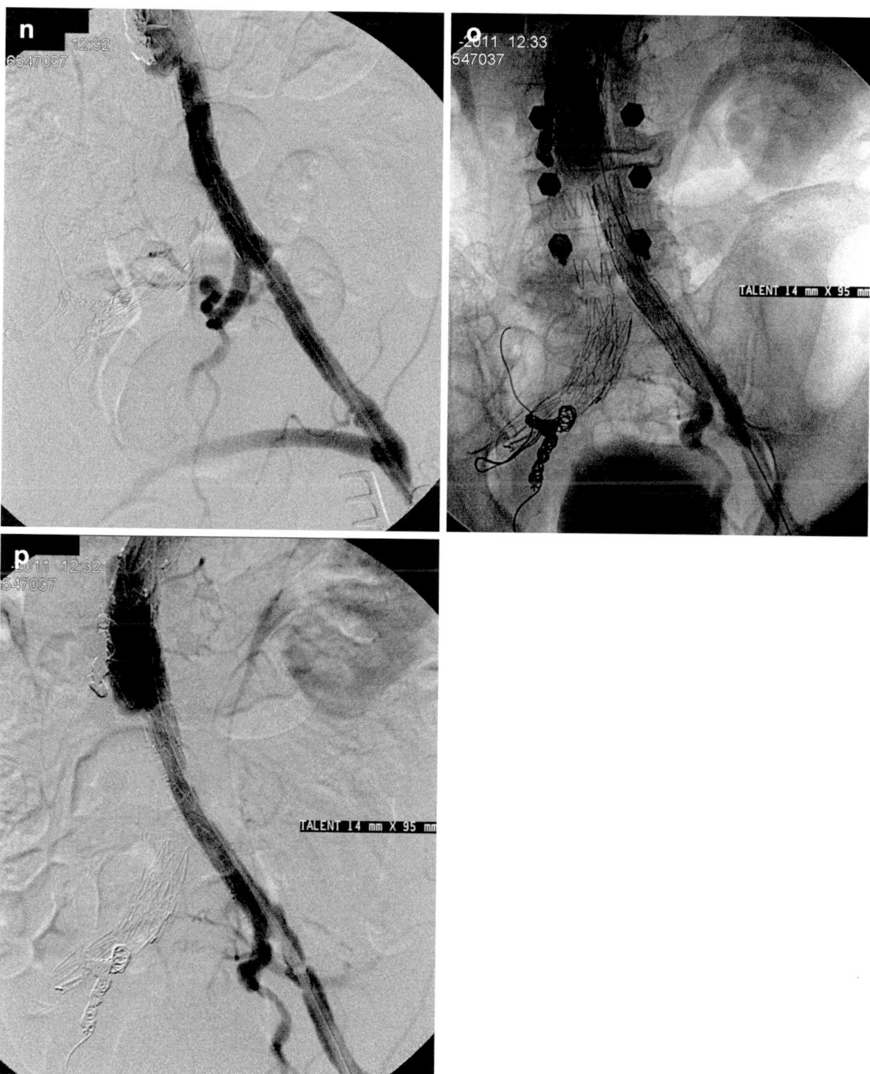

Fig. 17.3 (continued)

References

1. Becquemin JP, et al. Outcomes of secondary interventions after abdominal aortic aneurysm endovascular repair. J Vasc Surg. 2004;39(2):298–305.
2. Ohki T, et al. Increasing incidence of midterm and long-term complications after endovascular graft repair of abdominal aortic aneurysms: a note of caution based on a 9-year experience. Ann Surg. 2001;234(3):323–34; discussion 334–5.
3. Baum RA, et al. Aneurysm sac pressure measurements after endovascular repair of abdominal aortic aneurysms. J Vasc Surg. 2001;33(1):32–41.
4. Veith FJ, et al. Nature and significance of endoleaks and endotension: summary of opinions expressed at an international conference. J Vasc Surg. 2002;35(5):1029–35.
5. White GH, et al. Type III and type IV endoleak: toward a complete definition of blood flow in the sac after endoluminal AAA repair. J Endovasc Surg. 1998;5(4):305–9.
6. White GH, et al. Type I and Type II endoleaks: a more useful classification for reporting results of endoluminal AAA repair. J Endovasc Surg. 1998;5(2):189–91.
7. White GH, Yu W, May J. Endoleak – a proposed new terminology to describe incomplete aneurysm exclusion by an endoluminal graft. J Endovasc Surg. 1996;3(1):124–5.
8. Wain RA, et al. Endoleaks after endovascular graft treatment of aortic aneurysms: classification, risk factors, and outcome. J Vasc Surg. 1998;27(1):69–78; discussion 78–80.
9. Dias NV, et al. Intraoperative proximal endoleaks during AAA stent-graft repair: evaluation of risk factors and treatment with Palmaz stents. J Endovasc Ther. 2001;8(3):268–73.
10. Stavropoulos SW, et al. Inferior vena cava traversal for translumbar endoleak embolization after endovascular abdominal aortic aneurysm repair. J Vasc Interv Radiol. 2003;14(9 Pt 1):1191–4.
11. Baum RA, et al. Translumbar embolization of type 2 endoleaks after endovascular repair of abdominal aortic aneurysms. J Vasc Interv Radiol. 2001;12(1):111–6.
12. Sheehan MK, et al. Effectiveness of coiling in the treatment of endoleaks after endovascular repair. J Vasc Surg. 2004;40(3):430–4.
13. Zanchetta M, et al. Intraoperative intrasac thrombin injection to prevent type II endoleak after endovascular abdominal aortic aneurysm repair. J Endovasc Ther. 2007;14(2):176–83.
14. Martin ML, et al. Treatment of type II endoleaks with Onyx. J Vasc Interv Radiol. 2001;12(5):629–32.
15. Conrad MF, et al. Secondary intervention after endovascular abdominal aortic aneurysm repair. Ann Surg. 2009;250(3):383–9.
16. Sampram ES, et al. Nature, frequency, and predictors of secondary procedures after endovascular repair of abdominal aortic aneurysm. J Vasc Surg. 2003;37(5):930–7.
17. Baum RA, et al. Treatment of type 2 endoleaks after endovascular repair of abdominal aortic aneurysms: comparison of transarterial and translumbar techniques. J Vasc Surg. 2002;35(1):23–9.
18. Nevala T, et al. Type II endoleak after endovascular repair of abdominal aortic aneurysm: effectiveness of embolization. Cardiovasc Intervent Radiol. 2010;33(2):278–84.
19. Marty B, et al. Endoleak after endovascular graft repair of experimental aortic aneurysms: does coil embolization with angiographic "seal" lower intraaneurysmal pressure? J Vasc Surg. 1998;27(3):454–61; discussion 462.

Suggested Reading

Becquemin JP, et al. Outcomes of secondary interventions after abdominal aortic aneurysm endovascular repair. J Vasc Surg. 2004;39(2):298–305.

Conrad MF, et al. Secondary intervention after endovascular abdominal aortic aneurysm repair. Ann Surg. 2009;250(3):383–9.

Veith FJ, et al. Nature and significance of endoleaks and endotension: summary of opinions expressed at an international conference. J Vasc Surg. 2002;35(5):1029–35.

Part VII
Situations and Strategies: Female Pelvis

Chapter 18
Postpartum Hemorrhages

Pascal Chabrot, Abdoulaye Ndoye Diop, Denis Gallot, Isabelle Brazzalotto, and Louis Boyer

18.1 Background

Postpartum hemorrhage (PPH) occurs in the 24 h following birth. It is defined by a blood loss equal or greater than 500 ml in the case of a vaginal delivery, or greater than 1,000 ml in the case of cesarean sections. It is considered as severe when the loss is more than 1,000 ml. An early diagnosis therefore depends upon a rigorous quantification of the loss in each collecting pouch. PPH is the leading cause of maternal mortality in France, among which 2/3 of evitable deaths.

After excluding the obvious causes for bleeding (episiotomy, perineal wound), an artificial delivery and a uterine revision must be carried out as well as an instrumental examination of the birth canal, associated with the administration of uterotonics (oxytocics drugs and/or prostaglandins). The persistence of an externalized bleeding beyond 30 min, a uterine atony, or the occurrence of a hemodynamic instability requiring blood volume expansion and/or vasoconstrictors are all signs of a severe PPH, which requires an instrumental hemostasis by embolization or surgery. If the suitable strategy is not available on place and if the hemodynamic conditions allow it, patient transfer must be considered.

Surgical ligation of the hypogastric arteries or their branches does not always allow hemostasis. More recently, various suture techniques have been proposed to

P. Chabrot, MD, PhD (✉) • L. Boyer, MD, PhD
Department of Radiology, University Hospital of Clermont-Ferrand, Clermont-Ferrand, France
e-mail: pchabrot@chu-clermontferrand.fr; lboyer@chu-clermontferrand.fr

A.N. Diop, MD
Department of Radiology, University Hospital, Dakar, Senegal

D. Gallot, MD, PhD
Department of Obstetrics and Gynecology,
University Hospital of Clermont-Ferrand, Clermont-Ferrand, France

I. Brazzalotto, MD
Department of Anesthesia, University Hospital of Clermont-Ferrand, Clermont-Ferrand, France

P. Chabrot, L. Boyer (eds.), *Embolization*,
DOI 10.1007/978-1-4471-5182-1_18, © Springer-Verlag London 2014

compress the uterus, such as Cho or B-Lynch techniques. Hemostatic hysterectomy, preferentially subtotal, presents a high morbi-mortality rate.

18.2 Relevant Radiological Anatomy

The uterus is mainly supplied by the uterine arteries (UA) issuing from the internal iliac arteries (IIA).

The IIA (hypogastric) present many variations. The most frequent configuration (55–77 %) is the bifurcation into an anterior and a posterior trunk, at the level of the superior part of the greater sciatic notch. But there are many other division patterns: a single trunk (≅4 %), three trunks (≅15 %), four trunks, or more (≅3 %); the branches can also come about at once and form a bouquet (≅2 %). In 90 % of cases the mode of division is symmetric. The absence of IIA is rare: all of its branches hence arise from the common iliac artery.

In most of the cases, the uterine artery (UA) originates from the anterior trunk of the IIA, but in different ways depending on its division pattern: in 56 % of the cases, it arises alone from the anterior trunk of the IIA; in 40 % of the cases, from a branch which is common with the umbilical artery; in 2 % of the cases, from the internal pudendal artery; in 2 % of the cases, from a common stem with a long vaginal artery. When the UA emerges from the anterior trunk, its origin is usually correctly depicted on a contralateral anterior oblique view. When it branches off higher, it is best seen on an ipsilateral oblique view. Identifying the origin of the UA is the key to its catheterization.

The caliber of the UA, variable (2–5 mm), is particularly large during pregnancy and immediately after childbirth.

It describes a first descending segment against the pelvic wall, then a horizontal one crossing the ureter, and finally sinuously ascending along the uterus, thus easily recognizable.

Its terminal branches are:

- The artery of the uterine fundus.
- A medial tubal branch, coursing along the fallopian tube, confluent with the lateral tubal branch issuing from the ovarian artery (arising from the aorta at the level of L3).
- A medial ovarian branch coursing along the utero-ovarian ligament, anastomosed with a branch issuing from the ovarian artery. This medial ovarian branch provides the total ovarian supply in 4 % of the cases; it does not participate in the arterial feeding of the ovary in 40 % of the cases and provides it with the lateral ovarian branch in 56 %.

The UA gives several branches: peritoneal, ureteric, vesical, vaginal, and cervical, to the round ligament (anastomosed with the deep inferior epigastric artery).

Its uterine branches are anastomosed with those issuing from the contralateral UA. On the other hand, there are few anastomoses between the cervical and corporeal network. The UA is widely anastomosed with the ipsilateral ovarian and the inferior epigastric arteries.

The UA ensures most of the arterial supply of the uterus, to which the ovarian artery and the artery of the round ligament may contribute.

18.3 Technique

- Embolizations must be carried out in an angio suite with intensive care facilities.

Patient transfer may be necessary, ensured by the mobile emergency unit in agreement with the receiving team (anesthesiologists, gynecologists, vascular radiologists). The following are mandatory: the permanent supervision by an anesthesiologist, a permanent contact with the obstetrical team, as well as a permanent access to blood products, in a time delay of less than 30 min.

Discontinuation of sulprostone treatment upon arrival remains controversial.

- We do not prescribe any systematic prophylactic antibiotics.
- The arterial access is femoral; we prefer a bilateral femoral access, with two operators, to reduce the duration of the procedure and the irradiation.
- A clamped bladder catheter will maintain the bladder partly full and will contribute to hemostasis.
- An aortography specifies any participation of the ovarian arteries and depicts the distribution of the IIA branches. Selective catheterization of the UA is not absolutely necessary: the catheterization of the anterior trunk of the IIA is sufficient. Generally, microcatheters are not used.

A contrast extravasation is observed in less than 50 % of the cases; it is more frequent after a cesarean section.

In case of uterine atony, bilateral embolization of the UA or the anterior trunk of the IIA is performed. Cervico-uterine hemorrhages (placenta previa), vaginal thrombus, and vaginal tears may necessitate an additional embolization of cervico-vaginal branches.

Persistent bleeding or early recurrence after embolization must lead to an exploration of the ovarian arteries and the arteries of the round ligaments (branches of the external iliac artery).

Persistent bleeding or recurrences after surgical ligation must lead to catheterization through and beyond the ligatures or navigation via the collateral network (possibly using microcatheters). Embolization of the residual stump may be necessary.

- In case of atony and even in case of coagulopathy, absorbable gelatin sponge is used.

In the case of vascular wounds or of placenta accreta, microparticles of more than 500 μm diameter will be used.

In the case of an arterial rupture, a false aneurysm, or post-cesarean arteriovenous fistula, coils or glue can be used, if possible only on one side.

- In these young patients whose ovaries are located in the primary X-ray field, it is mandatory to limit irradiation by reducing fluoroscopy and angio series X-ray image rate, by road mapping, variations of angulation of the oblique views, and simultaneous bilateral catheterization, etc.
- Immediate follow-up: monitoring is carried out in an adapted unit (intensive care, recovery room, or resuscitation unit), in order to quickly perform a complementary embolization or surgery if necessary. The introducer sheaths will be removed only when hemodynamic and hemostatic stability is obtained.

18.4 Results

18.4.1 Immediate Results

- In the case of uterine atony or cervico-vaginal tear, primary success ranges from 73 to 100 %.

  A rebleeding during the first 24 h is possible: 12/194 during our 10 years of experience, for which we have established the main risk factors as primiparity, hemostasis disorders, and anatomic variants of the uterine arterial feeding. A second embolization is then possible and effective (10 successes out of 10 in our experience).

  A hysterectomy is necessary if embolization fails (4–10 % of the cases).

  In case of a consumption coagulopathy (about 60–90 % of patients), interruption of the bleeding leads generally to a normalization of the hemostasis.

  Only limited data are available to evaluate the results of an embolization after the failure of a surgical hemostasis (ligation, hysterectomy). Embolization is then effective, but with an increased ischemic risk if embolization of the collateral network is necessary.

- Complications: besides the nonspecific complications (puncture site, catheterization, iodine contrast medium), the following should also be noted:
  - Case reports of uterine necrosis, generally observed with particles of less than 600 μm or with powder gelatin
  - Endometritis (7 out of 113 cases in our personal series: 6 %) (Gaia)

18.4.2 Midterm Results

Few studies have investigated the gynecological and obstetrical follow-up of patients after embolization.

- We have observed (Gaia) six amenorrheas (5.4 %) among 110 patients who were followed up (12–84 months, average 46.4) after a successful embolization. In six of these patients, synechias were found at hysteroscopy.
- Pregnancies can occur in the months following embolization (60–100 %) in patients desiring such. However, we have observed a high rate of postpartum hemorrhages recurrences in patients treated by embolization, which makes us suspect that there might be an increased rate of placental abnormalities after embolization.

18.5 Indications

A multidisciplinary coordination (gynecologists-obstetricians, anesthesiologists, vascular radiologists) is essential and begins in the delivery room, according to a regularly updated protocol:

1. The obvious causes of bleeding must be eliminated (episiotomy +++).
2. Artificial delivery or uterine revision of the cavity, supplemented by an instrumental examination of the birth canal and uterotonics (oxytocics and prostaglandins).

   In some centers, intrauterine balloons are inflated, in order to obtain a hemostasis by packing.
3. If after 30 min, the following symptoms still exist, external bleeding, uterine atony, hemodynamic instability requiring large expansion volumes, and/or vasoconstrictors to maintain the hemodynamics, it becomes necessary to use a hemostatic instrumental therapy (embolization or surgery).

If the appropriate strategy is not locally available and if the hemodynamic conditions allow it, patient transfer must be considered, to carry out these hemostatic techniques.

If the patient is hemodynamically unstable, the transfer is contraindicated and thus a hemostasis surgery must be performed locally.

If the conditions for a transfer and for monitoring exist, an embolization is recommended in case of:

- Uterine atony resistant to medical treatment, particularly after vaginal delivery.
- Cervico-uterine hemorrhages (placenta previa).
- Vaginal thrombus.
- Already sutured or inaccessible cervico-vaginal tears, even in case of coagulopathy.
- Embolization can be considered in case of persistent bleeding after arterial ligation or hysterectomy.

When the interdisciplinary coordination is optimal, then surgery can be restricted to the patient who cannot be transferred for an embolization.

In case of childbirth by cesarean section, or if the optimal conditions to perform embolization are not met, vascular ligation, associated for some to uterine compression sutures, is the most appropriate first-line option. There is no available data which gives preference to ligation of uterine arteries, of arteries of the round ligaments and utero-ovarian ligament, over a bilateral ligation of the hypogastric arteries: this choice is essentially based on the experience of the surgeon.

Hemostasis hysterectomy, which is preferentially subtotal, generally takes place after failure of the embolization or the ligations, but it can be performed beforehand if the situation requires it.

18.6 Placenta Accreta, Ectopic Pregnancy

If an Anomaly in the Placental Cord insertion Is Diagnosed at the Time of Birth Explaining a PPH: refer to the standard care procedure, eventually with microparticles; the primary success rate of embolization in this particular case is evaluated from 60 to 100 %.

In Case of Prenatal Diagnosis of the Placenta Insertion Abnormality: these patients should be considered having a high risk of PPH, requiring antenatal planned strategy.

Some authors recognize the value of conservative treatment (placenta partially resected or leaved in plane), which may involve embolization, even in the absence of PPH. In this case the introducer sheaths can be set up before the cesarean section: this attitude has been adopted in our multidisciplinary group. Others proposed a prophylactic balloon temporary occlusion of the hypogastric arteries before the cesarean section and a planned hysterectomy, in order to reduce the blood losses.

Ectopic Pregnancy: preoperative embolization can diminish blood losses if a surgical intervention is necessary for a cervical or cornual pregnancy. UA methotrexate injection before, during, and immediately after the injection of gelatin sponge has been proposed for cervical pregnancy.

Key Points

- PPH=>500 ml; serious if >1,000 ml.
- About 20 % of maternal deaths.
- Multidisciplinary concertation (gynecologists-obstetricians, anesthesiologists, radiologists), as soon as the patient is in the delivery room.
- Persistent bleeding, atony, and hemodynamic instability lasting more than 30 min = serious PPH requiring a hemostatic treatment.
- If the appropriate strategy is not available locally and if the hemodynamic conditions allow it, patient transfer and embolization are considered; when the interdisciplinary coordination is optimal, surgery is restricted to patients who cannot be transferred for an embolization.
- Angiographic contrast extravasation occurs in less than 50 % of the cases.
- In the case of uterine atony, catheterization of the anterior trunk of the two hypogastric arteries is sufficient, and the embolization is carried out using absorbable gelatin sponge
- In the case of vascular wounds or of placenta accreta: microparticles.
- Technical success; 73–100 %; hysterectomy in case of failure, 4–10 %.
- Rebleeding can occur → monitoring mandatory.
- Complications: uterine necrosis (gelatin powder, particle < 600 μ), endometritis, and synechiae.
- Follow-up: fertility 60–100 %, but high risk of new PPH (abnormal placentation?).

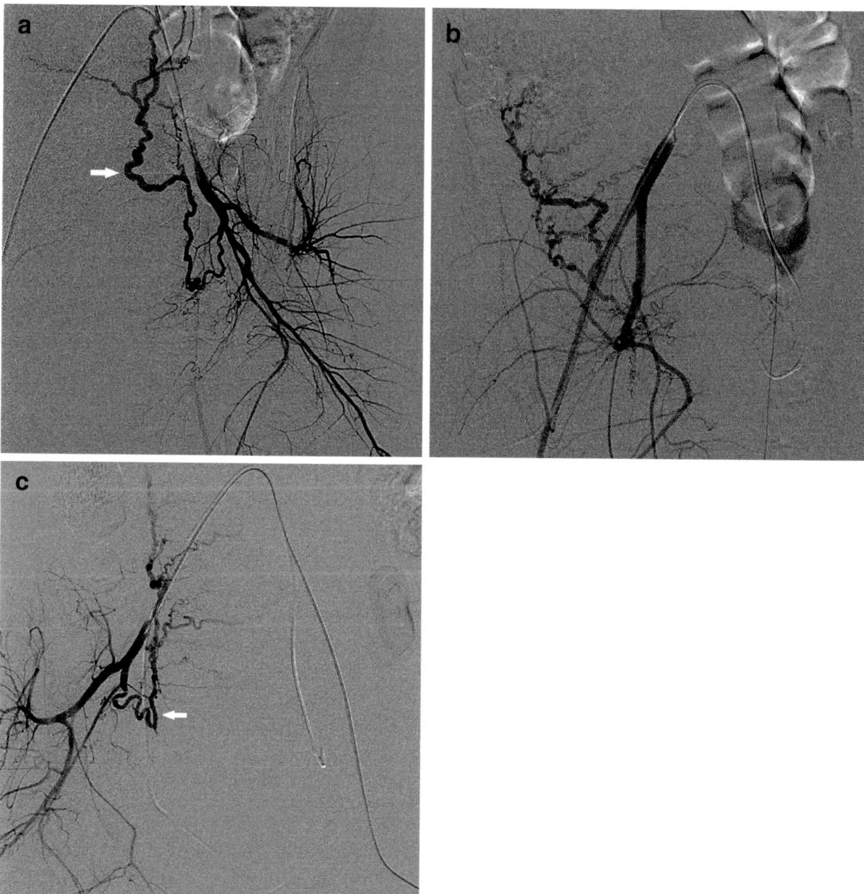

Fig 18.1 Postpartum hemorrhage: uterine arteries in late pregnancy. (**a**) Selective injection of the left hypogastric artery from a right femoral access (crossover), 27° RPO view. Modal termination of the hypogastric artery: bifurcation in anterior and posterior trunks; note the increased diameter of a very tortuous uterine artery (first branch of the anterior trunk) (*arrow*), usual in late pregnancy. (**b**) Injection at the end of the right common iliac artery (from a left femoral puncture: crossover catheterization), 30° RPO view, exposing the iliac bifurcation, before selective catheterization of the anterior trunk of the right hypogastric artery. (**c**) After selective catheterization of the hypogastric artery, selective injection (25° LPO view), to distinguish the posterior trunk from the uterine artery (a branch of the anterior trunk), often the largest branch in late pregnancy (*arrow*: ascending path of uterine artery, enlarged in late pregnancy)

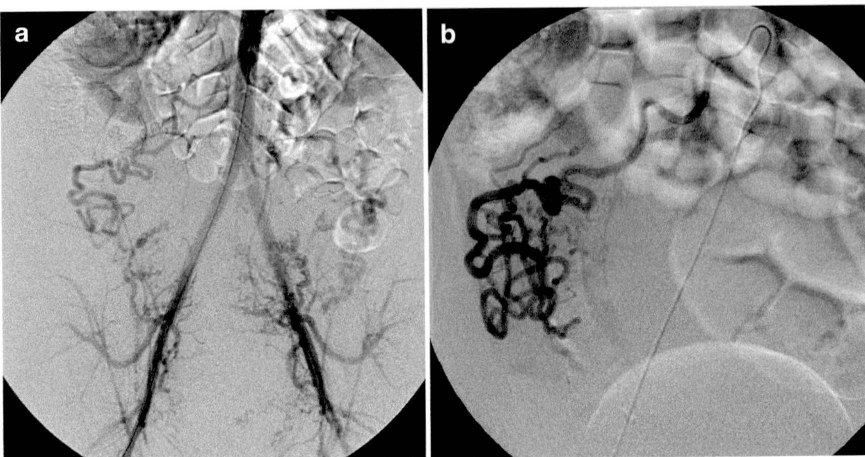

Fig. 18.2 (**a**) Postpartum hemorrhage, aortography, frontal view: right ovarian artery, arising from the right edge of the infrarenal aorta, enlarged and involved in uterine perfusion. (**b**) Selective injection before embolization by absorbable gelatin sponge

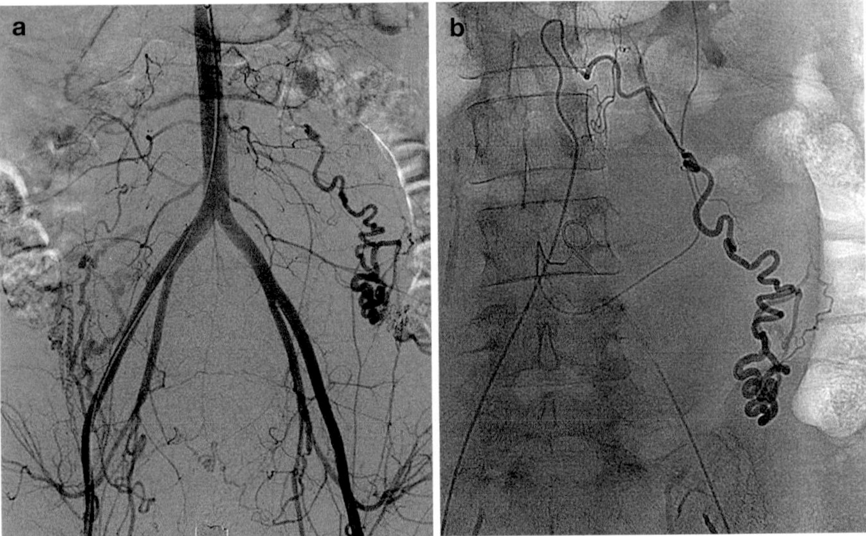

Fig. 18.3 Postpartum hemorrhage: enlarged left ovarian artery involved in the vascularization of an atonic uterus. (**a**) Aortography. (**b**, **c**) Selective catheterization

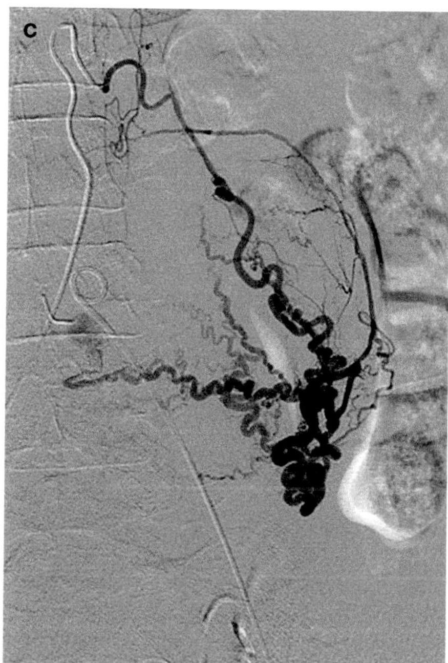

Fig. 18.3 (continued)

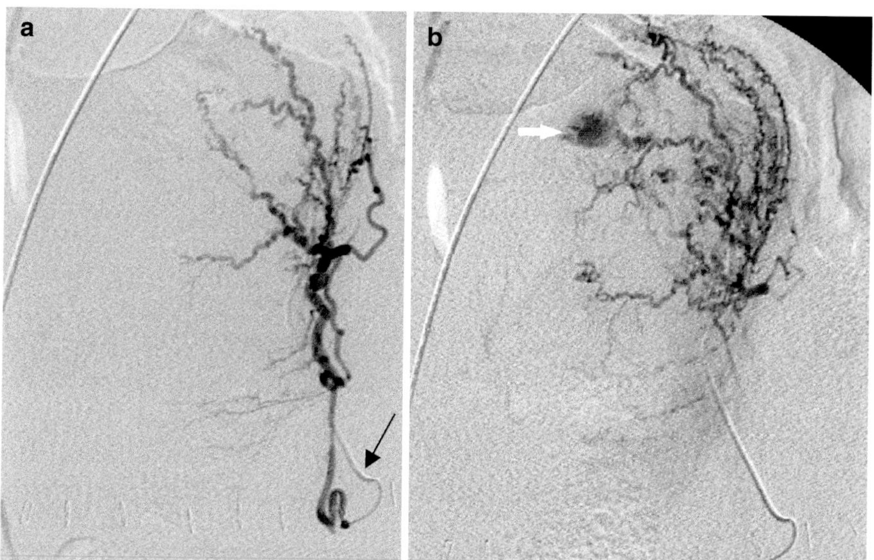

Fig. 18.4 (**a**) Frontal view, selective injection of the left uterine artery (4 F Cobra catheter) (*black arrow*) after right femoral puncture followed by a crossover. (**b**) Hypervascularization of the uterine fundus, with late extravasation (*white arrow*): PPH caused by uterine atony

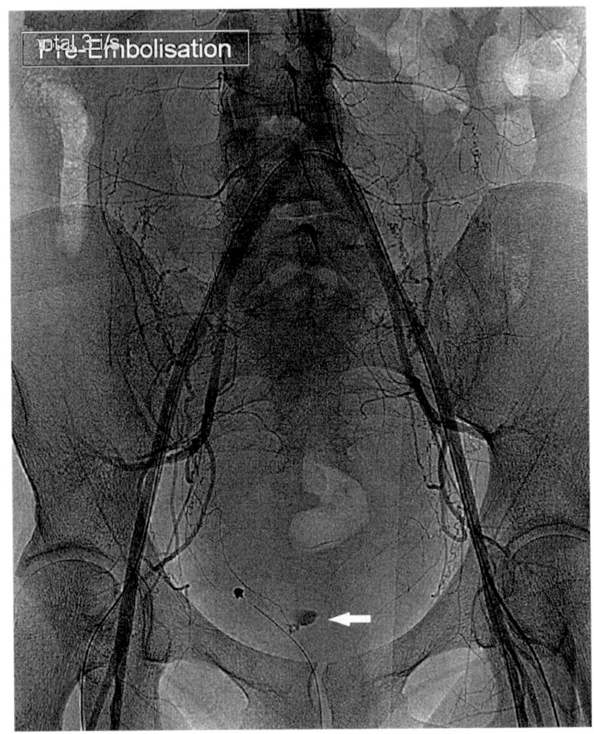

Fig. 18.5 PPH as a complication of a vaginal delivery (twin pregnancy): the bleeding was related to a long straight vaginal wound, easily seen on this aortographic injection (*arrow*), which will be embolized by gelfoam

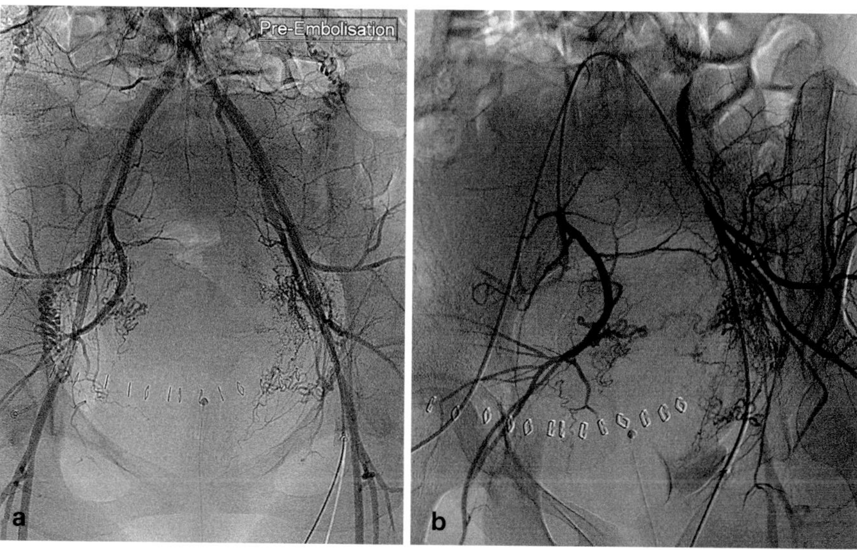

Fig. 18.6 A 21-year-old W, P4G1 (with a history of cervical ectopic pregnancy): hemorrhage during delivery (emergency C-section), due to a premature rupture of the amniotic sac, after two spontaneous preterm delivery threats; placenta accreta in over half of its surface. The persistence of bleeding after medical treatment and obstetric maneuvers led to the indication of embolization. (**a**) Bilateral femoral access; aortic end injection via the left femoral access, showing the arterial supply of the uterus by the right and left uterine arteries. (**b**) RAO view; simultaneously selective bilateral internal iliac injections, to identify the uterine arteries among the terminal visceral branches of the hypogastric arteries. (**c**) A hyper-selective catheterization of the right uterine artery was performed before an embolization using calibrated microparticles (700–900 μm). (**d**) Hyper-selective injection of the left uterine artery (from the right femoral access), before embolization by microparticles. In both two sides, this microparticles exclusion was completed by a very proximal embolization of the uterine arteries with resorbable gelatin sponge. (e1, e2 – late phase): Intermediate control aortoiliac opacification: rarification of uterine vascularization but the involvement of a right external iliac circumflex artery to the blood supply of the uterus (*arrows*, early phase then late phase) is demasked. (**f**) Selective catheterization of the right external iliac circumflex artery from the left femoral access (vertebral catheter), before embolization by gelatin. (**g**) Final aortoiliac opacification. (**h**) High juxta-renal aortic injection showing the participation of a small left ovarian artery (*arrows*) to the vascularization of the uterine fundus. The hemodynamic stabilization at this moment led us to not embolize. Introducer sheaths were left in place for 24 h

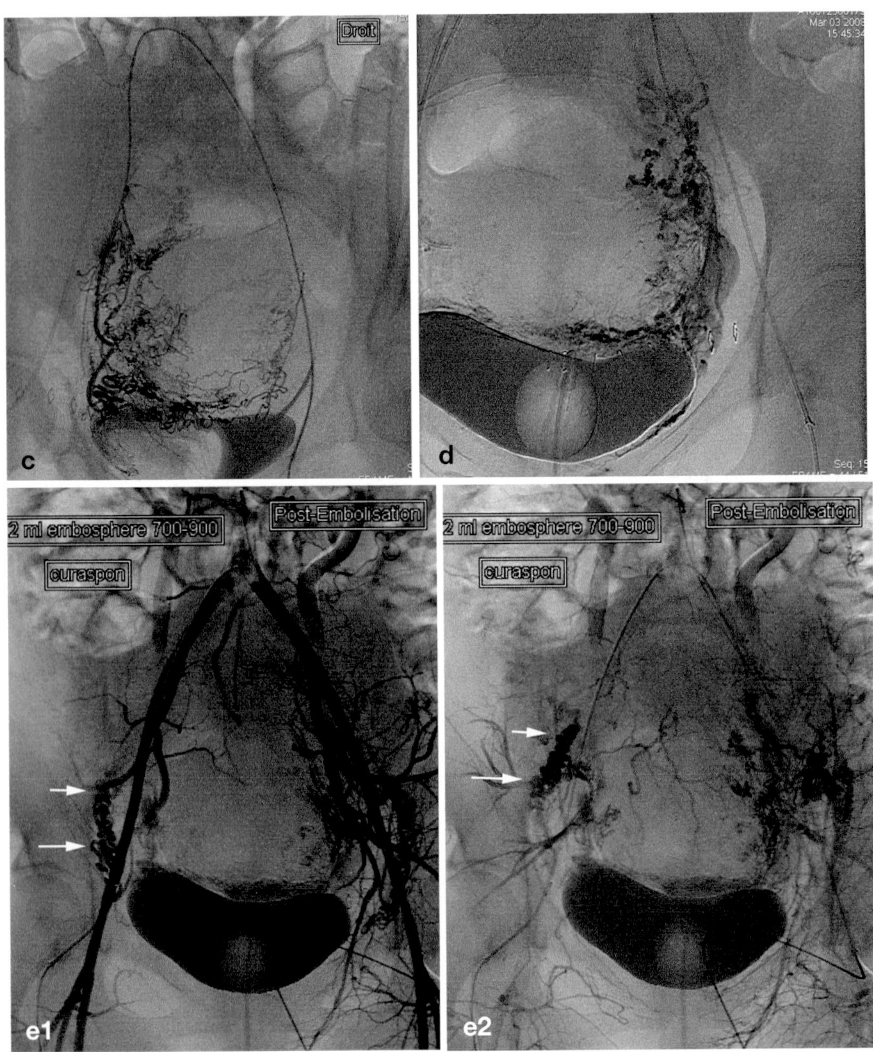

Fig. 18.6 (continued)

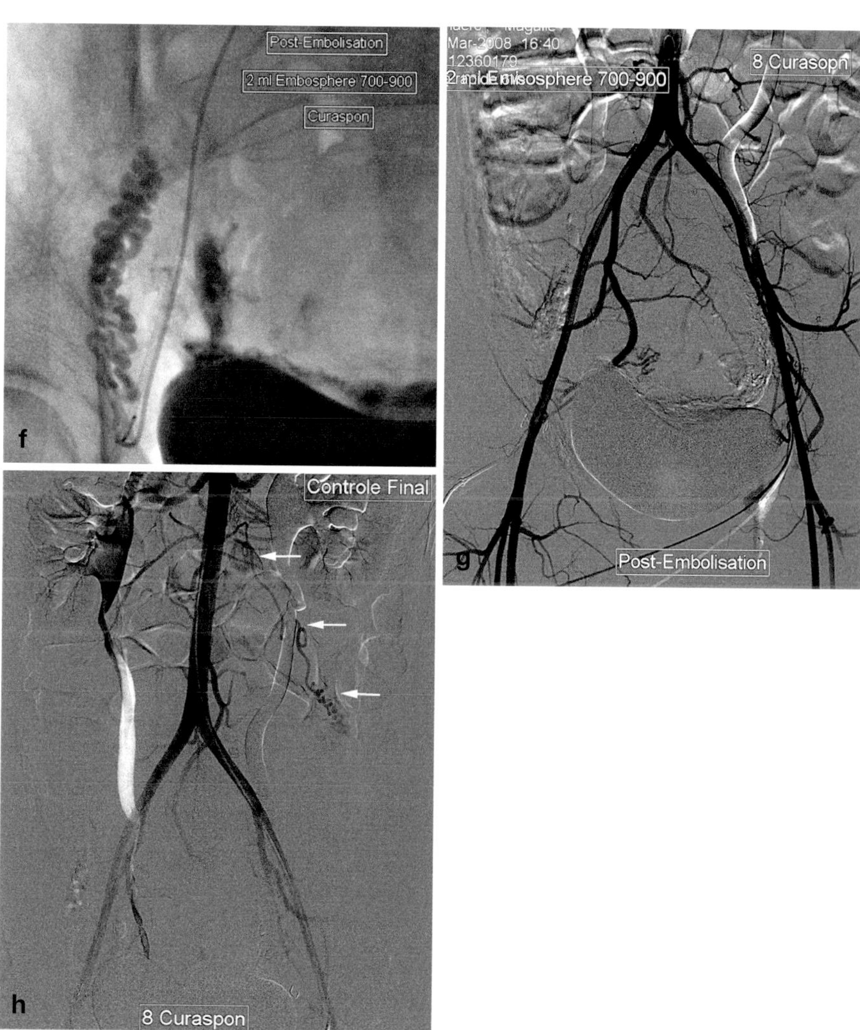

Fig. 18.6 (continued)

Suggested Reading

American College of Obstetricians and Gynecologists. ACOG practice bulletin: clinical management guidelines for obstetrics and gynecology: post partum hemorrhage. Obstet Gynecol. 2006;108:1039–47.

Bros S, Chabrot P, Kastler A, et al. Recurrent bleeding within 24 hours after uterine artery embolization for severe post partum hemorrhage: are there predictive factors? Cardiovasc Intervent Radiol. 2012;35(3):508–14.

Carnevale FC, Kondo MM, De Oliveira Sousa W, et al. Perioperative temporary occlusion of the internal iliac arteries as prophylaxis in cesarean section at risk of hemorrhage in placenta accreta. Cardiovasc Intervent Radiol. 2011;34:758–64.

Chabrot P, Vidal V, Louail B. Recommandations et bonnes pratiques en radiologie vasculaire interventionnelle. In: Vernhet H, editor. SFICV Ed. 2008, Paris.

Diop AN, Chabrot P, Bertrand A, et al. Placenta accreta: management with uterine artery embolization in 17 cases. J Vasc Interv Radiol. 2010;21:644–8.

Fargeaudou Y, Morel O, Soyer P, et al. Persistent postpartum haemorrhage after failed arterial ligation: value of pelvic embolisation. Eur Radiol. 2010;20:1777–85.

Gaïa G, Chabrot P, Cassagnes L, et al. Menses recovery and fertility after artery embolization for PPH: a single-center retrospective observational study. Eur Radiol. 2009;19:481–7.

Gonsalves M, Belli A. The role of interventional radiology in obstetric hemorrhage. Cardiovasc Intervent Radiol. 2010;33:887–95.

Jung HN, Shin SW, Choi SJ, et al. Uterine artery embolization for emergent management of postpartum hemorrhage associated with placenta accreta. Acta Radiol. 2011;52:638–42.

Pelage JP, Le Dref O, Soyer P, et al. Arterial anatomy of the female genital tract: variations and relevance to transcatheter embolization of the uterus. AJR Am J Roentgenol. 1999;172:989–94.

Recommandations pour la pratique clinique: HPP immédiat. J Gyn Biol Reprod. 2004;33 4S:130–6.

Chapter 19
Uterine Fibroid Embolization (UFE)

Louis Boyer, Eric Dumousset, Agaïcha Alfidja Lankoande, Nathalie Mazet, Anne Ravel, and Pascal Chabrot

19.1 Background

Fibroids are benign estrogen-dependant tumors which regress after the menopause and occur more frequently with ageing. Black women are more likely to have fibroids than white women, and they also are more frequent in nulliparous than in multiparous women. Often asymptomatic, they may be responsible for menorrhagia and in some cases anemia, pelvic heaviness, mass syndrome, urinary or intestinal symptoms, infertility, and miscarriages.

UFE were first carried out at the beginning of the 1990s, in preoperative situations (preopUFE), aiming to make the surgery (myomectomies, hysterectomies) less hemorrhagic and thus more conservative.

Very rapidly UFE as an exclusive treatment of fibroids (curUFE) was also performed. It is a simple and well-tolerated conservative treatment for symptomatic uterine fibroid, by an irreversible ischemia (and thus a gradual reduction in the volume of the fibroids), after occlusion of the perimyomatous arterial plexus, using particles, and preserving the branches feeding the ovaries and the cervicovaginal region.

L. Boyer, MD, PhD (✉) • E. Dumousset, MD • A. Alfidja Lankoande, MD
A. Ravel, MD • P. Chabrot, MD, PhD
Department of Radiology, University Hospital of Clermont-Ferrand,
Clermont-Ferrand, France
e-mail: lboyer@chu-clermontferrand.fr; pchabrot@chu-clermontferrand.fr

N. Mazet, MD
Department of Radiology,
CMC Beau Soleil, Montpellier, France

P. Chabrot, L. Boyer (eds.), *Embolization*,
DOI 10.1007/978-1-4471-5182-1_19, © Springer-Verlag London 2014

19.2 Relevant Radiological Anatomy

The uterus is mainly supplied by the uterine arteries (UA) issuing from the internal iliac arteries (IIA).

The IIA (hypogastric) presents many division variations. The most frequent configuration (55–77 %) is the bifurcation into an anterior trunk and a posterior trunk, at the level of the superior part of the greater sciatic notch. But a single trunk (≅4 %), three trunks (≅15 %), and four trunks or more (≅3 %) are also possible; the branches can also come about at once and form a bouquet (≅2 %). In 90 % of cases, the mode of division is symmetric. The absence of IIA is rare: all of its branches hence arise from the common iliac artery.

In most of the cases, the uterine artery (UA) originates from the anterior trunk of the IIA but in different ways depending on its division pattern: in 56 % of the cases, it arises alone from the anterior trunk of the IIA; in 40 % of the cases, from a branch which is common with the umbilical artery; in 2 % of the cases, from the internal pudendal artery; and in 2 % of the cases, from a common stem with a long vaginal artery. When the UA emerges from the anterior trunk, its origin is usually correctly depicted on a contralateral anterior oblique view. When it branches off higher, it is best seen on an ipsilateral oblique view. Identifying the origin of the UA is the key to its catheterization.

The caliber of the UA, variable (2–5 mm), is particularly large during pregnancy and immediately after childbirth.

It first describes a descending segment against the pelvic wall, then a horizontal one crossing the ureter, and finally sinuously ascending along the uterus, thus easily recognizable.

Its terminal branches are:

- The artery of the uterine fundus.
- A medial tubal branch, coursing along the fallopian tube, confluent with the lateral tubal branch issuing from the ovarian artery (arising from the aorta at the level of L3).
- A medial ovarian branch coursing along the utero-ovarian ligament, anastomosed with a branch issuing from the ovarian artery. This medial ovarian branch provides the total ovarian supply in 4 % of the cases, does not participate in the arterial feeding of the ovary in 40 % of the cases, and shares it with the lateral ovarian branch in 56 %.

The UA gives several branches – peritoneal, ureteric, vesical, vaginal, and cervical – to the round ligament (anastomosed with the deep inferior epigastric artery).

Its uterine branches are anastomosed with those issuing from the contralateral UA. On the other hand, there are few anastomoses between the cervical and corporeal network. The UA is widely anastomosed with the ipsilateral ovarian and the inferior epigastric arteries.

The UA ensures most of the arterial supply of the uterus, to which the ovarian artery and the artery of the round ligament may contribute.

Arterial feeding of uterine fibroids: the UF are not fed by a unique pedicle, but by a perimyomatous plexus. The presence of fibroids leads to an increased caliber and a distortion of the arterial branches of the UA feeding the uterus, which supply both the normal myometrium and the myoma. The myoma, which generally is poorly vascularized, is supplied by small centripetal arteries arising from a rich perimyomatous plexus, which is supplied by the two UA. The ovarian arteries contribute to the vascularization of the fibroid in 5–10 % of the cases and more frequently in patients who have a history of pelvic surgery and tubal or ovarian pathologies or in case of a large fundal fibroid. Pedunculated subserous fibroids can have an identified arterial pedicle. The fibroids that occur on a bicornuate uterus can be supplied by only one of the two UA.

19.3 Technique

19.3.1 Exclusive Curative Embolization (CurUFE)

- An analgesic protocol must systematically be planned by the anesthesiologist, during pre- and post-procedural phases, associating intravenous analgesics (paracetamol and nefopam, Acupan®), nonsteroidal anti-inflammatory drugs (ketoprofen, Profenid®), and morphine, by titration and then by PCA (PCA pump: patient-controlled analgesia). This therapeutic protocol must be continued for 24–36 h. Antiemetics can be added. We do not systematically administer antibiotics.
- Access: we prefer a bifemoral arterial approach (4F) to a uni-femoral one. It indeed allows the simultaneous catheterization of hypogastric arteries by crossing over the aortoiliac carrefour. This 4-hand procedure contributes to the reduction of radiation dose. A contralateral access can be helpful in case of catheterization difficulties and/or unusual anatomy. It also ensures the quality of the embolization by a global opacification before retrieving the selective catheterization.
- In these young patients whose ovaries are located in the primary X-ray field, it is mandatory to limit irradiation by reducing fluoroscopy and angio series X-ray image rate, by road mapping, variations of angulation of the oblique views, simultaneous bilateral catheterization, etc.
- Angiographic identification: the first step consists in performing a frontal view interrenal aortogram, to detect a large ovarian artery which may feed the uterus. Then, the division mode of the hypogastric artery is analyzed through aortoiliac injections of contrast medium on an oblique view (eventually with road mapping). Thirdly, a selective UA catheterization is performed using a 4F hydrophilic guide wire (we use a Cobra catheter) and then, possibly, should there be any difficulty, a large-lumen microcatheter, which is an interesting tool to prevent arterial spasm and dissection. The microcatheters' end is positioned in the

ascending segment of the UA, ensuring during embolization the visualization of a slowing down of the physiological flow, which helps determining more precisely the end point. It is obtained when a reflux is observed in the horizontal portion of the UA, while the patency of the cervicovaginal arteries and of the utero-ovarian anastomoses is respected. But for many authors, the use of microcatheters is not systematic.

A complete occlusion of the UA was carried out by the first operators; today by using microspheres, a distal occlusion and a simple slowing of the flow in the proximal segment of the UA (which is leaved patent) seem sufficient.

Catheterization difficulties and spasms may necessitate an injection of vasodilator drugs (in our group: Risordan, 1 mg).

- Embolization agents: curUFE are today carried out by using calibrated nonabsorbable microparticles of more than 500 μm diameter, to avoid any inopportune passage through the utero-ovarian anastomoses. We use diameters varying from 700 to 900 μm.

The Embospheres (BioSphere Medical) have been extensively evaluated. More recently other agents have been advocated, for which the end point is less formally defined, and without any comparative evaluation available: the choice depends on the habits of the physician and on the cost. Because of different compressibilities, PVA microspheres give a more distal occlusion than the tris-acryl spheres: with respect to the tris-acryl, a larger diameter must be chosen for PVA microspheres or hydrogel-polygene microspheres, in order to have the same equivalent effect (Embospheres 500–700 μ ≈ PVA 700–900 μ ≈ hydrogel-polygene 900 μ).

A unilateral embolization must be considered as a technical failure, except if one of the UA is absent.

A control angiography ensures the devascularization of fibroid(s), the interruption of the flow in the distal segment of the UA, the slowdown of the proximal flow, and the patency of the trunk of the UA, the cervicovaginal branches, and the utero-ovarian anastomoses. A uterine reperfusion after withdrawal of the selective catheter must lead to consider a vasospasm and to perform complementary embolization.

- Follow-up: the hospitalization is short (2–4 days). During 24–36 h, the combination of analgesics, anti-inflammatory drugs, and morphine (PCA) is used. The drug prescription given upon patient discharge combines paracetamol-type analgesics (Doliprane, 6 pills/day) or its derivatives and ketoprofen-type NSAI drug (Bi-Profenid, 3 pills/day). A work stoppage of 1 week is often enough.

Patients must be informed of the need to use a reliable contraception during the months after the embolization.

Post-embolization syndrome associates pelvic pain, febricula, nausea, vomiting, loss of appetite, and a general ill feeling, nonspecific and variable in intensity. It must not be considered as a complication, except in the case where the hospital stay is prolonged and/or a rehospitalization is necessary.

The telephone number of a referring physician must be given to the patient upon discharge.

A gynecological consultation must be planned 1 month after the embolization, for following up the symptoms and to make sure there is no complication. The quality of life should then be evaluated.

In the post-embolization care, imaging is interesting, even in the case of a favorable evolution; there is no consensus on an ideal schedule. In our group, an MRI is proposed 1 year after the embolization, in order to evaluate the devascularization of the UF and/or to detect eventually non-embolized UF.

19.3.2 Technical Distinctive Features of Preoperative Embolizations (PreopUFE)

- Analgesics: in order to avoid post-embolization pain, preopUFE must be performed immediately before surgery – in our group, the preopUFE takes place early in the morning, and surgery is then carried out 2 h later.
- PreopUFE must systematically be bilateral.
- Embolization agents: even though some authors use microparticles (with a diameter of at least 500 μm), we prefer absorbable gelatin sponge, which guarantees a better preservation of the uterine trophicity and future fertility and avoids an ovarian ischemia while producing a satisfactory uterine ischemia, should the surgical operation be carried out without any delay.

19.4 Results

19.4.1 CurUFE

- A technical success rate superior to 95 % is expected.
- Tolerance: nearly 80 % of the patients having had an embolization would be ready to have another embolization should it be necessary [1].
- Complications
  - Lesions of the structures involved in the conception, implantation, or fetal growth are rare: ovarian dysfunction may occur in patients older than 45 years; there is probably no significant impact on ovarian function before 40 years. The myometrium is rarely involved. Atrophy of the endometrium after curUFE is also considered as rare, although we do not have any precise data. An endometrial atrophy can cause of chronic vaginal losses after curUFE. However, for the majority of the patients, an evacuation of fibromatous debris is observed, which does not allow assessment of the endometrial damage.

An exceptional case of uterine rupture during labor has been reported; to our knowledge, there are no reports of placental insufficiencies after curUFE.

- Endometritis is inflammation and/or infection of the endometrium that can cause pelvic pain, leucorrhea, fever, and hyperleukocytosis in the weeks following the procedure. It can occur without any infection, sometimes at the same time than fibroid expulsion, or be due to an infection, requiring then a specific treatment. The infection can be more severe, concerning the embolized fibroid (local infection or hematogenous) and the uterus (where the infection can complicate an extensive necrosis, with pain, often purulent leucorrhea, fever, and hyperleukocytosis). The initial treatment associates analgesics, anti-inflammatory drugs, and antibiotics. A surgical treatment is sometimes necessary.

Submucosal fibroids, particularly the pedunculated ones, can be ejected, typically within the first weeks/months, and cause leucorrhea, bleeding, abdominal and pelvic expulsive pain associated to fever, nausea, and vomiting. A hysteroscopy is sometimes necessary in cases of retention, infection, or persistent pain.

The hysterectomy rate for complications of UFE is 1–2 %. The thresholds of the SIR-CIRSE 2009 common recommendations [2] are transient amenorrhea, 5–10 %; permanent amenorrhea before 45 years, 0–3 %; after 45 years, 7–14 %; cervical expulsion of debris, 0–3 %; noninfectious endometritis, 1–2 %; endometrial or uterine infection, 1–2 %; uterine necrosis, <1 %; thromboembolic disease, <1 %; and out-of-target embolization, <1 %.

To summarize, the published trials, randomized or not, do not show any significant difference in major complications rate between surgery and UFE. The hospital length of stay and recovery times are shorter for UFE than for the surgery (hysterectomy or myomectomy); the cost for UFE is lower [3, 4].

- Morphological results: on early (24–72 h) MRI controls (with Gd), infarction of more than 90 % of the leiomyomatous tissue allows a better clinical outcome and less re-interventions than with a lower percentage of infarction. A volume reduction of the dominant fibroid of 40–60 % in a year can be expected, but it is not immediate.
- Clinical results: bleeding, heaviness, and compression are improved in 75–95 % of the cases, with a quality of life comparable to that observed after surgical treatment. Five years after a curUFE, Spies [5] found, among 181 patients followed up, 73 % had maintained this improvement, while in 20 % of the cases, there was a recurrence of the symptoms, among which 13.7 % had a hysterectomy.

If the symptoms persist after 4 months, a clinical work-up and a MRI should be carried out.

A clinical recurrence is due either to the development of new fibroids or else to a persistent vascularization of treated UF. However, when compared to surgery, embolization requires more re-intervention procedures even after initial technical and clinical successes.

- Fertility: pregnancies are quite possible after curUFE, but the data still remains too limited to establish definitive conclusion with respect to their safety. Globally it seems that there is little difference with respect to the quality of the pregnancy obtained after a laparoscopic myomectomy: no extra miscarriages and no extra premature births (even though embolized patients are often older).

- *Particular cases: associations of "adenomyosis + fibroid" and "pelvic endometriosis + fibroids,"* a lower efficiency of embolization and a higher recurrence rate are to be expected.

19.4.2 PreopUFE

- Technical success is to be expected.
- The complications are not specific (puncture site, catheterization, iodine contrast medium) but rare in women who are often young.
- Our experience [6] gives similar results to other data available: simplified surgical dissection in case of myomectomy, shorter surgical interventions, and less blood loss thus avoiding transfusions.

To our knowledge, the number of potentially avoided hysterectomies with preopUFE (substitution with simple myomectomies) has not been determined.

PreopUFE concerns the myomas planned for surgery as well as the remainder of the myometrium, which can shelter other smaller myomas: the long-term effects of embolization followed by myomectomy on the remaining uterus, on myomatous recurrences, and on fertility are not well known; this is one of the reasons why we choose to use resorbable embolic agents, to preserve the trophicity of the remaining uterus.

- To our knowledge, there is no medico-economic data comparing "preopUFE + surgery" to surgery or curUFE alone.

19.5 Indications

19.5.1 CurUFE

All indications must systematically be preceded by a pelvic clinical examination performed by a gynecologist and imaging to confirm the diagnosis. Suprapubic and/or endovaginal ultrasound is often of interest. However, should the slightest doubt persists, then an MRI should be realized: to eliminate a pelvic tumor or an associated lesion (and particularly hydrosalpinx, which exposes to post-embolization infectious risk, and endometriosis); to confirm the existence of fibroids; to determine their size, position, and enhancement; and ideally to precisely define the pelvic arterial anatomy. But no predictive radiological criterion related to the clinical success of a curUFE has been established. Pelvic MRI must systematically include frontal, sagittal, and axial T2-weighted sequences and T1 axial and sagittal sequences and with/without fat saturation, before and after injection of gadolinium, and possibly an angio MR.

A multidisciplinary discussion is mandatory for the indications. The patient must be informed of the different therapeutic options, with their advantages and their risks, and with precise details concerning the impact on fertility for those who wish to become pregnant. Concerning curUFE, the following must be taken into account: the clinical status (age, fertility, parity, desire to become pregnant, surgical risk) and the fibroids features (size, number, and topography).

1. *Contraindications*:

   - Pregnancy.
   - Genital and/or urinary infection.
   - Abnormality on the pelvic clinical examination.
   - Recent injection of LHRH analog, which can cause a diffuse vasospasm: a therapeutic window of at least 6 weeks is recommended.
   - Pedunculated subserous UF.

2. *Indications* for symptomatic UF (bleeding, pain, compression), after failure of medical treatment:

   - CurUFE can be considered:

     – In case of a refusal for surgery
     – In the case of surgical risk (anesthesia, multi operations, obese patients)
     – As an alternative to hysterectomy
     – As an alternative to multiple myomectomies, in patients who already had one or for whom the myomectomy presents a high risk (many fibroids, anemia, surgical history, etc.)

   Great care must be taken in the case of very large fibroids (the threshold size varies: in our group = 12 cm greater diameter) or in the case of large submucosal fibroids.

   - In young women with a desire for pregnancy, multiple myomectomies are often preferred; for most of the authors, curUFE is not an alternative to a unique myomectomy (laparoscopy, endoscopic resection).
   - Particular cases: adenomyosis without fibroids or adenomyosis as the dominant uterine pathology, curUFE must be discussed, due to the fact that it is less efficient and that there are more frequent recurrences.

3. *UFE, desire for pregnancy and fertility*:

   - CurUFE indications for infertility are marginal.
   - Young women with a desire for pregnancy: as the effects on fertility remains uncertain, the standard approach should be a cautious one. If myomectomy is possible, surgery is preferred. CurUFE is an alternative to hysterectomy and to some cases of multiple myomectomies; single myomas are not an indication for embolization.

The radiologist must be particularly careful about radiation protection for these indications.

19.5.2 PreopUFE Indications

- Large fibromatous uterus with important hemorrhagic risk
- Surgical treatment of multiple myomas and/or enlarged uterus, to avoid hysterectomy
- Patients wishing to keep their uterus or patients refusing any blood transfusion (in particular Jehovah's witnesses) for whom curUFE is an alternative

Key Points

- Uterine fibroid treatment requires a multidisciplinary approach.
- CurUFE: microspheres >500 μm; PreopUFE: absorbable gelatin sponge.
- UFE: very few technical failures; it is relevant to use microcatheters.
- CurUFE is reliable and safe to treat some symptomatic uterine fibroids: 75–95 % improvement concerning the bleeding and the mass syndrome but recurrences are possible – alternative to hysterectomy and to multiple myomectomies.
- Patients should be advised of the non-frequent but possible complications after a curUFE (amenorrhea after 45 years, endometritis).
- Effects on fertility remain uncertain: caution is needed if the patient has a desire for pregnancy, but the embolization is a therapeutic alternative to preserve the uterus.
- The preopUFE reduces blood loss and facilitates the surgery, and thus contributes to achieve a conservative surgery.
- Unanswered questions:
  - Effects on the fertility and the progression of pregnancy: caution remains the rule.
  - The threshold size of fibroids for which an embolization is possible/reasonable (curUFE) (necrosis and infection) continues to vary depending on the authors.
  - CurUFE versus preopUFE + myomectomy and curUFE + medical treatment versus curUFE only: no comparative evaluation data available.

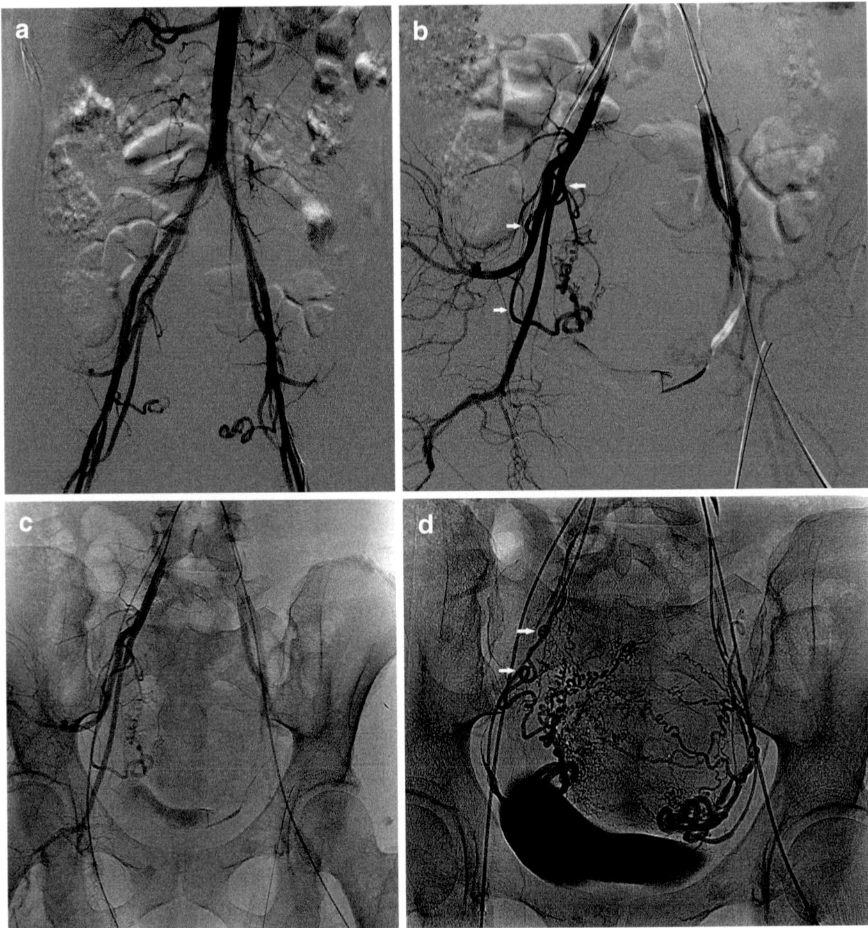

Fig. 19.1 Menometrorrhagia in a 45-year-old W caused by a poly-myomatous uterus, with a main interstitial-fundic 6-cm myoma. MRI showed that all myomas look uncomplicated. (**a**) Aortography: injection at the level of L2, showing a normal aortoiliac network and the 2 uterine arteries with symmetric and large diameter, without any large ovarian artery. (**b**, **c**) After crossing the aortoiliac bifurcation from a contralateral access, a selective injection was performed in the right hypogastric artery, of which the distribution of the branches was not modal (early phase, 1–2; later phase, 1–3): note that the right uterine artery originates from the first centimeter of the posterior trunk, on its internal edge. (**d**) Simultaneous injection of both uterine arteries after selective catheterization until their horizontal segment (Cobra hydrophilic 4F catheter): heterogeneous hypervascularization of the uterine fundus, relatively symmetrically provided from the left and right uterine arteries. Note the retro-opacification of the right ovarian artery via the utero-ovarian anastomosis (*arrow*). (**e**) End of procedure aortography, showing marked depletion of the arterial vascularization of the uterus

Fig. 19.1 (continued)

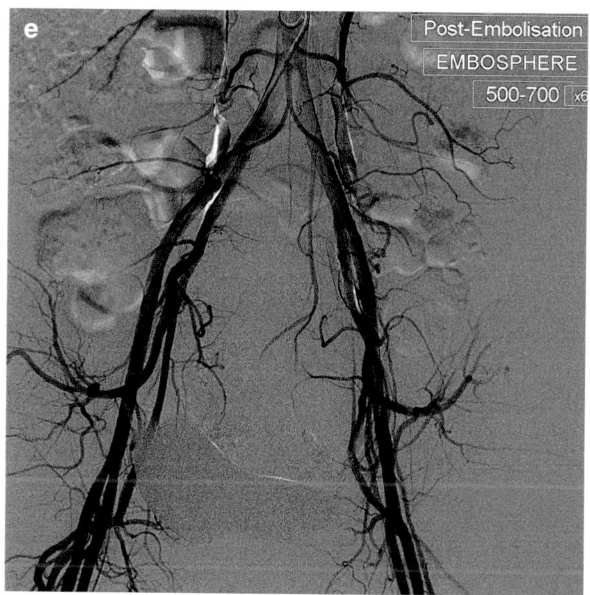

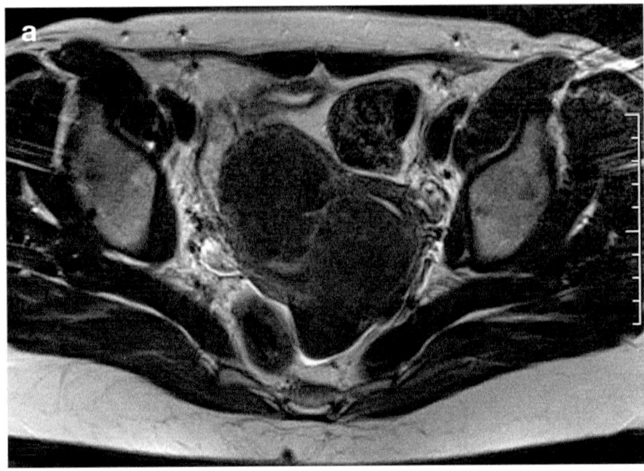

Fig. 19.2 A 40-year-old W, P3, suffering from menometrorrhagia, pollakiuria, constipation, and anemia caused by a myomatous uterus; not any efficacy of progestin treatment. (**a–c**) Sagittal and transverse T2-weighted MR scans: 3 interstitial low-signal myomas, the largest measuring 5 cm, distorting the contours, and displacing the uterine lumen. (**d**) T1WI, fat suppression, after gadolinium injection: the three myomas are enhanced. After a multidisciplinary consultation, taking into account the wishes of the patient to preserve her uterus, curative arterial embolization was proposed. (**e1**, **e2**) Aortography: normal aortoiliac network; hypervascularization of the uterus. (**f**) Opacification of the aortoiliac bifurcation (RAO view), showing the hypogastric bifurcation into anterior and posterior trunks (*black arrow*). It is also possible to identify the uterine artery, originating from the anterior trunk (*white arrow*). (**g1**, **g2**) Hyperselective catheterization of the uterine artery (4 F hydrophilic Cobra catheter), early and late phase: the extremity of the catheter is in the horizontal segment. Uterine hypervascularization, but there is not any specific pedicle nor any utero-ovarian anastomosis. (**h**) A catheter is in place in the left uterine artery, then tracking the right uterine artery by a crossover from the left femoral artery puncture, followed by an injection at the end of the right hypogastric artery (*black arrow*) (LAO view): bifurcation into anterior and posterior trunks, very early origin of the uterine artery (*white arrow*) from the anterior trunk. (**i**) Selective catheterization of the uterine artery: the right artery seems to be less involved in the vascularization of the uterus (this asymmetric pattern is frequent). Note the mass effect on the bladder. (**j1**, **j2**) Aortographic control after embolization: on the right side, 0.5 ml of 700- to 900-μm-diameter microparticles and then 1 ml of 900–1,200-μm particles were injected and, on the left side, 3.5 ml of 700–900 and then 1 ml of 900–1,200 μm. Note the retention of contrast in the myomatous uterus, while only the first few centimeters of the uterine arteries are injected. (**k–n**) MRI performed 1 year later, while pelvic heaviness disappeared, as well as bleeding and anemia; menorrhagia stays nevertheless described. Compared to pre-embolization MRI: reduction of over 50 % of the diameters of the three fibroids (axial and sagittal T2W, sagittal and axial T1W post gadolinium, fat suppressed); the low T2W signal is unchanged, but the T1W enhancement is significantly reduced

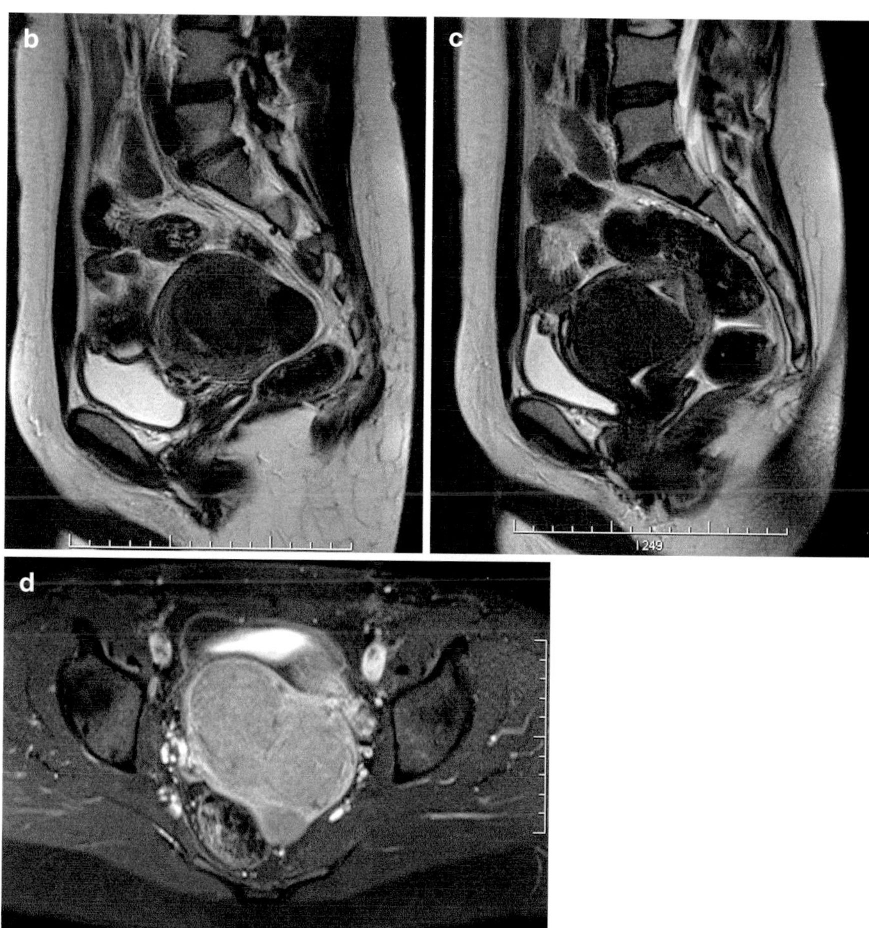

Fig. 19.2 (continued)

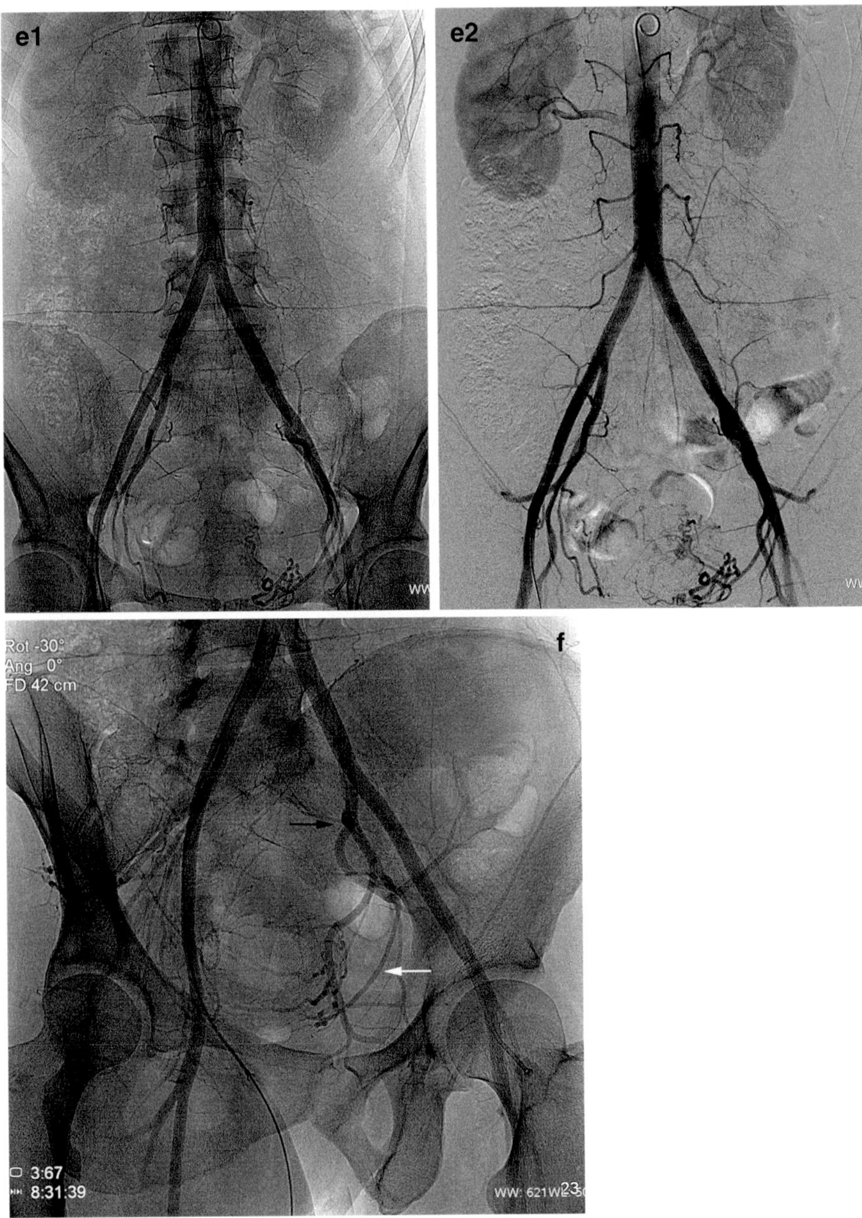

Fig. 19.2 (continued)

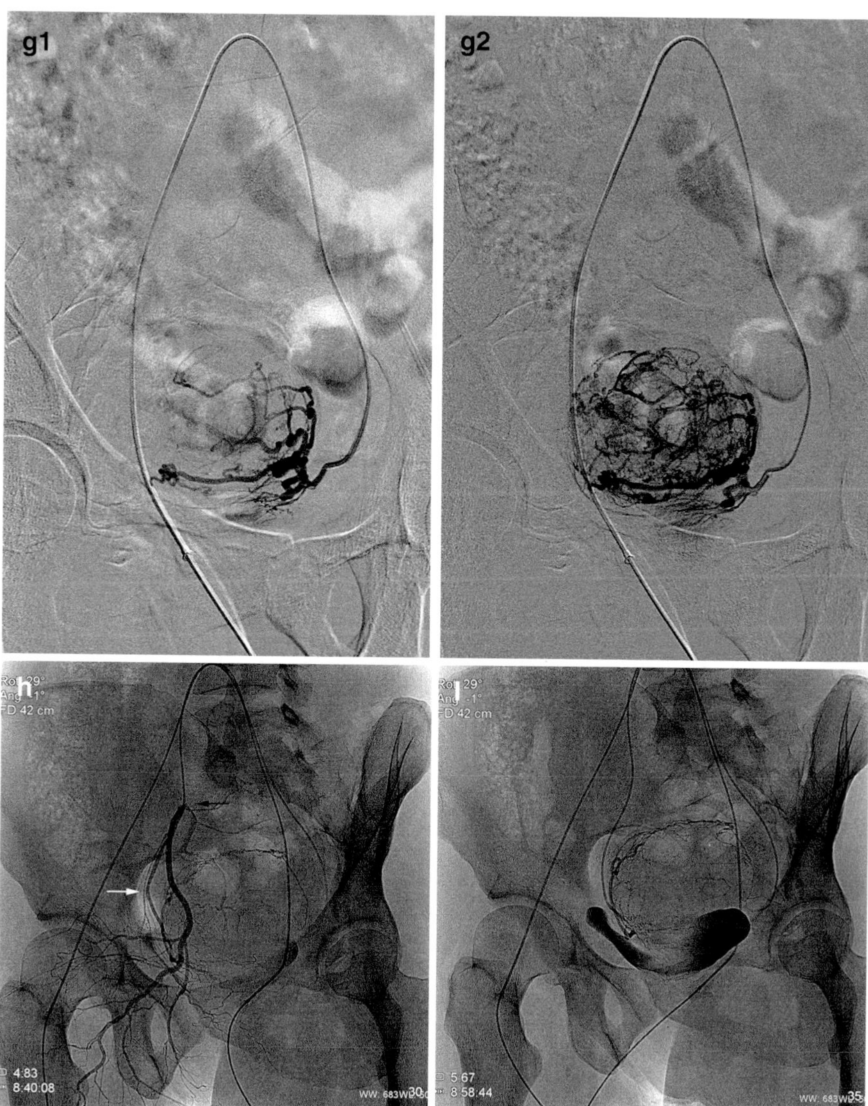

Fig. 19.2 (continued)

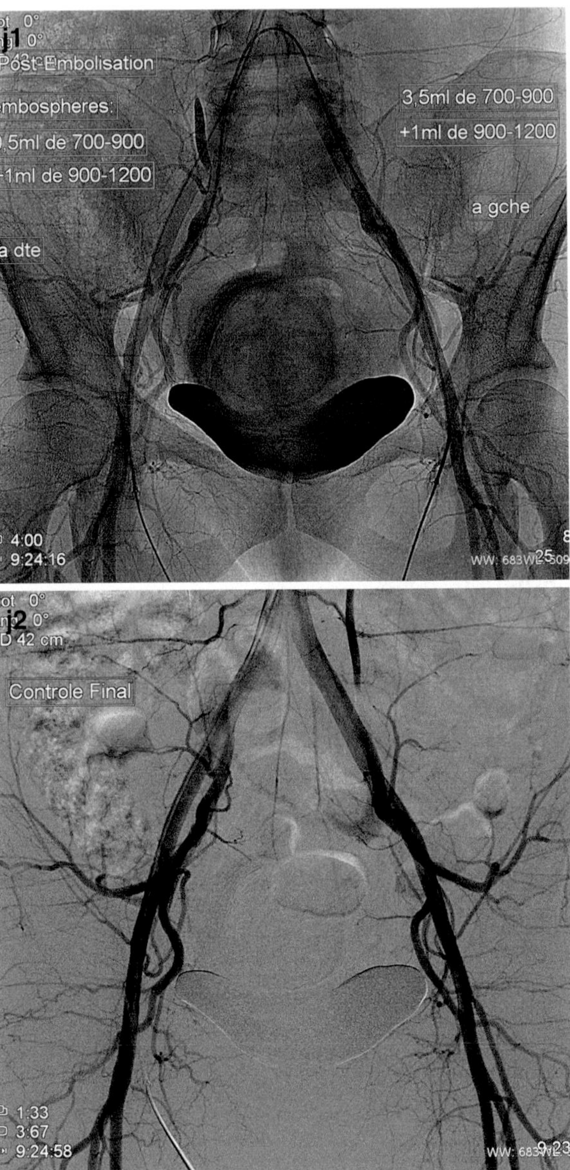

Fig. 19.2 (continued)

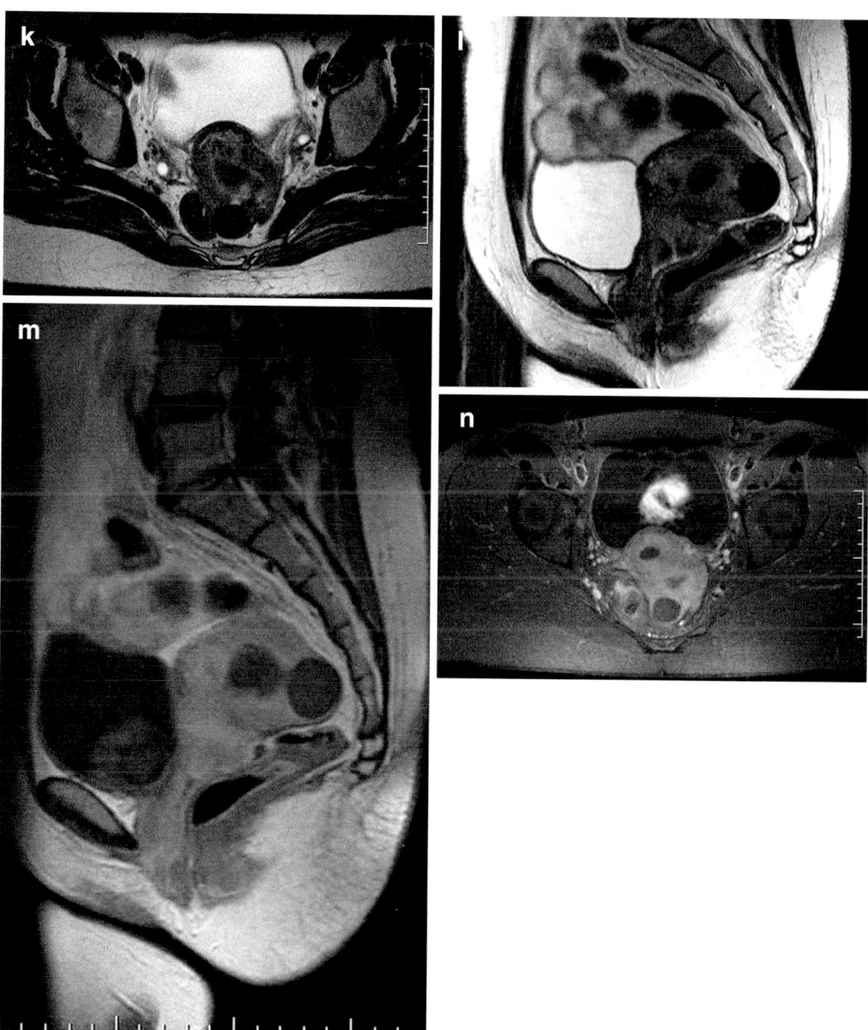

Fig. 19.2 (continued)

References

1. Worthington-Kirsch RL, Hutchins FL, Popky GL. Uterine arterial embolization for the management of leiomyomas: quality of life assessment and clinical response. Radiology. 1998;208:625–9.
2. Hovsepian DM, Siskin GP, Bonn J, et al. Quality improvement guidelines for uterine artery embolization for symptomatic leiomyomata. J Vasc Interv Radiol. 2009;20:193–9.
3. Pinto I, Chimeno P, Romo A, et al. Uterine fibroids: uterine artery embolization versus abdominal hysterectomy for treatment. A prospective, randomized, and controlled clinical trial. Radiology. 2003;226:425–31.
4. Mara M, Maskova J, Fucikova Z, Kuzel D, Belsan T, Sosna 0. Midterm clinical and first reproductive results of a randomized controlled trial comparing uterine fibroid embolization and myomectomy. Cardiovasc Intervent Radiol. 2008;31:73–85.
5. Spies JB, Ascher SA, Roth AR, Kim J, Levy EB, Gomez-Jorge J. Uterine artery embolization for leiomyomata. Obstet Gynecol. 2001;98:29–34.
6. Dumousset E, Chabrot P, Rabischong B, et al. Preoperative uterine artery embolization before uterine fibroid myomectomy. Cardiovasc Intervent Radiol. 2008;31:514–20.

Suggested Reading

Costantino M, Lee J, McCullough M, et al. Bilateral versus unilateral femoral access for uterine artery embolization: results of a randomized comparative trial. J Vasc Interv Radiol. 2010;21:829–35.

Dumousset E, Chabrot P, Rabischong B, et al. Preoperative uterine artery embolization before uterine fibroid myomectomy. Cardiovasc Intervent Radiol. 2008;31(3):514–20.

Hovsepian DM, Siskin GP, Bonn J, et al. Quality improvement guidelines for uterine artery embolization for symptomatic leiomyomata. J Vasc Interv Radiol. 2009;20:193–9.

Kroencke TJ, Scheurig C, Poellinger A, et al. Uterine artery embolization for leiomyomas: percentage of infarction predicts clinical outcome. Radiology. 2010;255:834–41.

Mara M, Maskova J, Fucikova Z, Kuzel D, Belsan T, Sosna 0. Midterm clinical and first reproductive results of a randomized controlled trial comparing uterine fibroid embolization and myomectomy. Cardiovasc Intervent Radiol. 2008;31:73–85.

Pelage JP, Le Dref O, Soyer P, et al. Arterial anatomy of the female genital tract: variations and relevance to transcatheter embolization of the uterus. Am JR. 1999;172:989–94.

Pinto I, Chimeno P, Romo A, et al. Uterine fibroids: uterine artery embolization versus abdominal hysterectomy for treatment. A prospective, randomized, and controlled clinical trial. Radiology. 2003;226:425–31.

Popovic M, Puchner S, Berzaczy D, Lammer J, Bucek RA. Uterine artery embolization for the treatment of adenomyosis: a review. J Vasc Interv Radiol. 2011;22:901–9.

The REST Investigators. Uterine-artery embolization versus surgery for symptomatic uterine fibroids. N Engl J Med. 2007;356:360–70.

Spies JB, Ascher SA, Roth AR, Kim J, Levy EB, Gomez-Jorge J. Uterine artery embolization for leiomyomata. Obstet Gynecol. 2001;98:29–34.

Spies JB, Bruno J, Czyda-Pommersheim F, Magee ST, Ascher S, Jha RC. Long-term outcome of uterine artery embolization of leiomyomata. Obstet Gynecol. 2005;106:933–9.

Stokes LS, Wallace MJ, Godwin RB, et al. Quality improvement guidelines for uterine artery embolization for symptomatic leiomyomas. J Vasc Interv Radiol. 2010;21:1153–63.

Uterine fibroid embolization in "Clinical practice in Interventional Radiology". p. 87–93. Vienna: CIRSE; Ed. 2007.

Van der Kooj SM, Hehenkamp WJ, Volkers NA, Birnie E, Ankum WM, Reekers JA. Uterine artery embolization vs hysterectomy in the treatment of symptomatic uterine fibroids: 5-year outcome from the randomized EMMY trial. Am J Obstet Gynecol. 2010;203:105, e1–13.

Worthington-Kirsch RL, Hutchins FL, Popky GL. Uterine arterial embolization for the management of leiomyomas: quality of life assessment and clinical response. Radiology. 1998;208:625–9.

Chapter 20
Pelvi-perineal Venous Insufficiency

Louis Boyer, Agaïcha Alfidja Lankoande, Antoine Maubon, Anne Ravel, Cristi Gageanu, Abdoulaye Ndoye Diop, and Pascal Chabrot

20.1 Pelvic Congestion Syndrome

20.1.1 Background

Chronic pelvic pain is defined as inferior abdominal and/or pelvic cyclic or noncyclic pain, lasting for more than 6 months. It accounts for 10–40 % of the reasons for gynecological visits, a third of the indications for diagnostic celioscopy, and 15 % of hysterectomies.

Pelvic congestion syndrome (PCS), one of its causes, results from a retrograde flow into an incontinent ovarian vein, thus causing pain. The stasis and the dilatation of the left ovarian draining vein are more important that on the right side.

Venous ovarian incontinence affects 10 % of women, among which 60 % can develop a PCS [1].

The mechanism of the PCS is most likely multifactorial: absence of valves on the ovarian vein; hormonal factors (dilated veins and PCS are more frequent in the cases of multiparity, occurring more willingly in the premenopause period, hence suggesting a link with ovarian activity); mechanical factors: venous stasis during pregnancy, kinking of the pelvic veins associated with an abnormal uterine position, and external

L. Boyer, MD, PhD (✉) • A. Alfidja Lankoande, MD • A. Ravel, MD • P. Chabrot, MD, PhD
Department of Radiology, University Hospital of Clermont-Ferrand,
Clermont-Ferrand, France
e-mail: lboyer@chu-clermontferrand.fr; pchabrot@chu-clermontferrand.fr

A. Maubon, MD, PhD
Department of Radiology, University Hospital of Limoges, Limoges, France

C. Gageanu, MD
Department of Radiology, Issoire Hospital, University Hospital of Clermont-Ferrand,
Clermont-Ferrand, France

A.N. Diop, MD
Department of Radiology, University Hospital, Dakar, Senegal

P. Chabrot, L. Boyer (eds.), *Embolization*,
DOI 10.1007/978-1-4471-5182-1_20, © Springer-Verlag London 2014

compressions such as the nutcracker syndrome (renal vein compression between aorta and superior mesenteric artery); and lastly an ovarian venous congestion due to portal hypertension, an inferior vena cava syndrome, or a pelvic venous thrombosis.

PCS corresponds to unexplained, global, or left-predominant pelvic pain that can spread out to the buttock or the thigh and which is increased in premenstrual phase and during the pregnancy, or with tiredness, standing up position, effort, and after intercourse. It can be associated with pelvic heaviness, dysmenorrhea, anxiety, dyspareunia, irritable bladder, dysuria, etc. [2]. Uni- or bilateral vulvar varicosities can be observed, often spreading to the internal face of the thigh, with internal saphenous varicose veins in some cases. Varicose veins of the buttock can also be observed. The association of an ovarian and postcoital pain allows the diagnosis of a PCS with sensitivity and specificity rates of respectively 94 % and 77 % [3].

In case of chronic pelvic pain, ultrasound is the first-line imaging test. The performance of suprapubic and endovaginal ultrasound is improved with the standing up position and/or after the Valsalva maneuver. Four main criteria are to be looked for [4, 5]: tortuous pelvic veins of more than 6 mm in diameter; slow flow (3 cm/s) or inverted cranio-caudal flow; dilated intramyometrial arcuate veins communicating with bilateral pelvic varicose veins; and polycystic ovaries. It must be completed with a Doppler ultrasound examination of the lower limbs, as well as a renal and retroperitoneal venous exploration. Besides the assessment of these pelvic varicose veins, ultrasound also contributes to the differential diagnosis. It can be completed with a CT scan or more readily by an MRI (morphological exploration and angio-MR, including venous phase). CT or MR false negatives are possible, due to the supine position during the examination.

The Coakley criteria allow a diagnosis: presence of at least 4 tortuous para-uterine veins of variable size, among which one of more than 4 mm diameter, or an ovarian vein larger than 8 mm. The extension of the varicose veins to the broad ligaments and to paravaginal plexuses can be determined, as well as an abnormality in the renal venous return (nutcracker syndrome).

The nutcracker syndrome incidence has 2 peaks: the early stage (young patient), with continent ovarian valves – a reflux is not observed, but there is a retrograde hypertension in the left renal vein, with or without hematuria and lumbar pain – then, valvular incontinence and reflux, leading to PCS.

To summarize: The clinical symptoms of a PCS are evocative; it nevertheless requires noninvasive imaging that depicts the pelvic varicose veins and contributes to the differential diagnosis. A laparoscopy can then be proposed, in order to confirm the diagnosis, but invasive venography remains the gold standard and constitutes the first step before embolization.

20.1.2 Relevant Radiological Anatomy

Three vein networks ensure the venous drainage of the pelvis: on the first hand the femoral, external, and common iliac veins, and the inferior vena cava; on the second hand the internal iliac veins; and lastly the ovarian and the left renal veins. Anastomoses exist between the left and right pelvic veins, with the inferior mesenteric vein (in particular on the left side), between the right and left ovarian veins, and between the ovarian and the iliac veins.

The left ovarian vein drains into the left renal vein, while the right ovarian vein drains directly into the inferior vena cava.

20.1.3 Techniques

- Generally a local anesthesia to the Scarpa is sufficient.
- We do not prescribe systematic prophylactic antibiotherapy.
- It is helpful to tilt the angiography tabletop (tilting test); otherwise we use the Valsalva maneuver.

Pelvic venography and embolization present technical similarities with embolization of varicoceles:

- The venous access can be femoral or jugular.
- 4–7 F catheters are used. We do not use any guiding catheter and prefer precurved hydrophilic cobra-type catheters as well as hydrophilic guides.
- The opacification of the left renal vein allows the depiction of its compression between aorta and SMA. A selective catheterization of the left renal vein and then of the left ovarian vein is carried out, with a 4 French cobra hydrophilic catheter in our center. A reflux is detected with a manual test allowing the detection of a valvular incontinence of the ovarian vein. In case of suspicion of nutcracker syndrome, a left renal venous manometry is helpful.

A careful distal catheterization extending to the promontory then allows a manual injection to detect pelvic venous distension and ovarian or hypogastric venous reflux. The volume of contrast medium used for this manual injection must be recorded.

Catheterization of the right ovarian vein is then carried out, according to the same protocol. It will be disregarded only when it is very spindly or not seen.

A complete venous cartography is thus obtained and can be detected a valvular incontinence of the ovarian vein, a reflux into the ovarian vein with possible filling of the contralateral veins, a hypogastric venous drainage, and sometimes an extension of the venous congestion to the inguinal, vulvar, perineal, rectal, or inferior limbs veins. Criteria for the diagnosis of pelvic varicose veins are [4–6] diameter of ovarian or uterine veins and utero-ovarian arcade equal to or larger than 5 mm diameter; a free reflux in the ovarian vein, with valvular incontinence; filling by the contrast agent above the median line; vulva or thigh varicose veins; and a stasis of the contrast medium in the pelvic veins.

But venous morphological anomalies are not necessarily related to a PCS: dilatation of the ovarian vein networks is possible in asymptomatic patients, especially in the multiparous women.

- Embolization is generally carried out just after the invasive diagnostic venography. After the left ovarian venography, we use the Valsalva maneuver and if necessary tilt the tabletop by 45°, to inject a volume of the sclerosing agent identical to the volume of contrast agent previously injected manually to obtain a distal selective opacification (evaluation of the blood volume of the pelvic varicose veins).

The sclerosing agent chosen by many authors is a Gelfoam-sclerosant mixture (5 % sodium morrhuate or 3 % tetradecyl sodium sulfate).

Other authors use only coils, while others use biological glues.

Large coils (0.035 in., or even Amplatzer plugs for some) are then deployed all along the ovarian vein, up to its drainage into the left renal vein.

Liquid agents must not be used if a communication has been observed between ovarian and colic veins.

When it is possible, bilateral embolization is performed, using the same protocol with the right ovarian vein. But if on the right side there is no visible reflux, occlusion can be carried out using only coils [7].

- When there is the slightest doubt on a link between the ovarian venous plexus and internal iliac affluents, a venography of the internal iliac must be carried out as well before performing embolization. It should take place immediately after the ovarian embolization or else 4–6 weeks later [8]. The catheterization of the right and left hypogastric veins requires a femoral approach. We use a Berman-type catheter equipped with an occlusion balloon, to carry out manual injections in the hypogastric trunk and possibly in afferent varicose veins. When pelvic, vulvar, or upper-thigh varicose veins are discovered, a volume equivalent to that of the contrast medium used is manually slowly injected, just until a reflux is observed. A mixture of Gelfoam-sclerosant is used (identical to that injected in the ovarian veins). The occlusion balloon is left inflated for about 5 min, in order to avoid primitive iliac vein or vena cava reflux. Some authors prefer using coils (keeping in mind the problem of a possible migration); others use a combination of coils + sclerosing agent.
- Keeping a supine position for a few hours is then necessary. For some, this procedure can take place on an outpatient basis, with patient discharge on the same night and a prescription of anti-inflammatory drugs (Ketoprofen: Profenid®) and oral analgesics (paracetamol: Doliprane®, Nefopam: Acupan®). The use of an IV pain pump (patient-controlled analgesia pump) requires a short hospitalization.

Afterwards, physically demanding activities must be avoided for at least 10 days.

Even in the case of a favorable evolution, a medical visit is advised 3 months and 6 months after the procedure. The imaging follow-up is not codified: we recommend at least a Doppler ultrasound, and ideally an MRI, 6 months after the procedure.

20.1.4 Technical Results

Technical successes rates of 98–100 % are reported.

A recurrence rate of less than 8 % is reported [9]. But it is not always possible to catheterize the right ovarian vein.

The morbidity is limited (less than 4 %), predominantly due to puncture site complications. It is therefore pertinent to carry out embolization and the diagnostic venography during the same session.

There is no significant change in hormone assays and menstrual cycles during the follow-up.

Fifteen days after, 70–85 % of the patients are improved.

Few data are available on the long-term results. The most important series [10], with a 45 ± 18-month follow-up in 127 patients (127 bilateral venous ovarian embolizations and 108 embolizations of the internal iliac vein), reports 83 % improvement, 13 % unchanged, and 4 % deteriorated rates.

The results are more favorable in multiparous women, less favorable in the case of dyspareunia, and identical in the case of unilateral or bilateral involvement.

A favorable effect could even be observed after a hysterectomy.

However no control study is available. The results are most likely related to patient selection, many of them being treated after the failure of other therapeutic methods.

It must be noted that the technical protocols are regularly evolving.

20.1.5 Indications

- The medical treatment (medroxyprogesterone acetate) helps with the pain but its benefits are short lasting: it is a symptomatic treatment for short periods.
- Venous surgical interventions have been advocated (uterine suspension, extraperitoneal resection of the left ovarian vein, laparoscopic ligation of the left ovarian vein, hysterectomy), but embolization is preferred by a number of authors, due to its efficacy and to its limited morbidity.

Embolization should be considered only if a venous access is possible and in the absence of any active pelvic inflammation disease or any other infectious state that should be treated beforehand.

- In the case of the nutcracker syndrome at the valvular incontinence phase and with a reflux resulting in a PCS, an embolization can be proposed if the symptoms are severe, especially when the left ovarian vein is not the only drainage of the venous flow coming from the left renal vein. Else, in the absence of reno-azygo-lumbar trunk, an increased intrarenal venous hyperpressure (or spinal plexus venous pressure with a reno-lumbar trunk without hemiazygos vein) must be discussed, and the benefit/risk ratio must be evaluated as a high reno-cava pressure gradient is unfavorable.

At an earlier stage, the renal venous stenting of the nutcracker syndrome can be attempted as an alternative to surgical solutions (bypass, autotransplantation, etc.), but its long-term results are not known.

- In the case of an ilio-caval obstruction, the treatment of the cause is more important than the treatment of the reflux and of the pelvic congestion.

20.2 Varicoceles, Lower Limbs Varicose Veins, and Pelvic Varicose Veins

Fifteen percent of recurrences of lower limbs varicose veins and some varicose veins of atypical localization are caused by pelvi-perineal venous insufficiency (PPVI).

Doppler ultrasound examination searching for PPVI must be systematic in case of varicose veins of the lower limbs with perineal involvement.

Encouraging initial results concerning the lower limbs veins have been obtained after embolization of incontinent ovarian veins, but these results have to be confirmed in the long term: Lasry [11] has reported 30 venographies with embolization in patients with perineal varicose veins; after 6 months (2–20): all the symptoms had disappeared in 31 % of the cases, an improvement in the symptoms and/or a considerable reduction of the varicose veins was observed in 59 % of the cases, and in 10 % of the cases, there was no improvement.

These results make us discuss about the place of this technique compared to traditional treatments in case of recurrences or in case of primitive varicose veins.

Key Points

- PCS is a cause of chronic pelvic pain, resulting from a retrograde reflux in an incontinent ovarian vein.
- The mechanism is multifactorial: absence of venous valves, hormonal factors, and mechanical factors.
- A clinical selection is mandatory.
- Ultrasound is the first imaging test, possibly completed by MRI, rather than CT, to visualize the pelvic varicose veins and contribute to the differential diagnosis.
- Nutcracker syndrome, early stage: left renal vein hypertension ± hematuria, ± lumbar pain; then valvular incontinence and reflux: PCS
- Venography remains the gold standard to visualize the dilated ovarian veins: selective venography of the left ovarian vein via the renal vein, ± distal embolization using a sclerosing agent Gelfoam mix, then proximal coils up to the confluent in the renal vein; right ovarian vein: coils can be sufficient.

- When there is the slightest doubt on a link between the ovarian venous plexus and affluents of internal iliac veins: venography and possible internal iliac embolization (Gelfoam + sclerosing agent, through an occlusion balloon), during the same procedure or 6 weeks later.
- Supine position for several hours, then analgesics and anti-inflammatory drugs. Ambulatory care is possible.
- Technical successes: 98–100 %; recurrences: less than 8 %; very limited morbidity.
- Improvement of the symptoms after 15 days: 70–85 % of the patients.
- Long-term results: to be confirmed; after 45 months (Kim): improvement, 83 %; unchanged, 13 %; and worsening, 4 %.
- No controlled study; many indications correspond today to failures of other techniques.
- Fifteen percent of recurrences of lower limbs varicose veins and some varicose veins of atypical localization are caused by pelvi-perineal venous insufficiency (PPVI).
- Systematic research of PPVI using Doppler ultrasound must be carried out in case of lower limb varicose veins when the perineal region is involved.
- Invasive venography confirms the diagnosis and allows embolization of the incontinent ovarian veins.
- Encouraging initial results concerning the lower limb veins after embolization of pelvic varicose veins, but the indications of embolization versus traditional treatments for recurrences and primitive varicose veins are yet to be established.

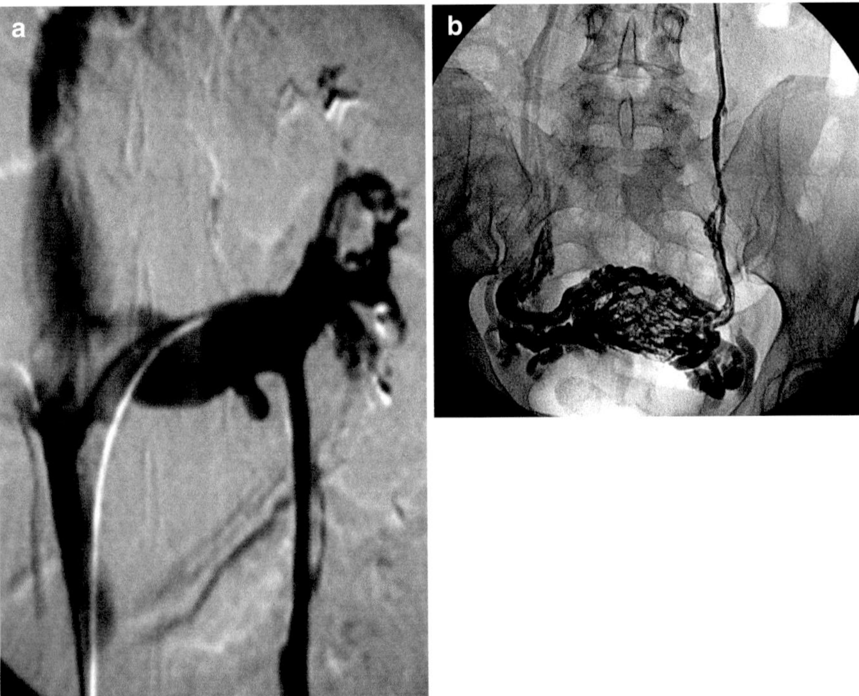

Fig. 20.1 Right venous femoral access, ilio-caval catheterization followed by left renal vein catheterization: venous drainage of a large left gonadal vein (**a**), in a context of chronic pelvic venous congestion, documented in this 48 y. o. W by noninvasive imaging (CT + Doppler) and confirmed by these selective catheterizations and injection in the lower left ovarian vein (**b**)

Fig. 20.2 A 45 y. o. W, clinical + radiological suspicion of chronic pelvic venous congestion syndrome. (**a, b**) Selective injection after catheterization of the left gonadal vein: pelvic venous congestion, opacification of the right gonadal vein (**b**) via the pelvic anastomosis. (**c**) Control after left ovarian vein embolization with tetradecyl sulfate + coils. (**d**) Right gonadal vein catheterization: coils + sclerosing agent embolization. (**e, f**) Additional pelvic embolization 4 weeks later: left hypogastric vein catheterization from a right venous femoral access (crossover) (**e**), followed by embolization beyond an occlusion balloon (**f**)

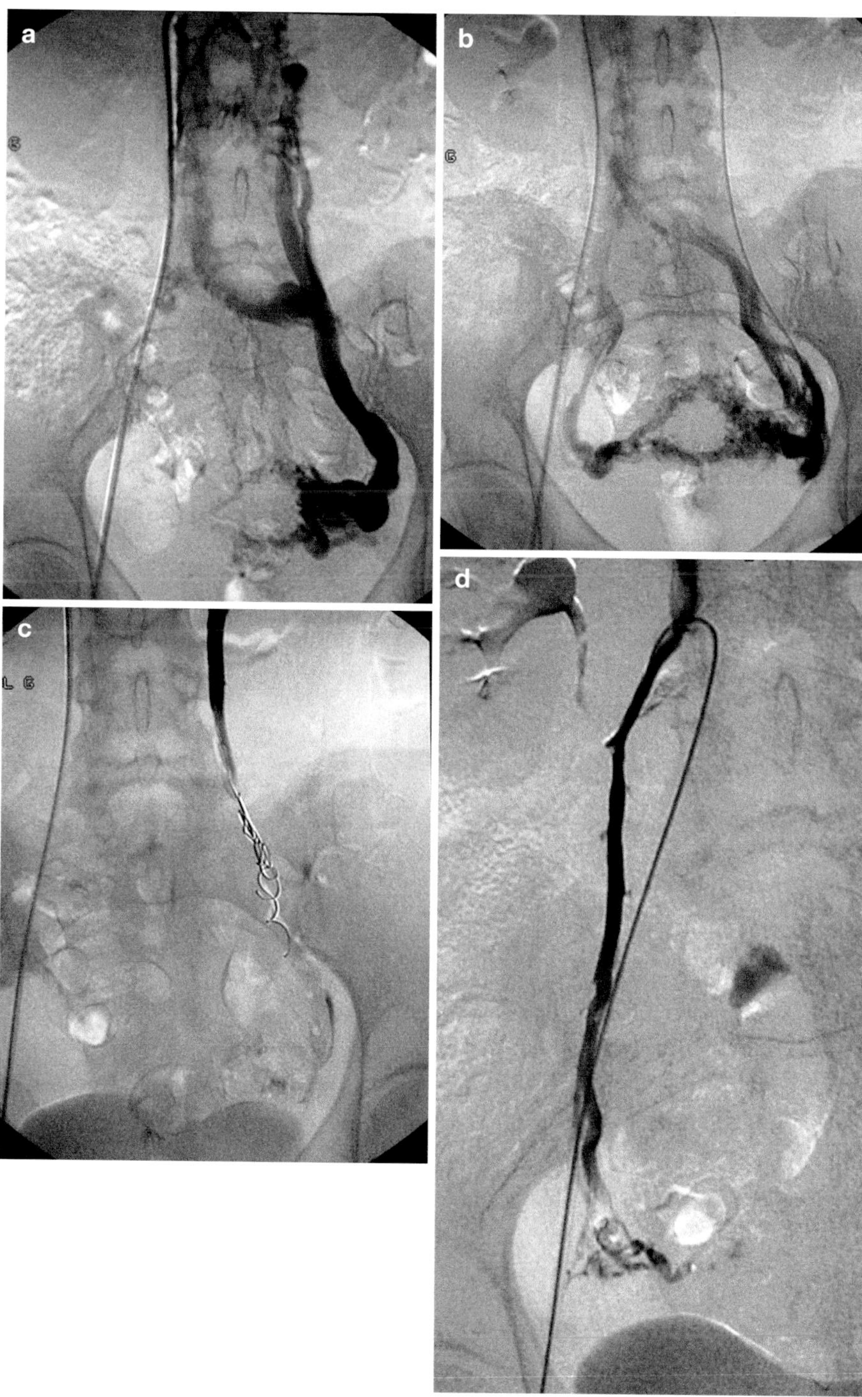

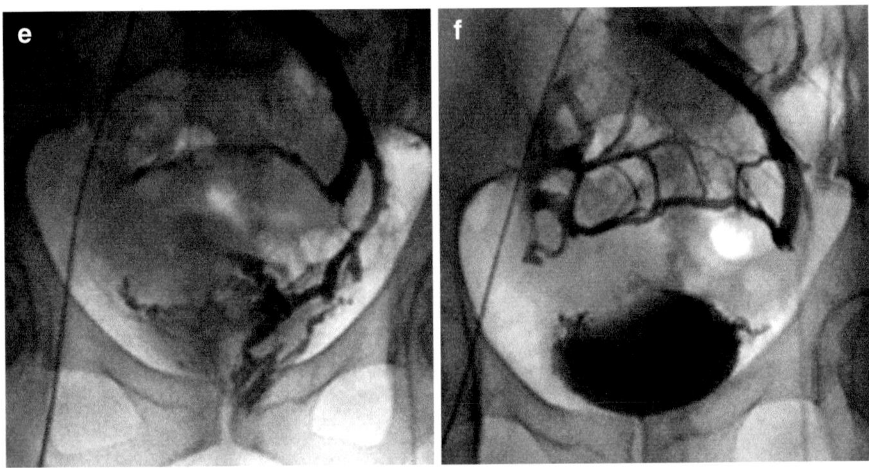

Fig. 20.2 (continued)

References

1. Belenky A, Bartal G, Atar E, Cohen M, Bachar GN. Ovarian varices in healthy female kidney donors: incidence, morbidity, and clinical outcome. Am J Roentgenol. 2002;179:625–9.
2. Kuligowska E, Deeds 3rd L, Lu 3rd K. Pelvic pain: overlooked and underdiagnosed gynecologic conditions. Radiographics. 2005;25:3–20.
3. Beard RW, Highman JH, Pearce S, Reginald PW. Diagnosis of pelvic varicosities in women with chronic pelvic pain. J Obstet Gynaecol. 1988;95:153–61.
4. Beard RW, Highman JH, Pearce S, et al. Diagnosis of pelvic varicosities in women with chronic pelvic pain. Lancet. 1984;2:946–9.
5. Park S, Lim J, Ko Y, et al. Diagnosis of pelvic congestion syndrome using transabdominal and transvaginal sonography. Am J Roentgenol. 2004;182:683–8.
6. Kennedy A, Hemingway A. Radiology of ovarian varices. Br J Hosp Med. 1990;44(1): 38–43.
7. Nicholson T, Basile A. Pelvic congestion syndrome: who should we treat and how? Tech Vasc Interv Radiol. 2006;9:19–23.
8. Ganeshan A, et al. Chronic pelvic pain due to pelvic congestion syndrome: the role of diagnostic and interventional radiology. Cardiovasc Intervent Radiol. 2007;30(6):1105–11.
9. Venbrux AC, Chang AH, et al. Pelvic congestion syndrome (pelvic venous incompetence): impact of vascular and interventional radiology. J Vasc Interv Radiol. 2002;13:171–8.
10. Kim HS, Malhotra AD, Rowe PC, Lee JM, Venbrux AC. Embolotherapy for pelvic congestion syndrome: long-term results. J Vasc Interv Radiol. 2006;17:289–97.
11. Lasry JL. Pelvi-perineal venous insufficiency and varicose veins of the lower limbs and endoluminal treatment in thirty females. J Mal Vasc. 2007;32:23.

Suggested Reading

Black CM, Thorpe K, Venbrux A, et al. Research reporting standards for endovascular treatment of pelvic venous insufficiency. J Vasc Interv Radiol. 2010;21:796–803.

Ganeshan A, et al. Chronic pelvic pain due to pelvic congestion syndrome: the role of diagnostic and interventional radiology. Cardiovasc Intervent Radiol. 2007;30(6):1105–11.

Kim HS, Malhotra AD, Rowe PC, Lee JM, Venbrux AC. Embolotherapy for pelvic congestion syndrome: long-term results. J Vasc Interv Radiol. 2006;17:289–97.

Lasry JL. Pelvi-perineal venous insufficiency and varicose veins of the lower limbs and endoluminal treatment in thirty females. J Mal Vasc. 2007;32:23.

Nicholson T, Basile A. Pelvic congestion syndrome: who should we treat and how? Tech Vasc Interv Radiol. 2006;9:19–23.

Venbrux AC, Chang AH, et al. Pelvic congestion syndrome (pelvic venous incompetence): impact of vascular and interventional radiology. J Vasc Interv Radiol. 2002;13:171–8.

Part VIII
Situations and Strategies: Traumatisms

Chapter 21
Embolization of Abdominal and Pelvic Trauma

Louis Boyer, Agaïcha Alfidja Lankoande, Cristi Gageanu, Isabelle Brazzalotto, Marie-Aude Vaz Tourret, Stéphane Boisgard, and Pascal Chabrot

21.1 Background

Polytrauma patients present with multiple injuries among which at least one is life threatening in the short term, justifying a team approach including radiologists, who contribute to the diagnosis, assessment, and endovascular management of the injuries, with a special mention to embolization of trauma-related bleedings.

An initial assessment and resuscitation are carried out during the *prehospital phase;* during patient *transfer*, the receiving hospital should be notified of patient condition to help in planning *in-hospital care* by a team coordinator (most logically: an intensive care doctor). Clinical assessment (airway, breathing, circulation, disability, events/environment) allows a patient categorization:

- Level 1: extreme hemodynamic or neurological distress
- Level 2: precarious state maintained by intensive resuscitation
- Level 3: unstable patient

L. Boyer, MD, PhD (✉) • A. Alfidja Lankoande, MD
M.-A. Vaz Tourret, MD • P. Chabrot, MD, PhD
Department of Radiology, University Hospital of Clermont-Ferrand, Clermont-Ferrand, France
e-mail: lboyer@chu-clermontferrand.fr; pchabrot@chu-clermontferrand.fr

C. Gageanu, MD
Department of Radiology, Issoire Hospital, University Hospital of Clermont-Ferrand, Clermont-Ferrand, France

I. Brazzalotto, MD
Department of Anesthesia, University Hospital of Clermont-Ferrand, Clermont-Ferrand, France

S. Boisgard, MD, PhD
Department of Orthopedic Surgery, University Hospital of Clermont-Ferrand, Clermont-Ferrand, France

P. Chabrot, L. Boyer (eds.), *Embolization*,
DOI 10.1007/978-1-4471-5182-1_21,

Imaging work-up must not delay patient resuscitation. Aside from the limbs, two radiological traumatic entities must be considered: the skull and the brain region and the trunk (thorax + abdomen + pelvis). If the polytrauma is severe, the two entities must be assessed, as lesion associations are frequent and because of the poor reliability of clinical examination. During this radiological assessment, it is important to limit patient mobilization, which exposes to hemodynamic and/or respiratory decompensation and/or to displacement of unstable bone fractures. A whole-body CT is the ideal imaging modality. For patients with non-compensated shock, a fast assessment in the emergency room is sometimes the only alternative, including a front-view chest plain film (is there pneumothorax requiring drainage?), a front-view pelvic plain film (is there an anterior pelvic fracture contraindicating bladder catheterization? a severe fracture explaining the hemodynamic collapse?), a lateral plain film of the cervical spine (is there an obvious and serious injury?), and a FAST-type ultrasound (Focused Assessment with Sonography for Trauma), to detect a hemoperitoneum. Secondary assessment with whole-body CT should be nonetheless considered for these cases. In all cases, conventional limb X-ray films will be performed on demand.

Patients presenting with *head trauma* should be considered as polytrauma patients until proven otherwise: this assumption must be confirmed or infirmed after the initial imaging work-up. Isolated head injuries are managed by the neurosurgical team.

The treatment of traumatic lesions of main large-caliber arteries (aorta, iliac arteries, subclavian arteries, etc.) is ideally performed with covered stents which restore vascular continuity.

In case of hemorrhage, precise criteria have yet to be established to define which patients should benefit from a *hemostasic embolization* and which patients should undergo *surgery*, but *three situations* can be schematically distinguished, after having formally excluded an exteriorized bleeding (cranial wounds, arterial wounds, and open fractures):

- Hemodynamically unstable hemorrhagic syndrome with hemoperitoneum on the ultrasound without any pelvic fracture is an indication of a laparotomy.
- Hemodynamically unstable hemorrhagic syndrome due to pelvic fractures should undergo pelvic arterial embolization.
- Hemodynamically stable abdominopelvic hemorrhagic syndrome controlled by intensive care resuscitation is an indication of a pelvic or solid organ embolization, as multiple bleeding sites can be treated during the same angiographic session.

Obviously, this strategy requires the participation of an anesthesiologist and round-the-clock availability of the interventional radiology team.

For terminal arterial tree organs (kidney, spleen), endovascular occlusion must be performed nearest to the bleeding site, in order to limit the parenchymal loss; however, should selective catheterization be too time consuming, a proximal embolization should be preferred.

When a rich anastomotic network exists, the goal is to occlude the small-size arterioles while preserving the distal anastomosis. Therefore, small fragments of gelatin sponge or large microparticles must be chosen instead of powders or fine granulates. A "sandwich" exclusion (upstream and downstream occlusion) of injured artery prevents "back door re-bleeding" which can be observed when only an upstream occlusion is performed (hepatic parenchyma, pelvic and buttock muscles, abdominal wall).

In all cases, patient's vital prognosis must be preserved: in a traumatic setting, too much embolization is often preferable to not enough embolization.

Often after multiple blood transfusions, these patients may present with progressive coagulopathy which must be taken into account when choosing embolic agents. Coils, for example, require a functioning coagulation pathway. In these cases, we prefer leaving the introducer sheath in place at the end of procedure until hemostasis disorders are corrected, instead of using closure devices.

As soon as vessel occlusion is obtained, a rapid stabilization of the blood pressure and of the cardiac frequency is generally observed, thus reducing the need for filling liquids and vasoconstrictors. If there is no improvement after embolization in spite of an efficient resuscitation, then another bleeding site must be looked for.

After the first-line treatment, a *secondary assessment* is mandatory including complete clinical examination, as well as a review of the laboratory work-up, and all the imaging data by a senior radiologist as missed or hidden injuries can decompensate secondarily (extradural hematoma, isthmic aortic injury, initially limited pneumothorax decompensating after ventilation, diaphragm rupture, peritoneal syndrome revealing a GI tract perforation, paraplegia due to an unstable fracture and/or dislocation of the spine, limb ischemia complicating a skeletal trauma, etc.)

(a) *Embolization of Solid Organs*

Embolization of traumatic injuries is exhaustively described in Chaps. 6, 9, and 13 which can be referred to.

The American Association for Surgery of Trauma (*AAST*) [1] classification of abdominal visceral injuries in five stages of increasing severity (Appendix 21.1) is the reference for the therapeutic strategy. Embolizations can be performed to treat hemodynamically stable patients or those with a controlled hemorrhagic shock, when there is an active blush (bleeding) on CT, a false aneurysm, an arteriovenous fistula. Embolization is a more conservative approach than surgery, but the vital prognosis must be taken into account before all.

(b) *Embolization of Pelvic Trauma*

Severe pelvic traumas most frequently occur in a polytraumatic setting. Vascular complications are observed in about 15 % of pelvic fractures, which can be responsible for severe hemorrhagic shocks, leading to death in 30–50 % of cases.

Retroperitoneal hematoma (RPH) is related to pelvic fractures in 55 % of cases. Other causes of RPH are pancreaticoduodenal and renal lesions in 15 % and upper abdominal trauma with large vessel injuries in 21 %. An infraperitoneal contrast extravasation in the soft tissues is usually due to an arterial hemorrhage.

Pelvic hematoma can be induced by variable injuries of the bones, the veins (peri-vesical and presacral plexus), and the arteries (hypogastric and its branches), and it can be increased in case of hemostasis disorders. An multiple-phase angioCT scan facilitates the distinction between venous and arterial bleedings. Many controversies remain with respect to the relation between these hemorrhages, the injury mechanism, and the type of fracture (unstable); however, arterial bleeding is a consequence of the most severe traumas and is sometimes located far from the bone lesions. The anterior branches of the hypogastric arteries that are most frequently concerned are the internal pudendal and the obturator arteries, while among the posterior branches, the most frequently concerned are the gluteal, lateral sacral, and iliolumbar arteries.

21.2 Embolization of Solid Organs: Indications and Results

The relevant radiological anatomy and the embolization techniques of solid organs are discussed in Chaps. 6, 9, and 13.

Indications and results for blunt abdominopelvic trauma are recapped here.

A targeted prophylactic antibiotic treatment is advocated whenever embolization induces an infarction with a significant parenchymal necrosis.

21.2.1 Hepatic Trauma

21.2.1.1 Indications

Hemorrhage stops spontaneously in at least 50 % of liver traumatisms.

Unstable patients (uncompensated hemorrhagic shock) require shortened laparotomy and hepatic packing. Surgery can also be required for associated visceral and retroperitoneal lesions.

Stable patients which are at risk of re-bleeding must be identified, so as to treat them with embolization.

- Embolization is indicated in case of active arterial bleeding on CT scan, in patients who are hemodynamically stable or who have had a compensated hemodynamic shock, no matter what the AAST injury grade is (see Appendix 21.1). Some authors even recommend arteriography for stable patients with AAST grade IV and V lesions.
- Gelatin sponge, coils, particles, or glues can be used.

Semi-proximal embolization using microcoils and/or gelatin sponge, sparing the anastomotic arterial network, reduces the risk of ischemic complication of the bile ducts. However, this anastomotic arterial network can also impair proximal embolization in case of centro-hepatic lesions.

- Combined radiological and surgical treatments may be necessary. A shortened laparotomy allows hemostasis by packing and if necessary the surgical treatment of other lesions. The resuscitated patient can then benefit from an arterial embolization.
- Embolization is not indicated in vena cava or portal vein bleeding, which is an indication for surgery.

21.2.1.2 Results

- The success rate of hepatic arterial embolization varies from 80 to 100 %; a second embolization is rarely needed.
- The mortality rate of treated isolated traumatic hepatic lesions does not exceed 10 % (but the mortality in case of polytraumatisms is obviously clearly higher).
- Ischemic cholecystitis is the main complication due to the embolization of the cystic artery; it is often asymptomatic.
- We perform as a rule a cross-sectional morphological imaging control with contrast injection (CT or MRI) before patient discharge (and no later than 8 days after) and then 1 month after the procedure.

21.2.2 Splenic Trauma

21.2.2.1 Indications

Surgery is used to be the treatment of first intention.

Currently, a nonsurgical conservative approach is often proposed in hemodynamically stable patients by attentive monitoring or by an arterial embolization. Patient selection is therefore the key step.

The advantage of an embolization is that it preserves the vitality of part of the parenchyma and thus the spleen functions. However, if the patient's vital prognosis is at stake, the surgery must be preferred.

- A systematic angiography, which was once advocated by some authors to help in selecting patients for embolization, is not nowadays recommended. The two factors that determine indications of embolization are the hemodynamic stability and the CT scan results (AAST-graded lesions (see Appendix 21.1), vascular blush (active contrast extravasation), false aneurysm, and arteriovenous fistula). Contrast extravasation can be intraparenchymal, subcapsular, or peritoneal.
  - According to most of the authors, patients suffering from a hemorrhagic shock and/or showing signs of peritonitis must undergo immediate explorative surgery, while for the hemodynamic stable patients, conservative treatment should be the standard. Hagiwara [2] has recently suggested to broaden embolization indications to hemodynamically unstable patients responding to

vascular filling and having high (IV and V) AAST scores, but this is contested by other authors.
- Besides surgical indications, all traumatic splenic lesions with a blush on the CT scan, or an abundant hemoperitoneum according to others, must undergo a selective arteriography and often an embolization. This arterial blush observed on CT has a positive predictive value, but it is depicted on arteriography only in 93 % of the cases [3]. Embolization is also indicated in case of arteriovenous fistula or post-traumatic false aneurysm.

The AAST grade I lesions (for which a blush is only rarely visible) require a strict clinical and radiological monitoring and active management should a lowering of red blood cell count occur.

AAST grade II lesions without any blush on CT also require monitoring for a number of authors; in case of a blush, an arteriography/embolization must be carried out.

Arteriography must be carried out for grades III and IV, irrespective of whether there's a blush or not.

For grade V, there is no consensus. We recommend, as a number of other authors, surgical management.

- In addition to splenic lesions which are categorized according to the AAST classification, the "Baltimore" codification has been proposed by Marmery [4] (Appendix 21.2) to take into account the associated vascular lesions. It helps in identifying patients requiring surgical treatment and those needing an embolization, when there is a blush and/or false aneurysms and/or post-traumatic arteriovenous fistulas (Baltimore grade IV).
  - There is no consensus on whether embolization should be proximal or distal. Both are performed in our team. Distal embolization which is technically more difficult obtains, however, a safer intraparenchymal hemostasis, while preserving the spleen's immune function.

For proximal embolization, coil sizing and positioning are fundamental; hemostasis is achieved by diminishing arterial flow and pressure. It has notably been proposed for high-grade traumas without extravasation. But it can lead to an incomplete hemostasis and a delayed re-bleeding (in these cases, re-embolization can be difficult). It is inefficient in the case of AVF, because of the collaterality.

In our team, we initially carry out distal embolization with microparticles of increasing diameter (firstly 300–700 μm, then 900–1,200 μm); if it fails, we carry out a proximal embolization (coils, even Amplatzer occluders). In the case of a pseudoaneurysm or of AVF, a distal embolization is our initial choice, with or without additional proximal embolization.

21.2.2.2 Results

- Embolization of active bleeding is technically successful in more than 90 % of the cases. The failures are linked to catheterization difficulties or to bleeding recurrences.

- Complications have been reported in nearly 5 % of the cases, notably partial splenic necrosis and abscesses (which occur more frequently after a distal embolization than with proximal ones).

  We have noted a lower morbidity rate when embolization is carried out within 24 h following the trauma.

  The nonoperative management has been compared with surgical management, considering intention to treat strategies:

  - Overall mortality rate is the same in both cases (5–10 %).
  - Complications are less frequent and the hospital stay shorter with the nonsurgical management.
  - Splenectomy rates vary from 26 to 43 % with the operative management versus 12–15 % with the nonoperative strategy; thus, embolization performed in case of active arterial blush, and systematically for high-grade lesions, would grant a global splenectomy gain of 7–19 %.

- We perform a cross-sectional morphological imaging control with contrast injection (CT or MRI) before discharge (and no later than 8 days after) and 1 month after.

21.2.3 Renal Traumatisms

21.2.3.1 Indications

Emergency Embolizations

An emergency embolization can be required for severe trauma with large parenchymal fractures and voluminous hematomas of the perinephric space.

Active bleeding is identified on CT as a contrast blush on the arterial phase scans. It is due to an injury or a rupture of the renal artery or its branch.

The higher the AAST grade is, the more severe are the vascular lesions, and bigger is the risk of post-embolization parenchymal loss. Therefore embolization and hemostasis nephrectomy benefits/risk ratio must always be compared. A massive embolization of the kidney (main branches, even truncal) can however be indicated in case of severe trauma, thus providing preoperative stability needed for surgery.

In some cases, bleeding due to renal parenchyma trauma amends spontaneously within a few hours because of the relative inextensibility of the space. A careful monitoring is thus essential. In a very large majority of the cases, hemodynamically stable patients with a CT evaluation can be managed by attentive monitoring. AAST grade IV and V lesions often require surgery but can also be managed nonoperatively if they are well evaluated, selected, and monitored [5].

In the hours following trauma, worsening of clinical condition and/or laboratory tests can lead to a CT reevaluation and to an arteriography with embolization.

- Embolization is indicated if an active bleeding is depicted on CT in hemodynamically stable patients or in case of a hemodynamic shock responding to resuscitation.
- Embolization has also been proposed in patients with uncontrolled shock, but whenever the patient's vital prognosis is compromised, then surgery should be preferred.

The treatment of AAST grade I to III is generally a conservative management; embolization can be indicated for active bleeding. For the AAST grade IV, the treatment is, if possible, conservative, with embolization in case of active bleeding. For the AAST grade V, the treatment can be conservative if the patient is stable; an embolization may be required if the patient is unstable.

Depending on the morphology of the lesions, coils, particles, and/or absorbable agents can be used.

- It must also be noted that in some favorable cases, covered stents can restore the lumen of a traumatic renal artery.

Secondary Period

Around the tenth day, an occlusive thrombus can break off and induce a sudden and severe bleeding. The patient is not always under medical surveillance at that moment. As in the acute phase, an emergency embolization is a good option in this case.

Delayed Hemorrhages

Delayed hemorrhages are not rare (see Chap. 13); they sometimes occur several weeks after the initial trauma, in relation with an AVF or a secondary rupture of a traumatic false aneurysm, especially in cases of penetrating trauma by stabbing wounds. Their treatment with coils allows a conservative management.

21.2.3.2 Results

- Embolization is effective in 70–100 % of cases, with a low re-intervention rate (0–10 %).
- Complications are rare (out of target embolization, abscess, etc.).

Parenchymal loss depends on the embolization extent; however, there is often no long-term consequence on the renal function if it was normal prior to trauma. A post-traumatic hypertension is possible (approximately 5 %), which may be due to the trauma itself or to an excessive embolization of normal renal parenchyma. Side effects in children (impairment of renal function and hypertension) seem negligible, even after severe renal trauma.

- A CT follow-up is recommended for all AAST grades, with a systematic reevaluation 5–7 days after trauma.

  For severe traumas, a scintigraphy or an MRI must be planned 6 months after, in order to evaluate the residual renal function of the traumatic kidney.

  On the follow-up imaging, the renal infarction created by the embolization is often less important than one would expect.

21.3 Embolization of Pelvic Traumas

The relevant radiological anatomy of the internal iliac arteries and their branches is detailed in Chap. 12 (hypogastric arteries—aneurysms and occlusion before stent graft).

21.3.1 Technique

- If the patient is transferred with a pressure suit, it can be taken off gradually only when embolization is completed.
- In the event of a catastrophic hemodynamic shock, an occlusion balloon will be first set up, using the Seldinger's technique, at the level of the lower abdominal aorta, before carrying out all the steps listed below. If necessary, this maneuver may be performed in the emergency room.
- Arteriography must be conducted in parallel with resuscitation measures including the correction of hemostasis disorders of metabolic acidosis and maintaining patient's temperature.

Depending on the type of lesions, a prophylactic antibiotic treatment may be necessary (open wound fractures, important parenchymal ischemia, etc.).

- The clamping of a bladder catheter increases the intrapelvic pressure by filling up the bladder and thus contributes to the hemostasis.
- Under local anesthesia, a femoral approach is the standard procedure. Whenever it is possible, we prefer a bilateral access via the femoral arteries which is valuable should the hemodynamic instability worsen and/or should catheterization difficulties arise.
- After carrying out a global aortoiliac aortography (targeting the celiac aorta, should any doubt exist about bleeding injuries on the liver, spleen, or kidney), selective injections (more sensitive for the detection of bleeding lesions) will be performed cautiously with limited injection pressure, guided by CT findings. Even if the bleeding is unilateral, both hypogastric arteries must be catheterized and injected, because of the rich vascular network. With a bilateral access, we prefer using the crossover technique to catheterize the contralateral hypogastric artery as it facilitates considerably the catheterization not only of the pudendal and obturator arteries but also of the epigastric and circumflex iliac arteries.

We use 4 or 5 F hydrophilic catheters; micro-catheters are rarely needed.

Contrast extravasation can be observed (delayed angiographic series—more than 15 s—are required to see them), as well as false aneurysms, arteriovenous fistulae, traumatic dissection or arterial rupture characterized by an interruption of vessel opacification, and vasospasms (frequent in case of severe hemorrhage): all of these lesions should be treated.

- When the arterial lesion can be crossed, a "sandwich"-type occlusion with upstream and downstream coils is ideally performed. Microparticles and liquid agents can also be used or frequently, for many authors, absorbable gelatin. The choice of the occlusion agents and eventually their combination depends on the severity of the bleeding, whether it is focal or is diffuse and if it is proximal or distal.

Embolization should be as selective as possible owing to the procedure length: it is however preferable to obtain a proximal occlusion of the hypogastric artery with coils and/or absorbable gelatin than to perform a time-consuming hyperselective embolization in unstable patients.

When selective injection of the hypogastric arteries does not depict any abnormality, then the collaterals of the common femoral and of the lumbar arteries should also be explored. If angiography fails to depict contrast extravasation, then other etiologies must be discussed such as hypovolemia or diffuse arterial and venous injuries; a bilateral proximal hypogastric embolization using gelatin sponge and a cavography can be helpful in these cases.

Lesions of the primitive iliac and the external iliac arteries are much less frequent (less than 2 %) and have a poor prognosis: they can be treated quickly and efficiently with covered endoprostheses.

- After embolization, a control aortoiliac angiography is recommended, completed by selective visceral injections should there be the slightest doubt about associated lesions. It allows the detection of other bleeding sites which may not have been initially seen and depicts an eventual residual arterial supply of the bleeding site through the collateral network.

Introducer sheaths are left in place for at least 24 h, in order to be able to perform another embolization should a re-bleeding occur.

21.3.2 Results

Published data is limited and not comparable as there is no established therapeutic gold standard.

- Technical success is obtained in 85–95 % of the cases, but re-embolizations have been reported in 5–22 %, due to the reversal of the vasospasm with restoration of the blood volume or by persistent hemostasis disorders; arteriography must be rapidly repeated in case of a persistent arterial hypotension after initial embolization. Persistent hemorrhagic shock, absence of other intra-abdominal injury, and uncompensated metabolic acidosis are the predictive factors of a re-embolization.

- The mortality rate after an embolization remains high (18–50 %), mainly due to associated injuries. The results are ameliorated when the delay between the trauma and embolization is short.
- Complications, usually minor, have been observed in less than 2 % of the cases: puncture site complications, renal failure, contrast medium-related complications; and/or complications due to embolization: ischemia, necrosis, sexual dysfunction, and buttock claudication: these complications are generally observed after bilateral embolization, while muscle necrosis, sciatic paralysis, and sexual dysfunction can also be caused by the trauma itself.

The periodic evaluation of the trauma medical care results, through multidisciplinary morbidity and mortality reviews, gives much more efficiency to the trauma team and contributes to the optimization of the protocols.

21.3.3 Indications

A multispecialty approach is indicated.

In the case of polytrauma, the most severe lesions (the most hemorrhagic ones or those that constitute an immediate vital risk) must be treated in first; embolization can treat multiple bleeding sites.

Setting up an aortic occlusion balloon is possible directly upon arrival in the emergency room, with or without X-ray guidance; this takes place initially in the case of very severe collapse, before carrying out embolization.

Embolizations of the hemorrhagic complications of pelvic fractures should be preferred over surgery: it can be achieved without pressure modification, whereas the surgical approach compromises the packing effect of the hematoma.

Stabilization by orthopedic external fixing is convenient; but it has little chance to significantly reduce an arterial hemorrhage, whereas it can contribute to the hemostasis of a venous hemorrhage. There is no consensus on when it should be undertaken with respect to arteriography and embolization, which must nevertheless be early, so as to limit as much as possible blood transfusions. In a hemodynamically stable patient, in the absence of extravasation, the fixation can be directly achieved. In our group, the stabilization by external fixation does not delay embolization: the external fixator is set up in the angiography room, directly after the embolization, under fluoroscopic guidance. The introducer sheaths are left in place, and if there is the slightest doubt, we carry out another angiographic control after the fixation.

To summarize, embolization can take place:

- In hemodynamically unstable patients as quickly as possible, in the absence of associated severe injuries (absence of hemoperitoneum).
- In hemodynamically stable or stabilized patients with a fractured pelvis, when a blush or an arterial occlusion is depicted; is another criterion, a poor hemodynamic response to the vascular filling.

Key Points

- The management of polytrauma patients must be undertaken by an experienced multidisciplinary team, among which the interventional radiologist who contributes to the diagnosis and the management.
- Repair of large-caliber arterial injuries (aorta, iliac arteries, subclavian arteries, etc.) by restoring vascular continuity ideally with covered endoprostheses.
- Therapeutic options for abdominal solid organ traumas are determined by AAST classification.
- Solid organ embolizations are conceivable among hemodynamically stable patients or in case of controlled hemorrhagic shock, when there is an active blush on CT, a false aneurysm, and an arteriovenous fistula, and depend on the severity of lesions.
- Embolization is a more conservative approach than surgery, but if the patient's vital prognosis is at stake, then surgery must be preferred.
- Hepatic trauma: arterial embolization is effective on arterial bleeding and is indicated in stable patients with active bleeding on CT. Caval or portal venous bleeding is an indication for surgery.
- Splenic trauma: embolization can be carried out in hemodynamically stable patients, in case of false aneurysm, AFV, or when there is a blush for AAST grade II lesions and with or without blush for grade III and IV lesions. We recommend whenever it is possible to carry out rapidly a distal embolization. The grade V lesions require surgery.
- Renal trauma (endoprostheses in some cases of truncal arterial ruptures); acute phase (hemostasis embolization); secondary treatment (the 10th day hematuria) of arterio-urinary fistula; exclusion of late false aneurysms or AVF; embolization is effective, with few complications; morphological sequels depend on the extension of injury; possible post-traumatic hypertension.
- Pelvic traumas are generally severe and very frequently associated to other lesions.
- CT assessment is valuable in defining therapeutic indications, but it may not always be feasible for hemodynamically unstable patients.
- Embolization of hemorrhagic complications of pelvic fractures must be preferred to surgery:
  - In hemodynamically unstable patients and in the absence of associated severe injury (absence of hemoperitoneum), as soon as possible, immediately after plain film.
  - In hemodynamically stable or stabilized patients with a fractured pelvis, when a blush or an arterial occlusion is depicted; a poor hemodynamic response to the vascular filling is a second criterion.
- Embolization is more efficient than the external fixator to stop arterial bleeding: we thereby undertake it first.
- An embolization is efficient and rarely complicated, but re-embolization is not rare (5–22 %), and in spite of a technical success, the mortality remains high (18–50 %).

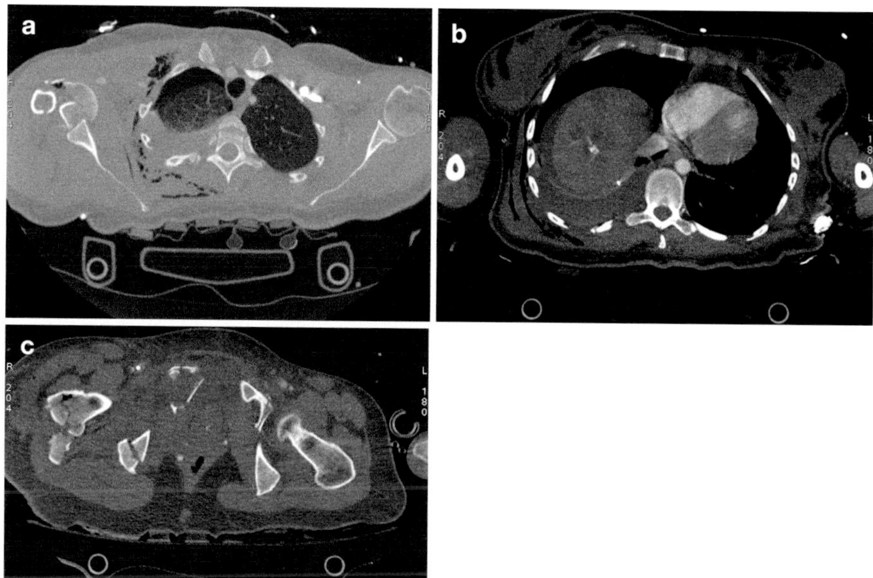

Fig. 21.1 Fifty-one-year-old male admitted with a very serious hemodynamic shock, after defenestration from 3rd floor. The mobile emergency medical unit (SAMU) conducted him directly to the CT room for a complete morphological assessment, because of multiple traumatic impacts, especially to the abdomen and pelvis. (**a**) Chest plain film: fractures of the right humeral head, thoracic flail, limited hemopneumothorax, and subcutaneous emphysema. (**b**) Hepatic blush; multiple foci of contusion of the liver. Enhancement of the kidneys and the spleen was decreased, but without apparent focal injury. (**c**) Multiple pelvic fractures, intrapelvic hematomas with blushes. (**d**) MPR reconstruction of the pelvis: multiple fractures. The critical hemodynamic status led the patient directly to the angiography room. (**e**) After bilateral femoral artery punctures (as pulse were even perceptible), aortography enabled a selective catheterization by crossover of the right and left internal iliac arteries. The selective injection of the right gluteal artery shows multiple extravasations that were treated by embolization with coils + gelatin. Extravasation in the anterior branches territories was also treated with coils. (**f**) Selective injection at the end of the left common iliac artery (from a right femoral access and crossover): massive vasoconstriction of the entire internal iliac network. The presence of a blush on the CT led us to inject resorbable gelatin in the trunk of the left hypogastric artery. (**g**) Left external iliac artery opacification: extravasation from the external iliac circumflex artery, a branch of the common femoral artery (*arrow*). (**h**) Selective catheterization of the iliac circumflex artery: massive extravasation, treated with coils. At this moment, the patient remained hemodynamically unstable, with abundant hemoperitoneum on ultrasound performed on the angio table: the opacification of the visceral arterial branches was then decided. (**i**) Abdominal aortography: vasoconstriction of renal and splanchnic arterial territories. Extravasation in the liver (*arrow*). (**j**) Selective catheterization of the common hepatic artery, which confirms massive blush in segment VIII. (**k**) Control injection after exclusion by particles and coils

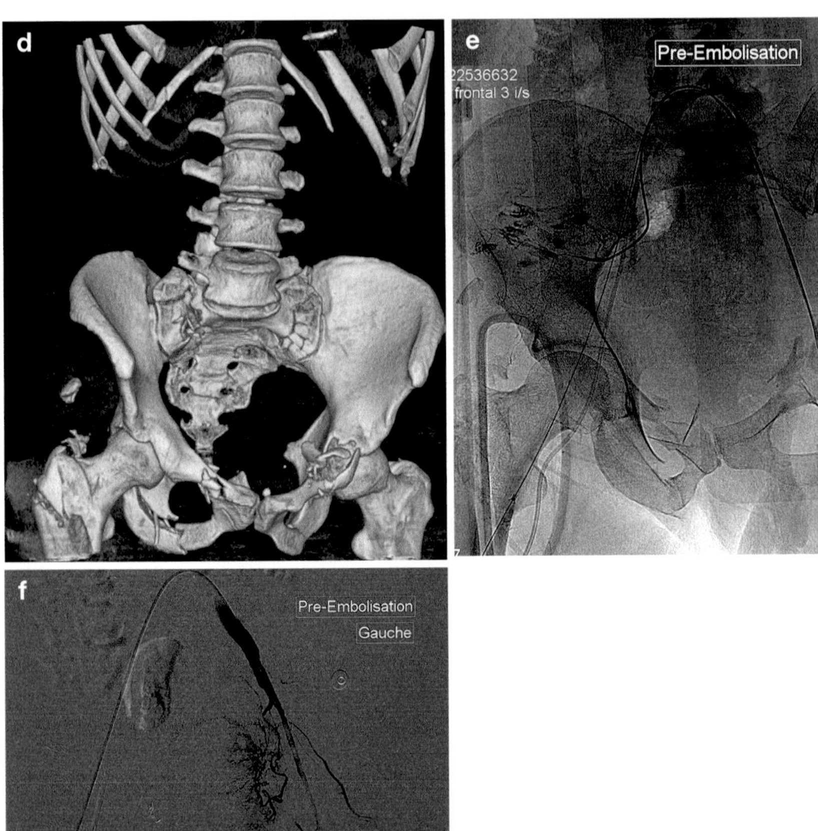

Fig. 21.1 (continued)

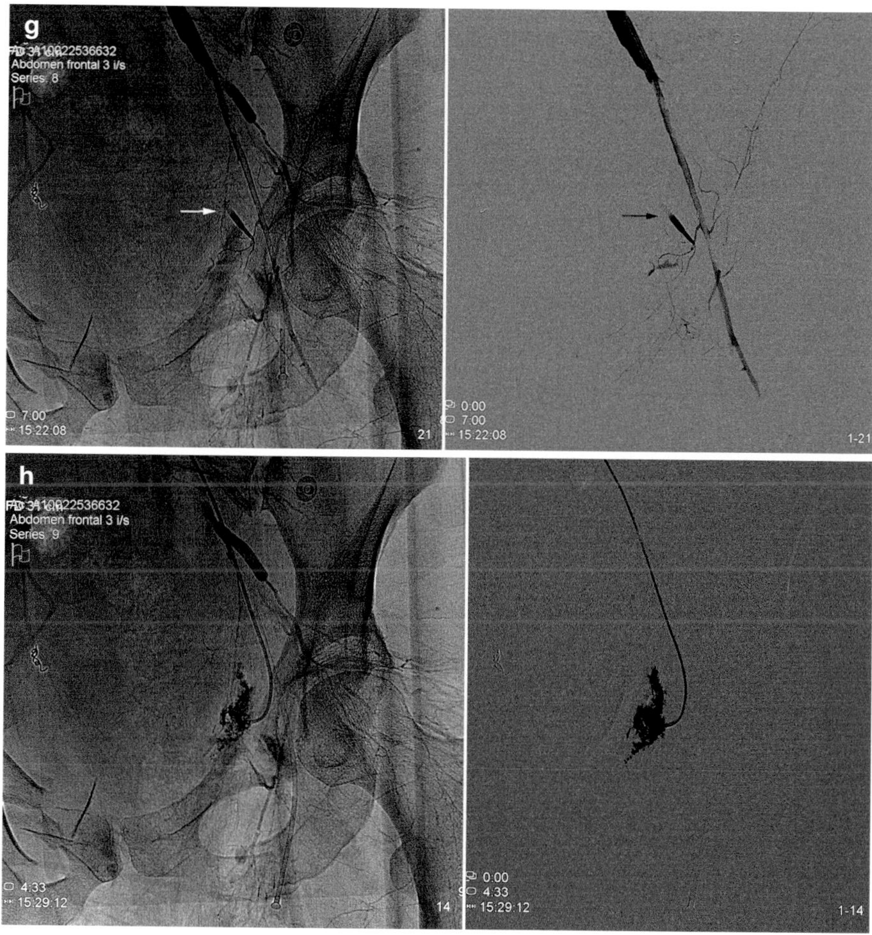

Fig. 21.1 (continued)

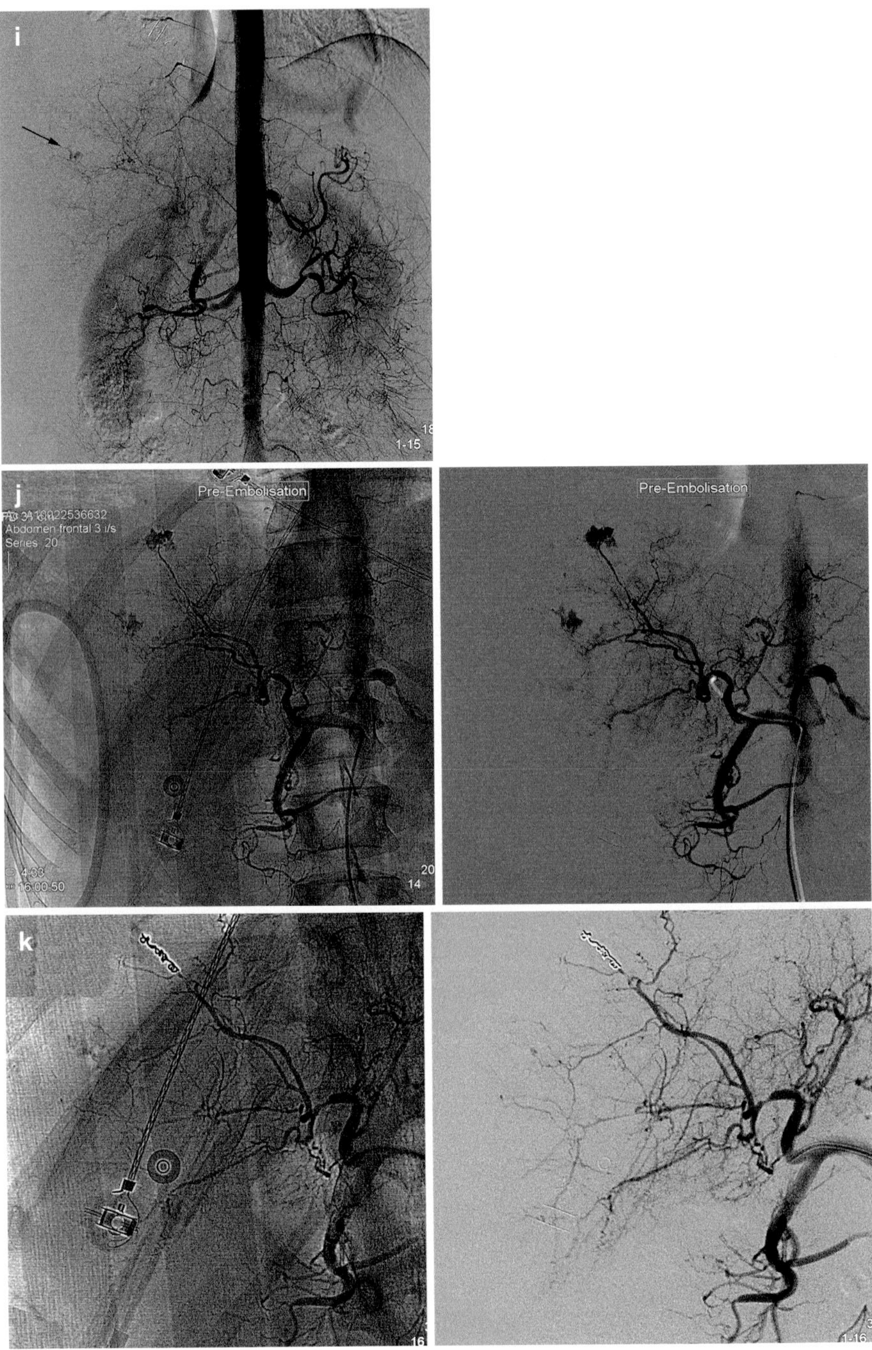

Fig. 21.1 (continued)

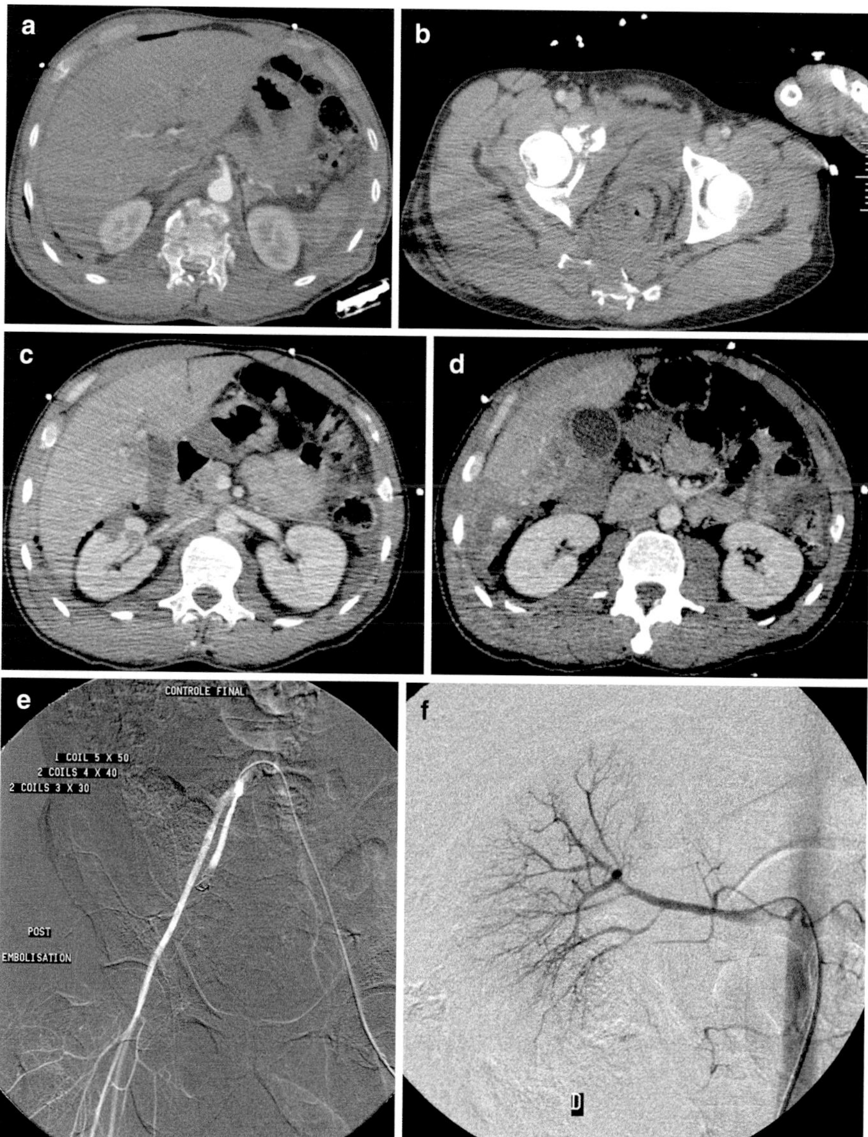

Fig. 21.2 Forty-six-year-old male, 8 m fall. (**a–d**) Initial CT: D12 fracture, pelvic fractures with large asymmetric pelvic hematoma; focal right renal contusion, important liver injury with blush. (**e**) Exclusion by coils of the right hypogastric artery because of multiple extravasations of anterior and posterior branches. (**f**) Selective injection of the right renal artery: no extravasation (no embolization). (**g**) Selective injection of the hepatic artery: diffuse vasoconstriction; important extravasation in segment VI, considered as the cause of the hemoperitoneum. (**h**) Hyperselective catheterization. (**i**) Control opacification after hyperselective exclusion by microparticles

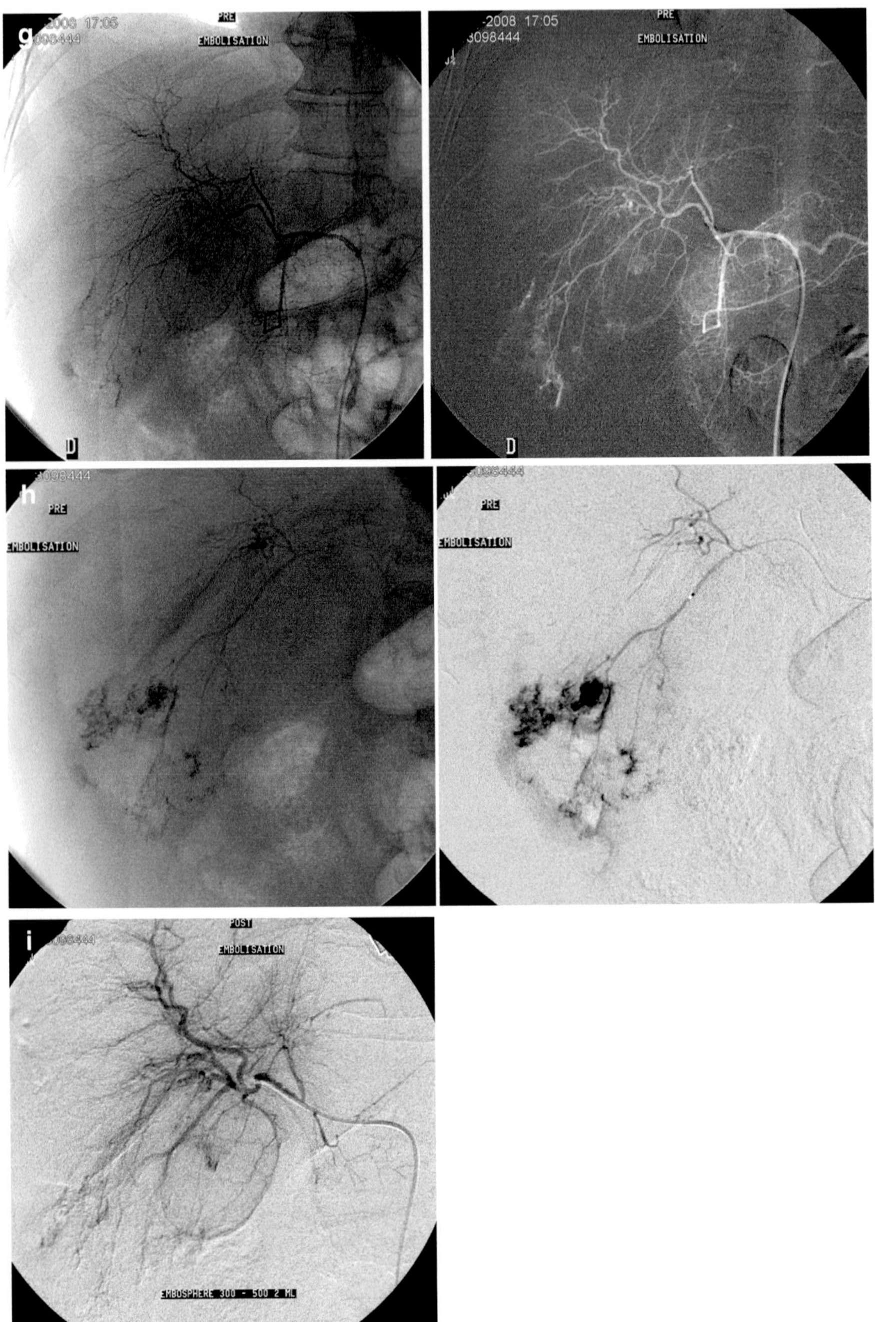

Fig. 21.2 (continued)

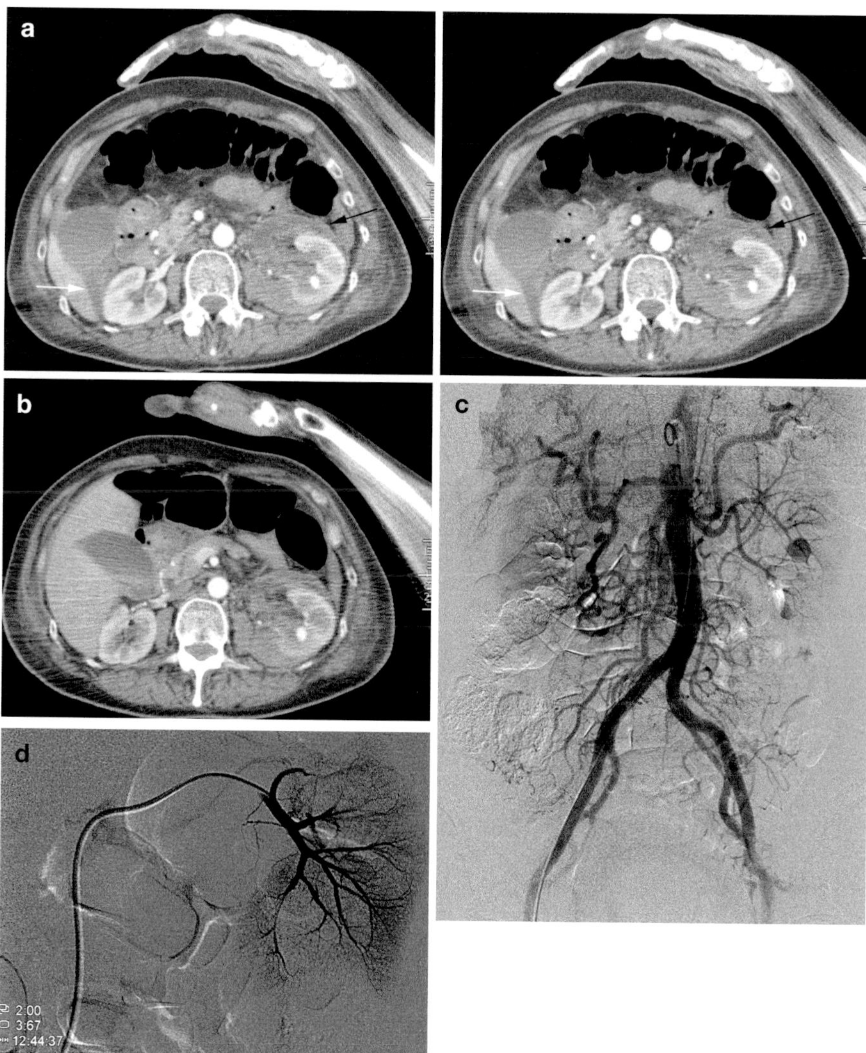

Fig. 21.3 Fall from horse: fracture of the left humerus, rib fractures, limited left pleural effusion, and left upper quadrant pain. (**a**) Intraperitoneal effusion (Morison pouch: *white arrow*), associated with a left limited perirenal hematoma (*black arrow*), with a blush localized in the sinus. The hemodynamic stability has led to abstention. (**b**) Four days later, during surveillance: abundant hematuria with deglobulization. New CT: the retroperitoneal effusion is partially absorbed; the perirenal hematoma had not significantly increased in size, but the parenchymal blush with the synchronous enhancement of the renal pelvis was suggestive of arterio-calyceal fistula. (**c**) Aortography: opacification of a left intrarenal arterialized cavity. (**d**) Hyperselective injection into the retro pelvic artery: this artery does not participate to the vascularization of the traumatic lesion. (**e, f**) Semi selective injection of the pre-pelvic artery: the first-order arterial branch supplies the traumatic cavity. (**g**) Control opacification after exclusion by coils of the arterial branch feeding the arterio-calyceal fistula

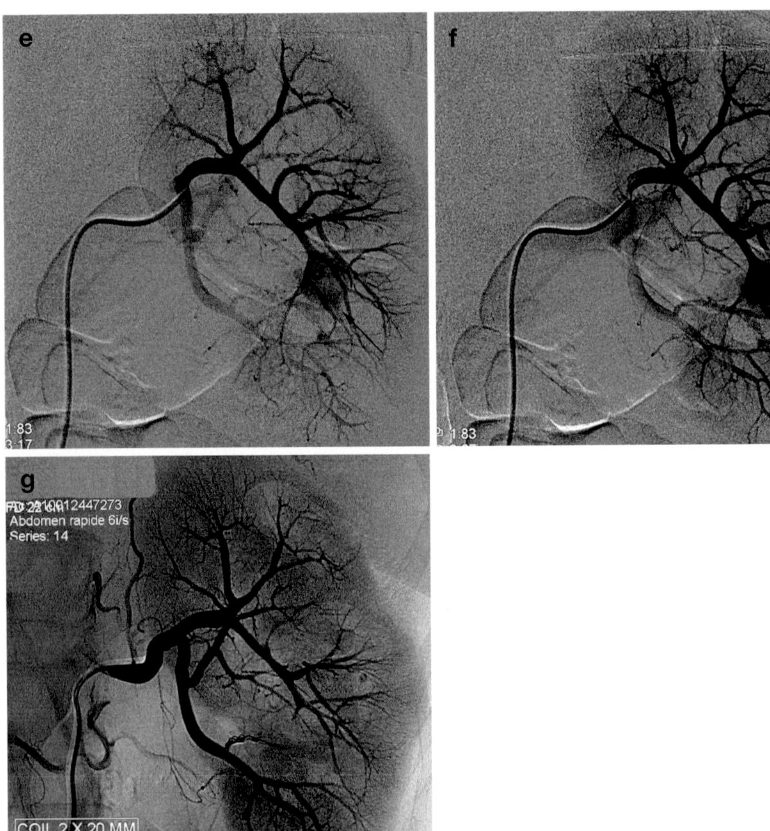

Fig. 21.3 (continued)

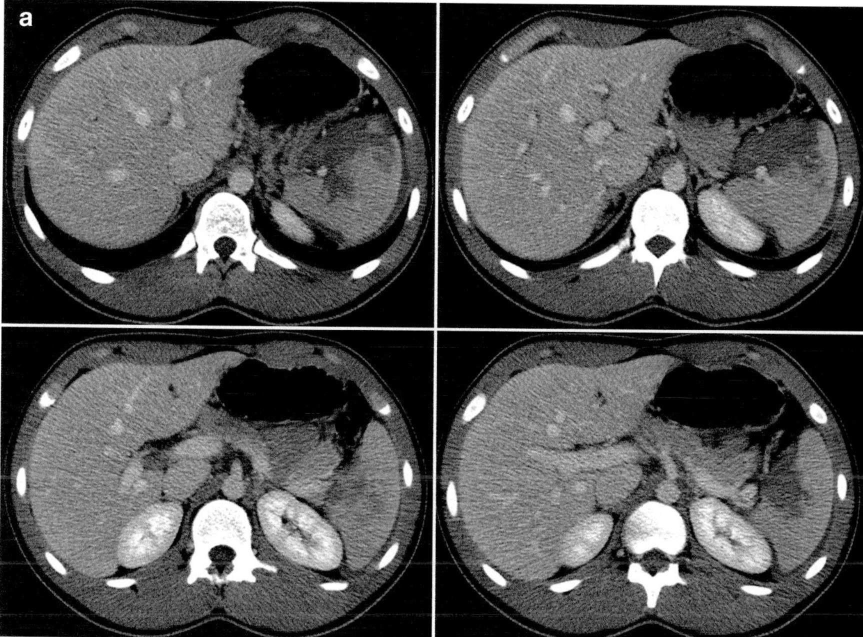

Fig. 21.4 Fall from bike with parietal cephalic impacts and abdominal pain: collapse. Brain CT was normal. (**a**) Abdominal CT: AAST III trauma of the spleen. (**b**) Frontal CT reconstruction. (**c**) Selective catheterization of the celiac trunk: displacement of the intrasplenic arterial tree, but without any obvious extravasation. (**d**) Hyperselective catheterization of the superior lobar branch, which shows a blush with extravasation. (**e**) Control opacification after exclusion by microcoils + gelatin of the inferior division branch of the superior lobar artery. (**f**) CT scan 6 months later, while the immediate aftermath and the clinical course were very simple: despite the artifacts caused by coils, the spleen appears correctly perfused

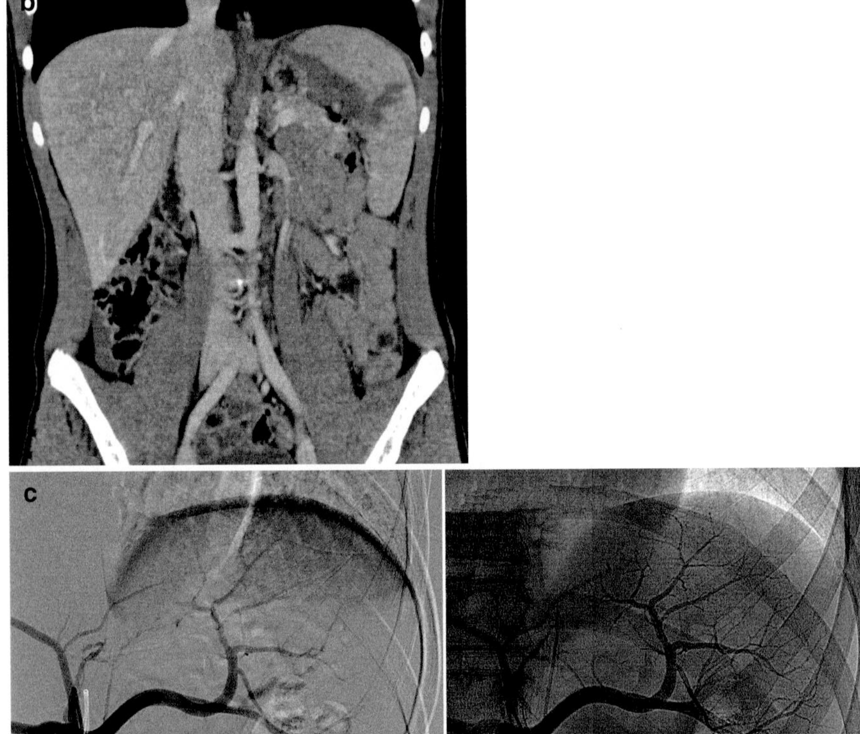

Fig. 21.4 (continued)

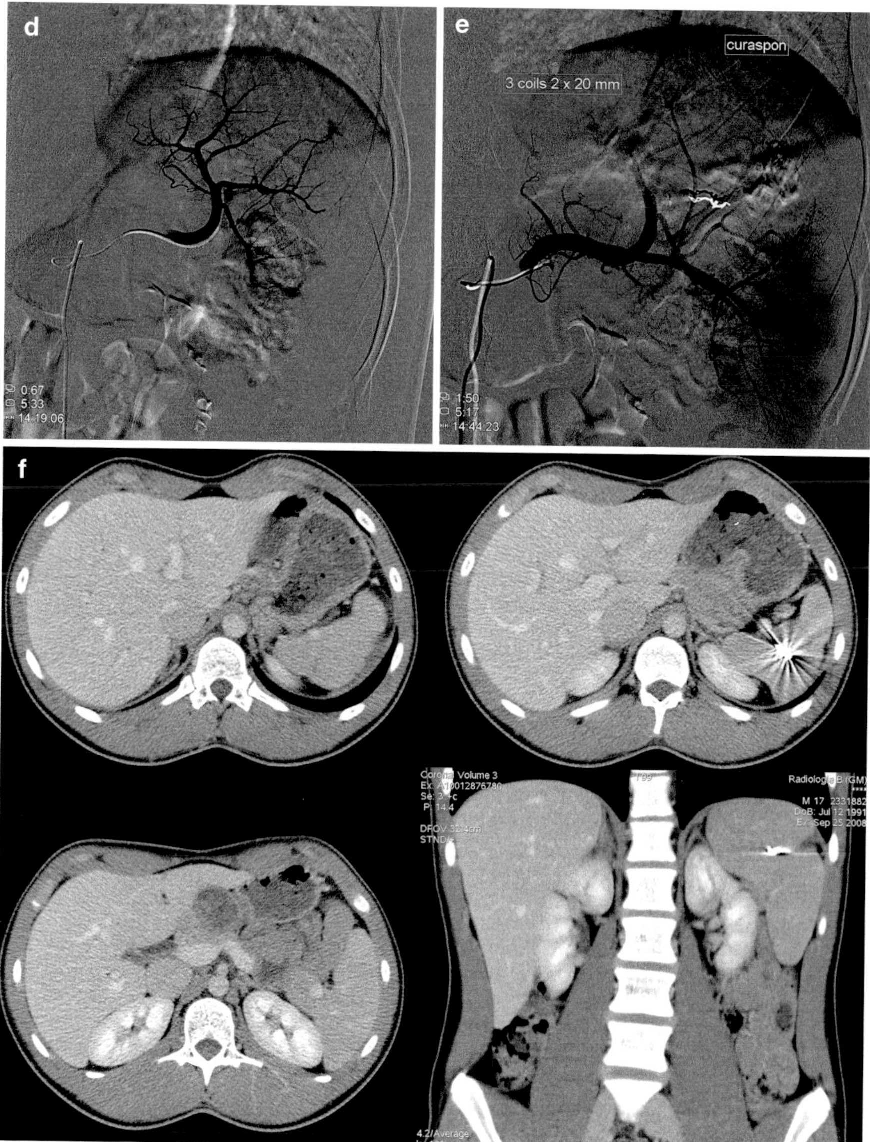

Fig. 21.4 (continued)

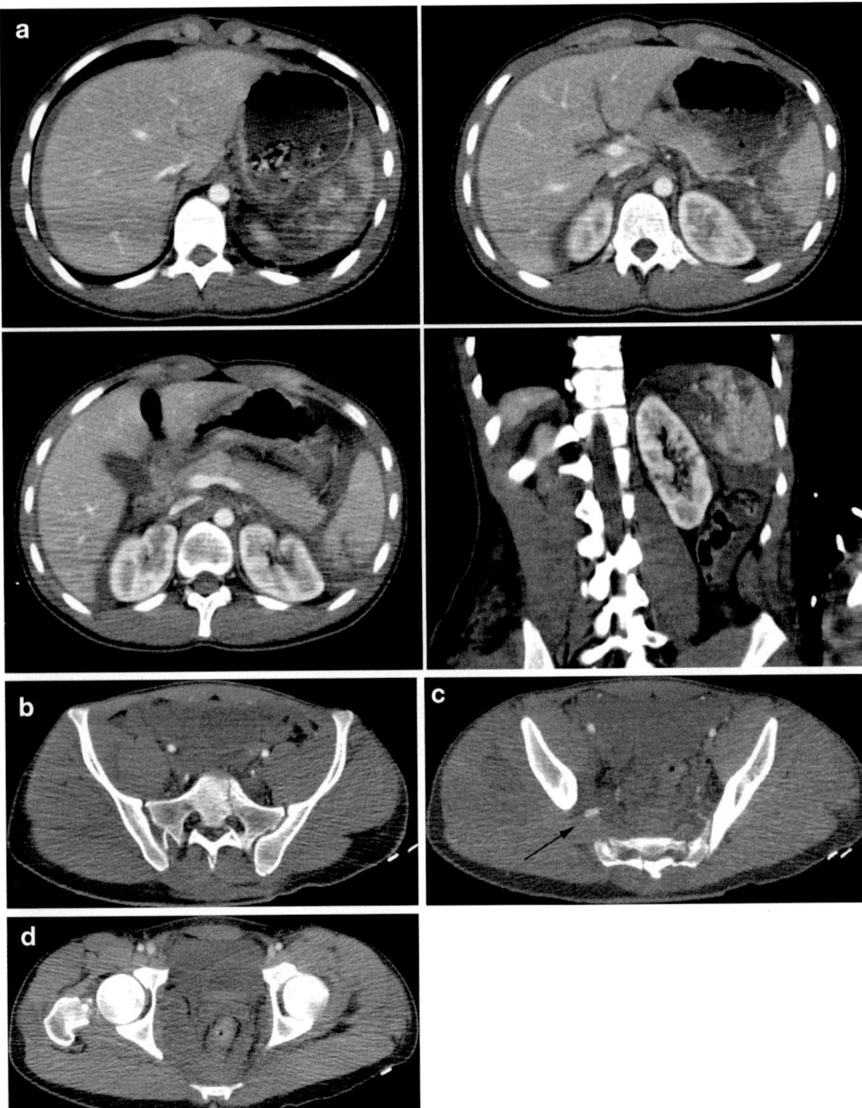

Fig. 21.5 Seventeen-year-old, ATV accident with head trauma without loss of consciousness; trauma to the chest, abdomen, pelvis, and left lower limb: hemodynamic collapse. Besides a fracture of the left femur, brain and spinal CT does not retain any lesion of concern. A diffuse bronchioloalveolar condensation of the left base was also noted. (**a**) Hemoperitoneum caused by a AAST grade IV–V splenic injury. (**b**) Multiple fractures of the sacrum and the ischiopubic branches with blush, consequence of the injury of the gluteal artery (**c**), responsible for an important intrapelvic hematoma. (**d**) An endovascular treatment was decided. (**e**) After arteriographic verification of the superficial femoral arteries, the localization of the arterial traumatic lesion at the right buttock has led to an initial balloon occlusion of the internal iliac artery, followed by a rapid hemodynamic stabilization. We then carried on the spleen trauma. (**f**) The splenic artery is selectively catheterized: a significant blush was found at the upper pole, leading to exclusion by resorbable gelatin supplemented by truncal coils (**g**). (**h**) The selective injection of the right hypogastric artery showed extravasations not only in the territory of the gluteal artery but also from intrapelvic arterial branches, leading to coil embolization (**i**) supplemented with gelatin in the hypogastric artery

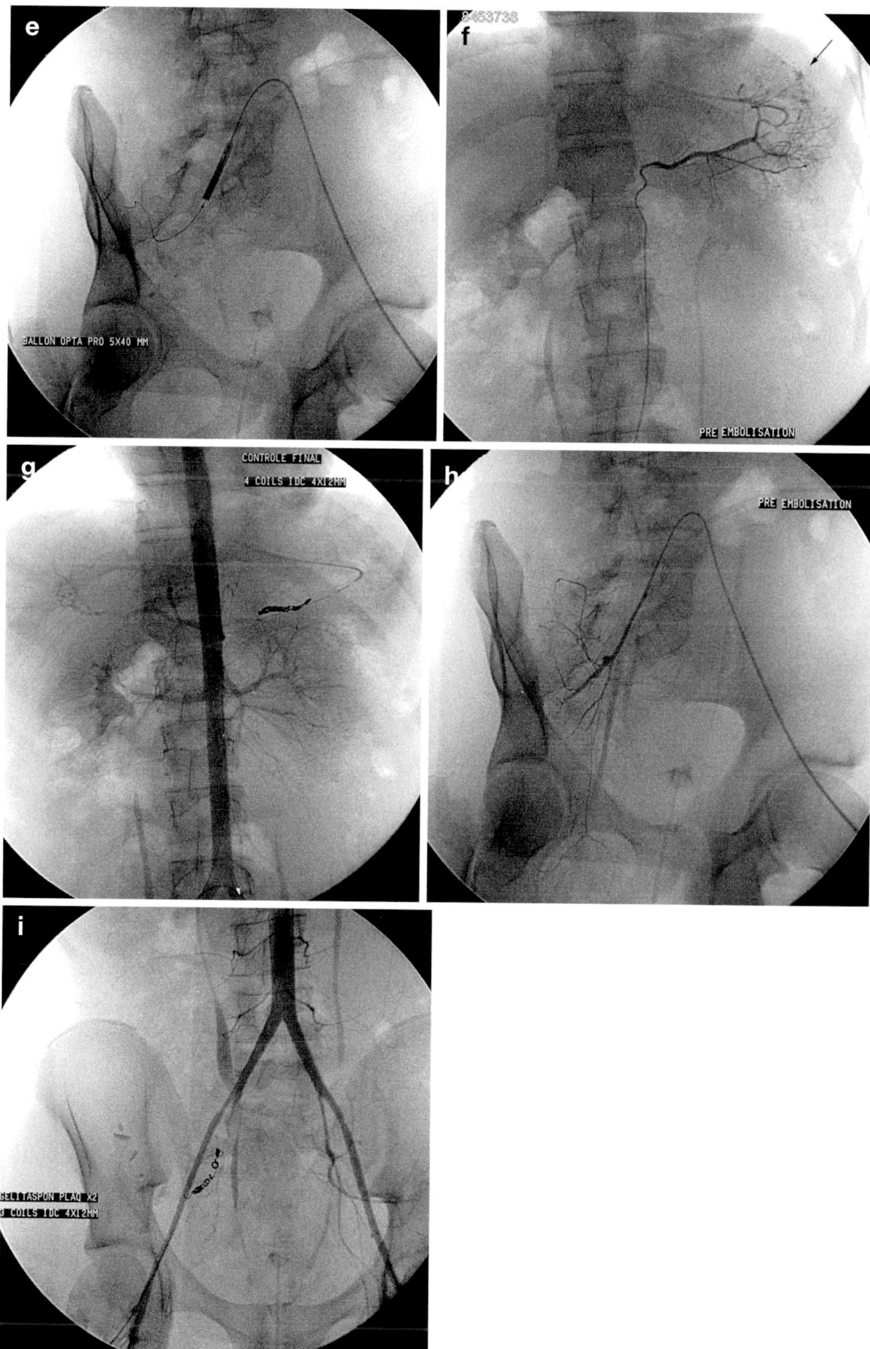

Fig. 21.5 (continued)

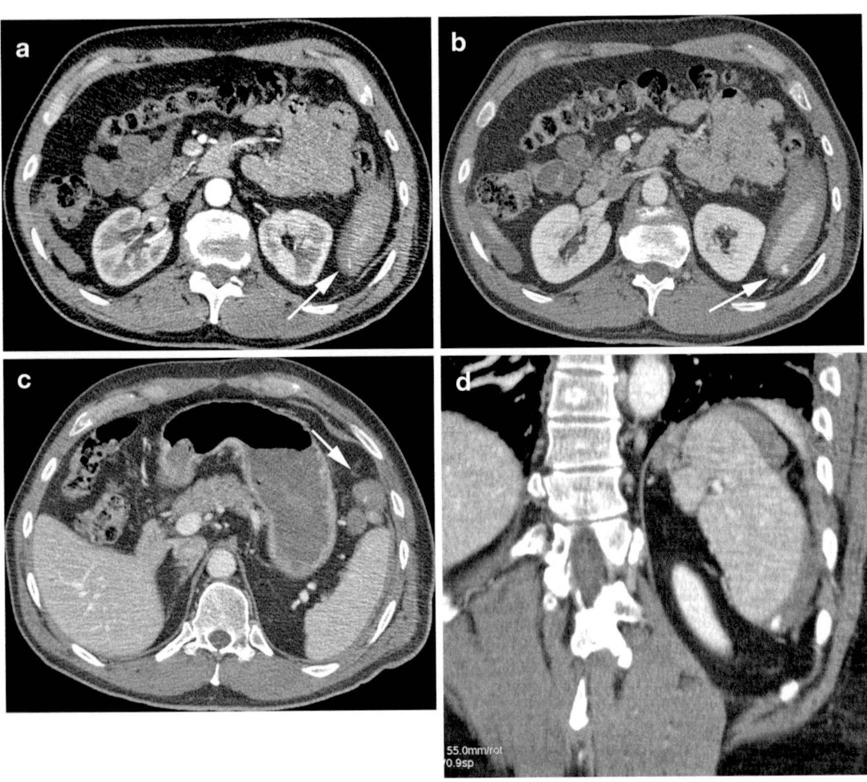

Fig. 21.6 Forty-nine-year-old; highway accident with limb fractures, basi-thoracic and left hypochondrial impact. (**a**–**d**) CT, AAST III splenic traumatic injury (ruptured subcapsular hematoma + blush); coronal reconstruction: no evident parenchymal lesion, but a ruptured subcapsular hematoma (*arrow*). (**e**–**f**) Selective injection of the splenic artery: modal distribution of branches. We found an inferomedial blush (*white arrow*), while the external contours of the spleen are deformed (*black arrow*). Hyperselective catheterization by micro-catheters led to the exclusion by coils + gelatin + particles (hyperselective control). (**g**–**h**) Semi-selective control after embolization

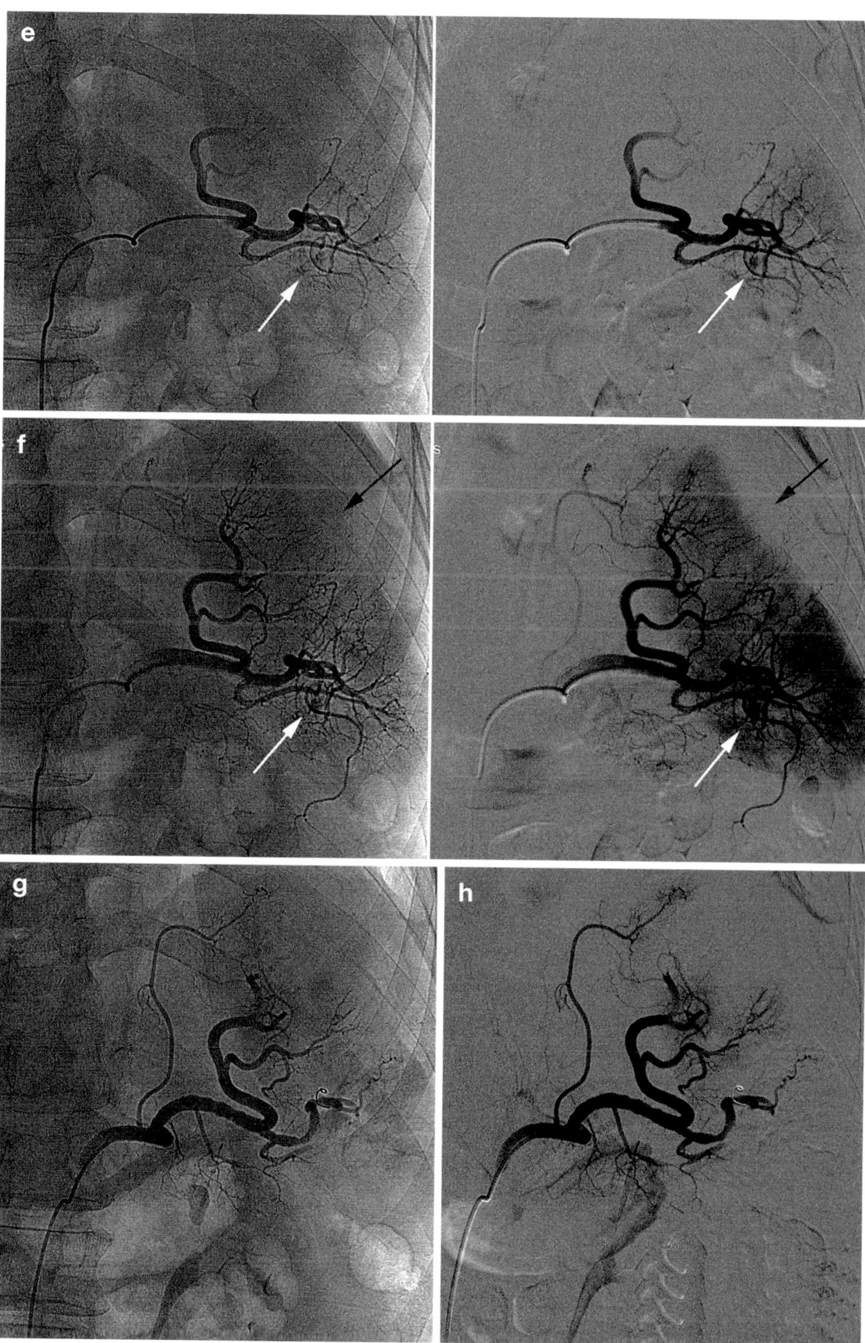

Fig. 21.6 (continued)

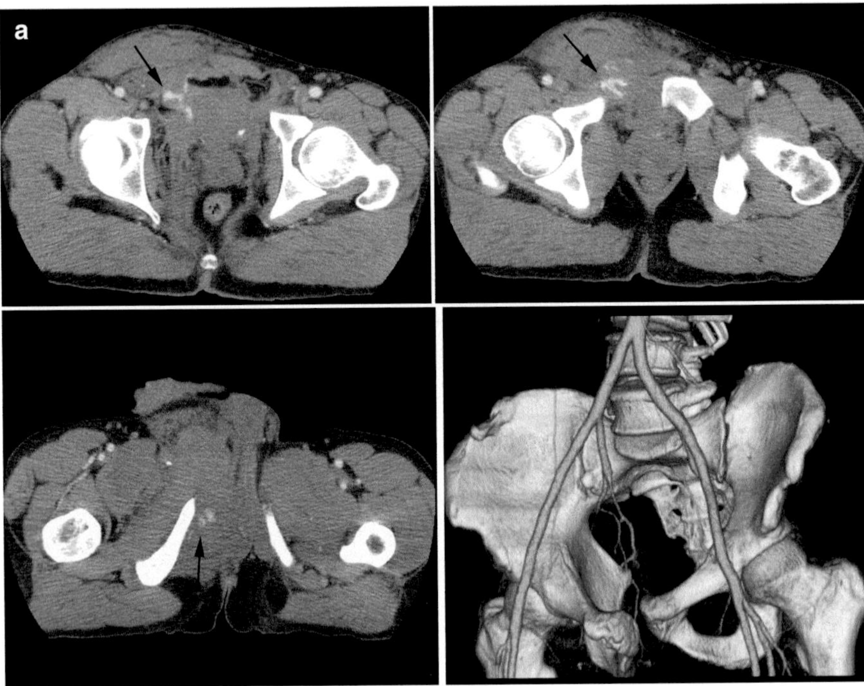

Fig. 21.7 Seventeen-year-old, car accident: pelvic trauma, patient in critical collapse. (**a**) CT: symphysary disjunction, very large pelvic and scrotal hematomas with blush (*arrow*). (**b**) Aortography: a good correlation with the CT topography. Important extravasation of the territory of the right pudendal artery. (**c**) Hyperselective catheterization before exclusion by resorbable gelatin and coils (**d**). (**e**) Selective control of the contralateral hypogastric artery: no traumatic lesion

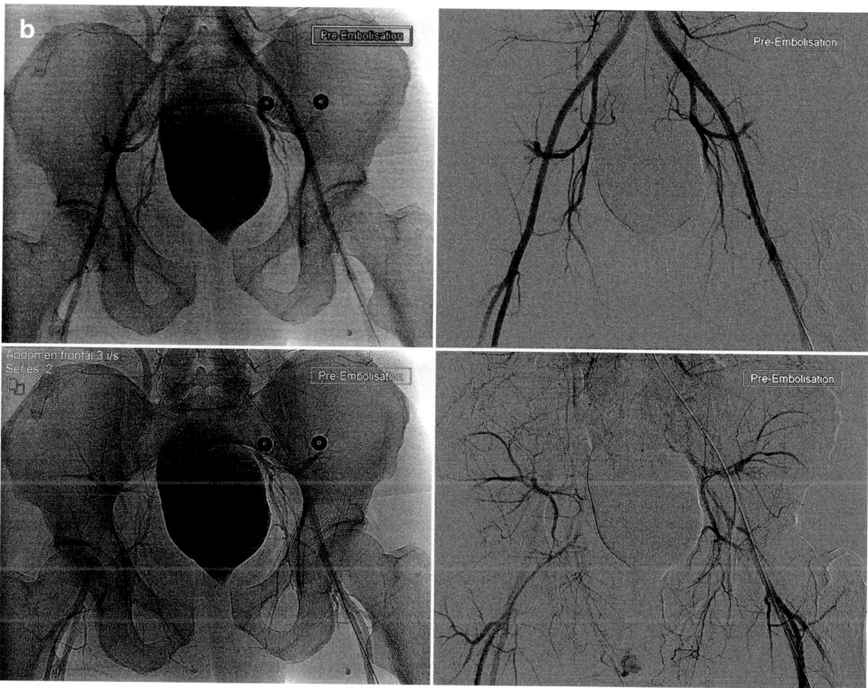

Fig. 21.7 (continued)

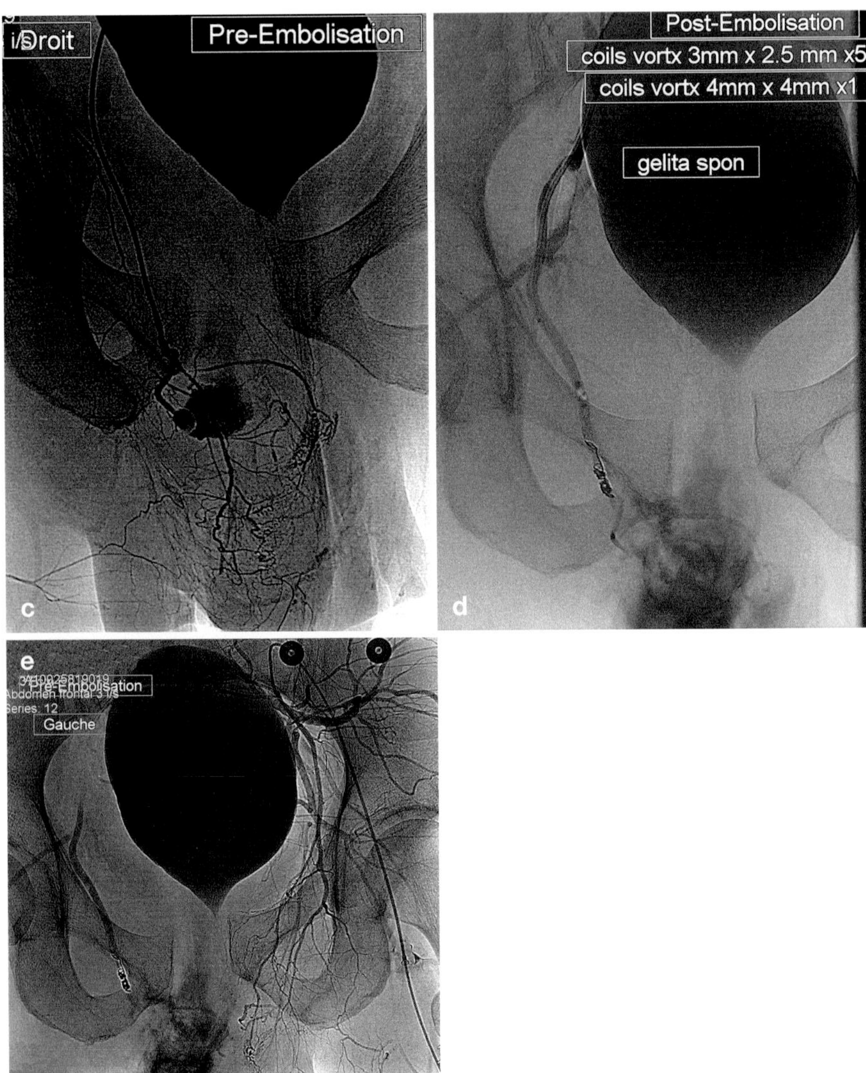

Fig. 21.7 (continued)

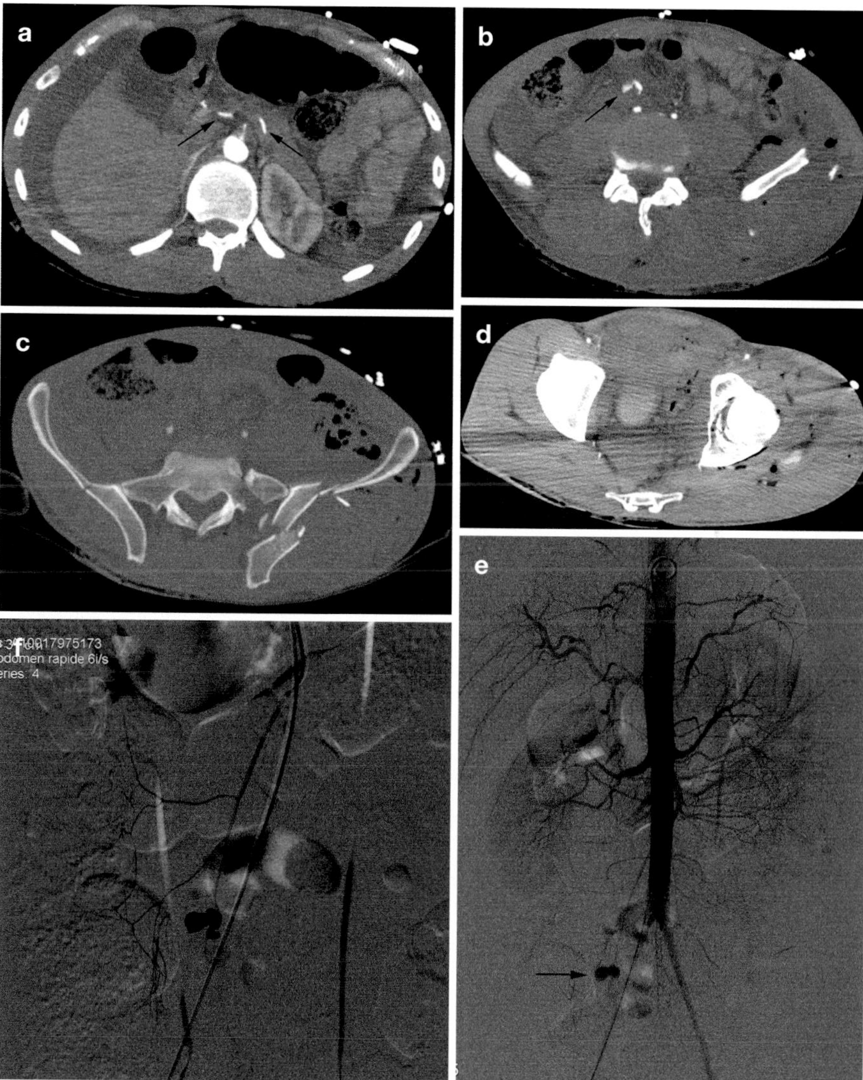

Fig. 21.8 Thirty-four-year-old: crushed by a beam (work accident), very severe hemodynamic collapse. Total body CT scan. (**a**) Hepatic and splenic arteries: generalized splanchnic vasoconstriction (*arrows*); important hemoperitoneum, no obvious solid organ injury. (**b**) But we see a very important arterial blush near the right common iliac artery. (**c**) Multiple pelvic fractures. (**d**) Intrapelvic hematoma. (**e**) Aortography: diffuse vasoconstriction with extravasation in the territory of the superior mesenteric artery (*arrow*). (**f**) Selective injection of the superior mesenteric artery: extravasation corresponding to the end of the ileocecum-appendicular artery. (**g**) Hemodynamic improvement after exclusion by coils, but the ileal branches are checked. (**h**, **i**) Early phase then late phase: the peripheral arterial arcade persistent feeding of the leak, leading to the release of additional microcoils (**j**). (**k**) Ultimate control opacification of the SMA. (**l**) Selective catheterization of the anterior trunk of the left hypogastric artery: massive blush, excluded by microparticles. (**m**) Control injection in the trunk of the left hypogastric artery. (**n**) Final aortoiliac control. (**o**) CT 1 year later: the orthopedic sequelae are important; the patient has lost a lot of weight, but the GI consequences were surprisingly simple

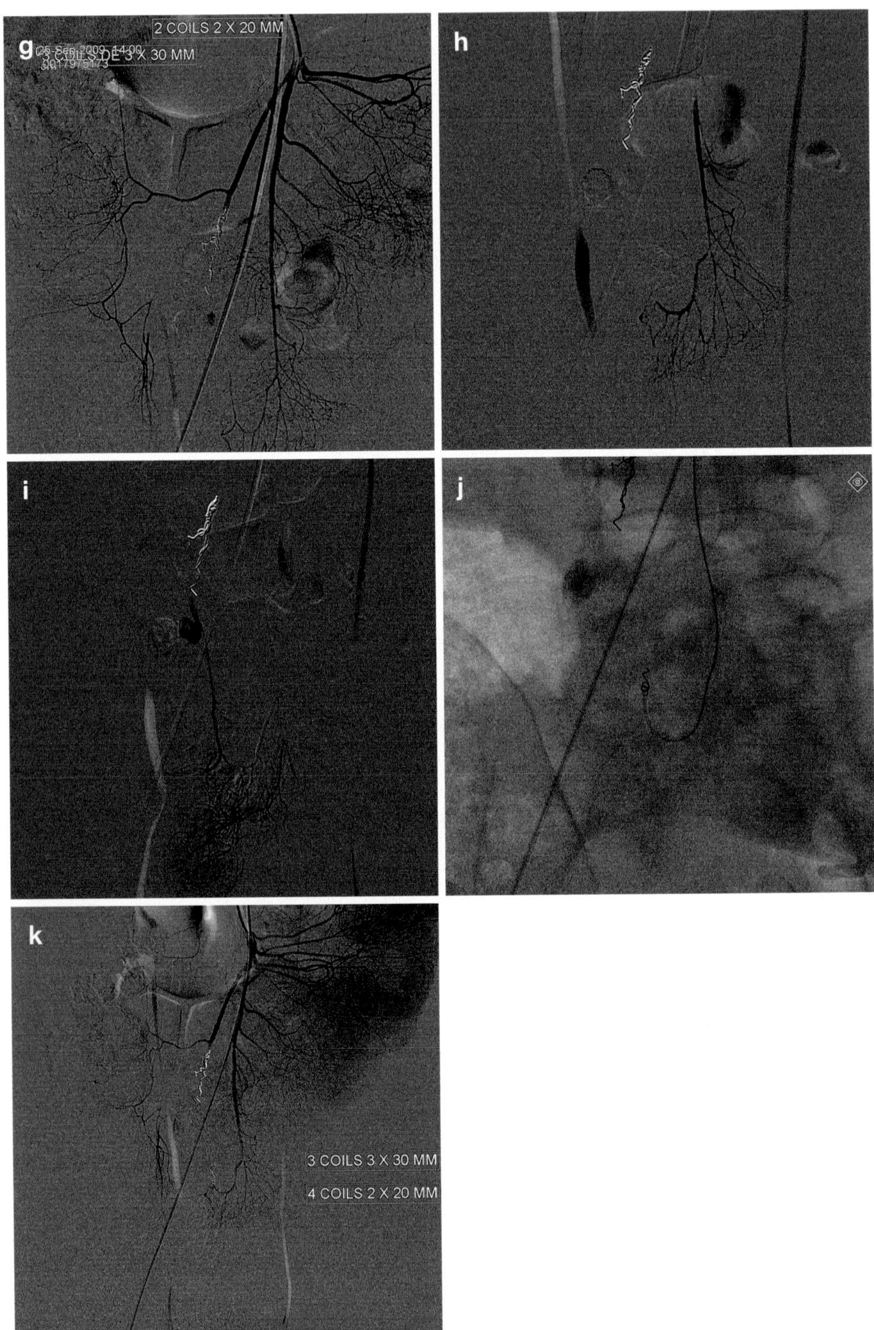

Fig. 21.8 (continued)

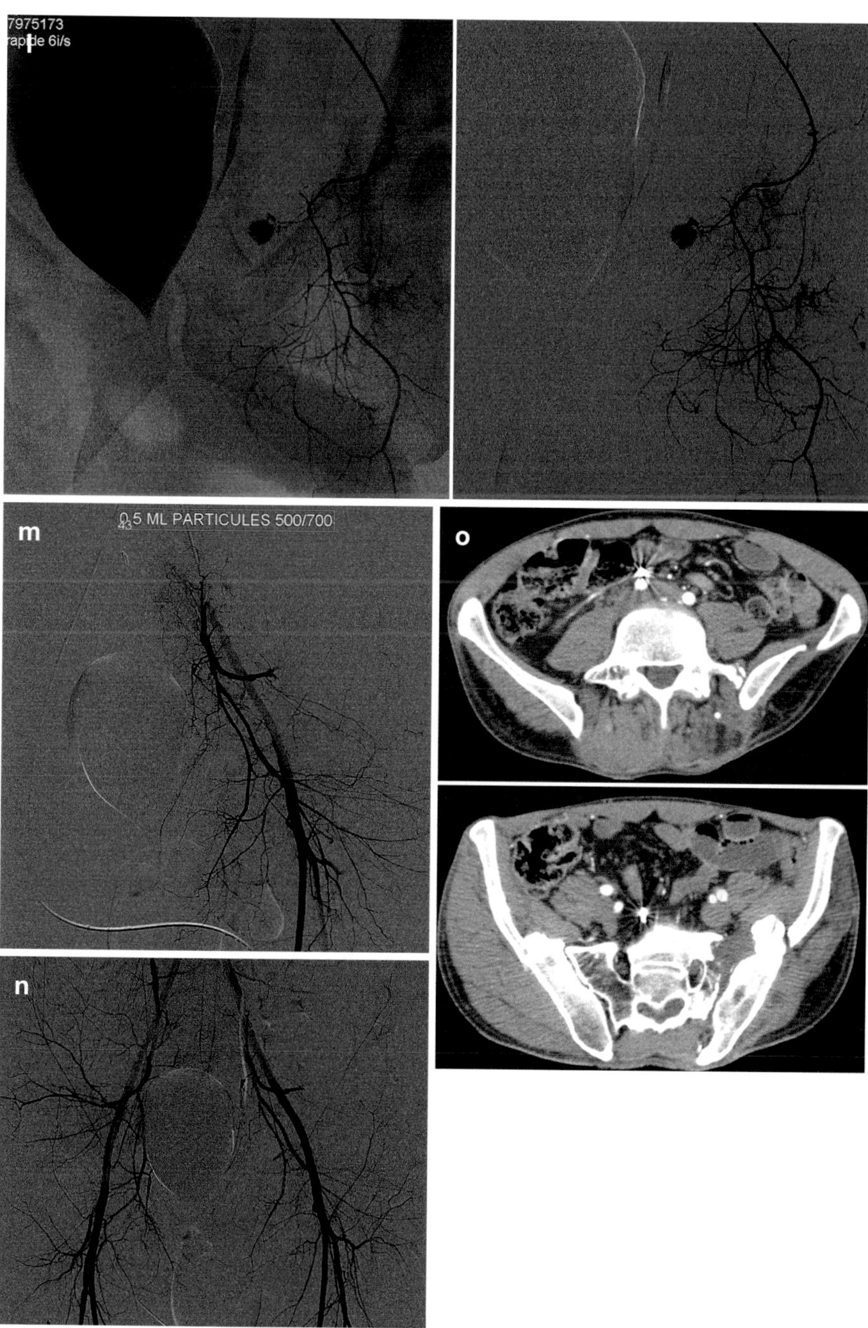

Fig. 21.8 (continued)

Appendix: AAST Organ Injury Scale for Spleen, Liver, and Kidney [1]

Organ, grade[a]	Injury type	Description of injury	AIS
Spleen			
I	Hematoma	Subcapsular, <10 % surface area	2
	Laceration	Capsular tear, <1 cm parenchymal depth	2
II	Hematoma	Subcapsular, 10–50 % surface area; intraparenchymal, <5 cm in diameter	2
	Laceration	Capsular tear, 1–3 cm parenchymal depth that does not involve a trabecular vessel	2
III	Hematoma	Subcapsular, >50 % surface area or expanding; ruptured subcapsular or parenchymal hematoma; intraparenchymal hematoma ≥5 cm or expanding	3
	Laceration	>3 cm parenchymal depth or involving trabecular vessels	3
IV	Laceration	Laceration involving segmental or hilar vessels producing major devascularization (>25 % of spleen)	4
V	Hematoma	Completely shattered spleen	5
	Laceration	Hilar vascular injury devascularizes spleen	5
Liver			
I	Hematoma	Subcapsular, <10 % surface area	2
	Laceration	Capsular tear, <1 cm parenchymal depth	2
II	Hematoma	Subcapsular, 10–50 % surface area: intraparenchymal <10 cm in diameter	2
	Laceration	Capsular tear 1–3 cm parenchymal depth, <10 cm in length	2
III	Hematoma	Subcapsular, >50 % surface area of ruptured subcapsular or parenchymal hematoma; Intraparenchymal hematoma >10 cm or expanding	3
	Laceration	>3 cm parenchymal depth	3
IV	Laceration	Parenchymal disruption involving 25–75 % hepatic lobe or 1–3 Couinaud's segments	4
V	Laceration	Parenchymal disruption involving >75 % of hepatic lobe or >3 Couinaud's segments within a single lobe	5
	Vascular	Juxtahepatic venous injuries, i.e., retrohepatic vena cava/ central major hepatic veins	5
VI	Vascular	Hepatic avulsion	6
Kidney			
I	Contusion	Microscopic or gross hematuria, urologic studies normal	2
	Hematoma	Subcapsular, nonexpanding without parenchymal laceration	2
II	Hematoma	Nonexpanding \hematoma confirmed to renal retroperitoneum	2
	Laceration	<1 cm parenchymal depth of renal cortex without urinary extravasation	2
III	Laceration	>1 cm parenchymal depth of renal cortex without collecting system rupture or urinary extravasation	3
IV	Laceration	Parenchymal laceration extending though renal cortex, medulla, and collecting system	4
	Vascular	Main renal artery or vein injury with contained hemorrhage	4
V	Laceration	Completely shattered kidney	5
	Vascular	Avulsion of renal hilum that devascularizes kidney	5

AIS, Abbreviated Injury Scale
[a]Advance one grade for bilateral injuries up to grade III

Appendix: "Baltimore" Classification of Spleen Traumas (Marmery) [4]

Grade	1	2	3	4a	4b
Subcapsular hematoma	<1 cm	1–3 cm	>3 cm		
Intraparenchymal hematoma	<1 cm	1–3 cm	>3 cm		
Laceration	<1 cm	1–3 cm	>3 cm	Shattered spleen	
Other lesions			Capsular tear	Active intraparenchymal and subcapsular splenic bleeding, splenic vascular injury	Active intraperitoneal bleeding

References

1. Tinkoff G, Esposito TJ, Reed J, et al. American Association for the Surgery of Trauma organ injury scale 1: spleen, liver and kidney, validation based on the national trauma data bank. J Am Coll Surg. 2008;207:646–55.
2. Hagiwara A, et al. Blunt splenic injury: usefulness of transcatheter arterial embolization in patients with a transient response to fluid resuscitation. Radiology. 2005;235(1):57–64.
3. Hagiwara A, et al. Nonsurgical management of patients with blunt splenic injury: efficacy of transcatheter arterial embolization. AJR Am J Roentgenol. 1996;167(1):159–66.
4. Marmery H, Shanmuganathan K, Alexander MT, Mirvis SE. Optimization of selection for nonoperative management of blunt splenic injury: comparison of MDCT grading systems. AJR Am J Roentgenol. 2007;189:1421–7.
5. Santucci RA, McAninch JW. Diagnosis and management of renal trauma: past, present and future. J Am Coll Surg. 2000;191(4):443–51.

Suggested Reading

Otal P, Auriol J, Chabbert V, et al. Radiologie interventionnelle et traumatismes thoraco-abdomino-pelviens. J Radiol. 2008;89:1855–70.

Pilleul F, De Queiros M, Durieux M, et al. Prise en charge radiologique des lésions vasculaires secondaires aux traumatismes du bassin. J Radiol. 2007;88:639–46.

Thony F, Gaubert JY, Varoquaux A, pour la SFICV: Embolisations en urgence In recommandations 2007 pour la pratique de la radiologie interventionnelle, sous la direction d'H. VERNHET KOVACSIK, Paris: SFICV; Ed. 2007.

Thony F, Rodière M, Monnin V, et al. Radiologie interventionnelle en pathologie traumatique lecture JFICV 2009, Lille 05.06.09.

Van Der Vlies CH, Van Delden OM, Punt BJ, et al. Literature review of the role of ultrasound, computed tomography, and transcatheter arterial embolization for the treatment of traumatic splenic injuries. Cardiovasc Intervent Radiol. 2010;33:1079–87.

Chapter 22
Traumatisms of the Limbs

Louis Boyer, Antoine Roche, Lucie Cassagnes, Grégory Favrolt, Hatem Gobara, and Pascal Chabrot

22.1 Background

Arterial and venous lesions are observed more readily in penetrating and high-velocity traumas. The development of endovascular techniques and mini invasive approaches also explains the increasing occurrence of iatrogenic injuries.

The upper limbs would be involved in 25 % of cases among civilians versus 34 % in the military.

The immediate consequence can be external or internal bleedings but also limb ischemia which can lead to irreversible damage if not managed rapidly.

Crushing, wrenching, and stretching produce limb contusions and/or lacerations which can involve long vascular segments sometimes resulting in a dissection. An extensive thrombosis can occur and sometimes be complicated by peripheral embolisms.

Traumatic hemorrhages can be exteriorized or contained within pulsatile hematomas, constituting false aneurysms, with the risk of delayed rupture. Concomitant arterial and venous injuries can bring about an arteriovenous traumatic fistula, which is at risk of rupture but also of cardiac complications and downstream ischemic consequences.

Finally, an isolated spasm can be depicted; in these cases associated lesions must be looked for to explain ischemia.

L. Boyer, MD, PhD • A. Roche, MD • L. Cassagnes, MD (✉) • P. Chabrot, MD, PhD
Department of Radiology, University Hospital of Clermont-Ferrand, Clermont-Ferrand, France
e-mail: lboyer@chu-clermontferrand.fr; pchabrot@chu-clermontferrand.fr

G. Favrolt, MD
Department of Radiology, Clinique de Fontaine, Dijon, France

H. Gobara, MD
Department of Radiology, Riom Hospital, University Hospital of Clermont-Ferrand, Clermont-Ferrand, France

P. Chabrot, L. Boyer (eds.), *Embolization*, DOI 10.1007/978-1-4471-5182-1_22,

If the peripheral vascular traumatism occurs in a polytrauma context, the diagnostic and therapeutic strategies depend on the overall patient assessment (see also Chap. 21).

In patients with isolated limb traumas, the diagnosis is primarily based on the clinical work-up. However, a normal clinical examination does not formally exclude any vascular injury, so should the slightest doubt exist, a complementary noninvasive imaging (ultrasound or CT) will be carried out.

In case of clinical suspicion of limb traumatism with associated vascular injury, bones X-rays plain films are very often carried out as the first-line investigation. Doppler ultrasound can easily and quickly explore the peripheral vessels. Angio CT also depicts the bones and the soft tissues, with a good negative predictive value. But invasive arteriography remains the Gold Standard, because it is very sensitive and specific. Its indications were until recently very large, in substitution for systematic surgical exploration; nowadays in many teams they are more elective, exposing to a higher rate of missed injuries and delayed diagnosis, and making follow-up crucial.

Moreover, diagnostic arteriography has now become more often the first step to an endovascular treatment.

22.2 Techniques

The ideal strategy is to work in a hybrid room, in conformity with the requirements for surgery and radiology (radioprotection, image quality), and allowing combined therapeutic strategies.

The arteriography can be carried out in the angiographic suite or in the operating room, according to the organization of the trauma team and the initial patient assessment. It can constitute the first step of endovascular treatment.

In resuscitated patients, sedation and anesthesia are administered according to their clinical status.

The Seldinger technique is the easiest percutaneous access. The puncture site is chosen according to the topography of the lesions, so as to be able to carry out opacifications upstream to the presumably injured segments, and must depict a non-traumatic upstream arterial segment. As a rule for the lower limb, we choose to puncture the contralateral femoral artery.

A high-frame-rate image acquisition will be carried out if there is the slightest doubt of arteriovenous fistula; late-phase images are necessary to detect extravasations. Arterial lesions must be depicted on two orthogonal projections. More views should be acquired in the presence of foreign bodies.

Angiographic findings include lacerations with active bleeding, occlusions, pseudoaneurysms, arteriovenous fistula, and/or the presence of foreign bodies. A narrowing of the lumen can be caused by a spasm, a wall hematoma, an intimal lesion, an extrinsic compression, or a preexistent atheromatous lesion.

In the event of vascular laceration with active bleeding inducing a rapidly increasing hematoma, embolization of nonvital branches in the area of the bleeding can be performed using microparticles, coils, glues, and/or gelatin sponge. The choice of the embolization agent depends on the bleeding site, the vessel diameter and flow, as well as the coagulation status. The use of microcatheters is very helpful, allowing a very distal catheterization and while avoiding spasms and reflux.

In favorable cases, a stent graft allows a less invasive restoration of the arterial continuity with minimal blood loss. A "sandwich" occlusion with coils can also be carried if the lesion can be crossed. Thrombin injection has also been proposed to treat false aneurysms.

An intramural hematoma or a dissection can be treated by angioplasty, with balloons and/or non-covered stents.

False aneurysms and AVF can be treated by covered stents. Coils can be used for the upstream occlusion of a nonvital arterial branch feeding these lesions when they occur on arteries of lesser diameter.

In case of arterial occlusion, especially if bone fractures are associated, the prognosis is severe and depends highly on the delay of ischemia. A very rapid revascularization by stent or stent graft is an alternative to the surgical bypass.

After an endovascular treatment, we prefer maintaining the percutaneous arterial access for 12–24 h, thus allowing delayed angiographic controls and avoiding the immediate compression of the puncture site.

If the arteriography is carried out in the angiographic suite prior to patients' surgical management, then an angioplasty balloon can be inflated upstream of the hemorrhagic lesions before the transfer to the operating room.

22.3 Results

When it is technically possible, endovascular treatment for traumatic arterial lesions gives very good technical results; post procedure pain is less intense and lasts less than after surgical treatment.

The main complication of embolization is off-target occlusion of the vascular branches which can be limited with the use of microcatheters.

Long-term results are generally also satisfactory. We carry out a morphological and/or hemodynamic follow-up which includes an assessment of the puncture site and the injured vessel which at 1 month and 1 year after the procedure, with Doppler ultrasound or CT, even if clinical work-up is satisfactory, to detect false aneurysms and/or in-stent restenosis. Long-term patency of the stents must be followed up (in our group: 1 year later).

However, the outcome of these injuries does not solely depend on the endovascular procedures; delayed patient management and associated extravascular injuries may also lead to complications and sequelae (ischemia, compartment syndrome, neurological sequelae, etc.).

Concomitant injuries may also require complementary treatments and have an impact on follow-up.

22.4 Indications

Indications have to be established in a multidisciplinary management approach, according to the clinical work-up and by the radiological assessment (bone plain films and/or CT, or first step arteriography).

Compared to a surgical approach, endovascular techniques management carried out immediately after diagnostic angiography allow an often easier access to the injured vessels.

The embolization of the bleeding sources is often possible and is a valuable alternative to a surgical hemostasis which can sometimes be very dilapidating; thus, limb amputations could be avoided.

Key Points

- The initial clinical work-up determines the diagnostic and therapeutic strategies; Doppler can provide false reassurance by depicting flow signal while physical examination detects no palpable pulse.
- In the case of limb ischemia, an arterial spasm must not be considered as the unique etiology and other lesions must be looked for.
- Arteriography, which can be carried out in the operating room, is the first step before embolization, stenting, and stent grafting.
- Careful follow-up is mandatory for patients who do not undergo initial radiological or surgical exploration, in order to detect minor initially missed vascular injuries.

Fig. 22.1 Tibiofibular open fracture treated by osteosynthesis with an intramedullary nailing of the tibia. Supra-malleolar sudden swelling 8 days after the injury. (**a**, **b**) CT: axial sections and reconstructions: large vascular pouch, which enhancement is synchronous to the arterial network enhancement. (**c**) Arteriography (groin antegrade puncture of the right common femoral artery), view of the lower third of the leg: the posterior tibial artery is normal; the middle third of the tibiofibular trunk is very thin and responsible of the feeding of the pouch (*arrows*). (**d**) Selective injection of the anterior tibial artery: the artery is interrupted at the site the fracture, while its collateral branches are not involved in the supply of the pouch. (**e**) Super selective injection of the posterior tibial artery, which is not involved in the supply of the traumatic vascular lesion. (**f**) Hyper selective injection of the fibular artery, which supplies the large traumatic pseudoaneurysm. (**g**) Control opacification after occlusion by coils of the fibular artery

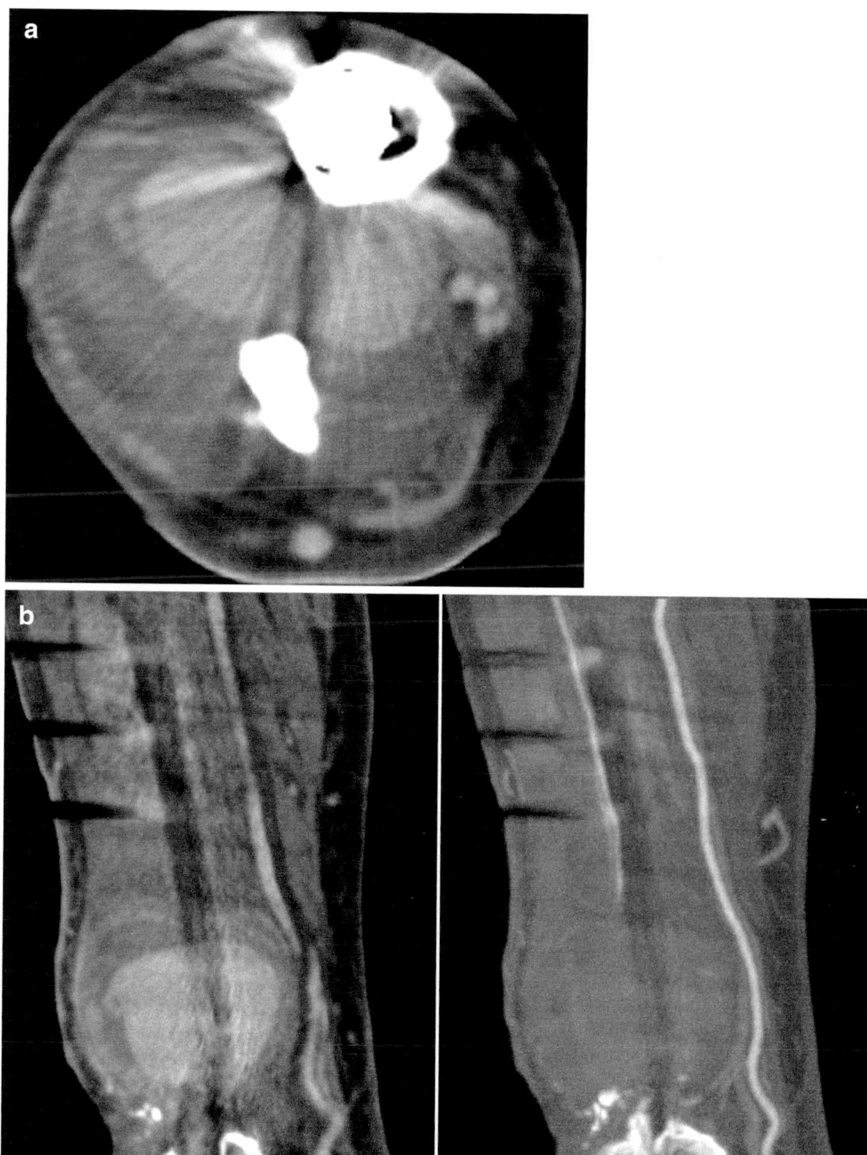
a
b

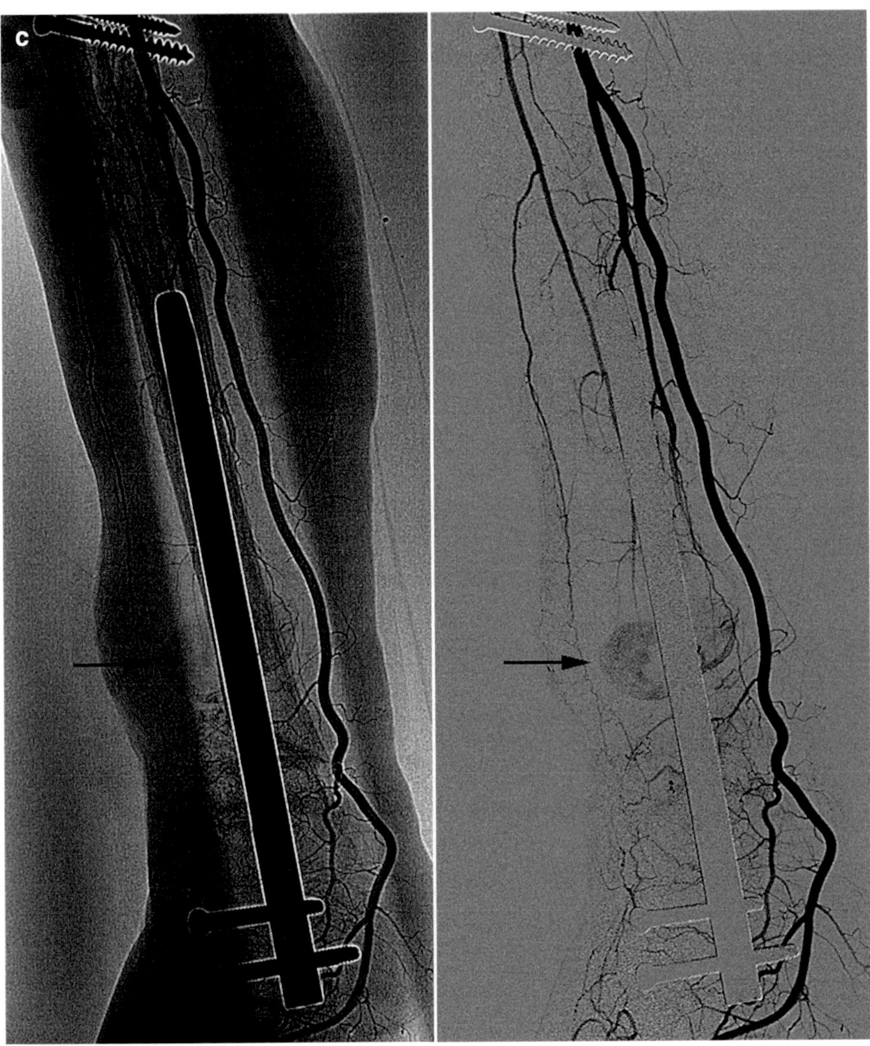

Fig. 22.1 (continued)

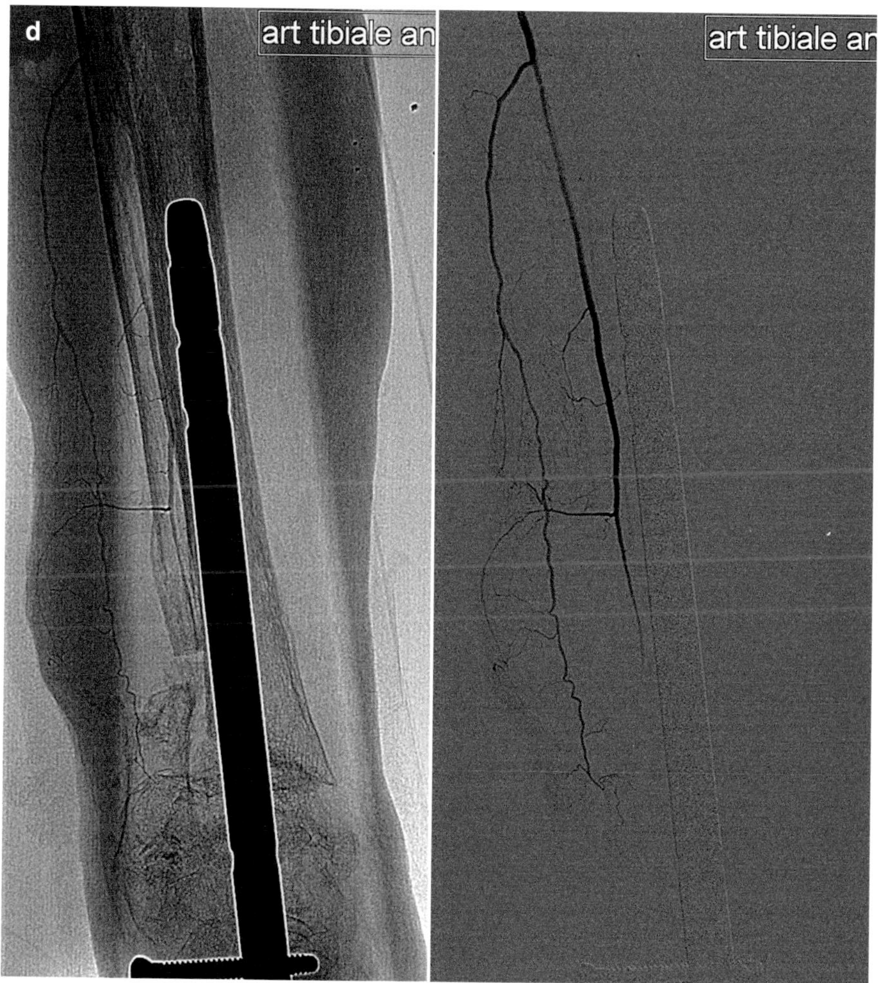

Fig. 22.1 (continued)

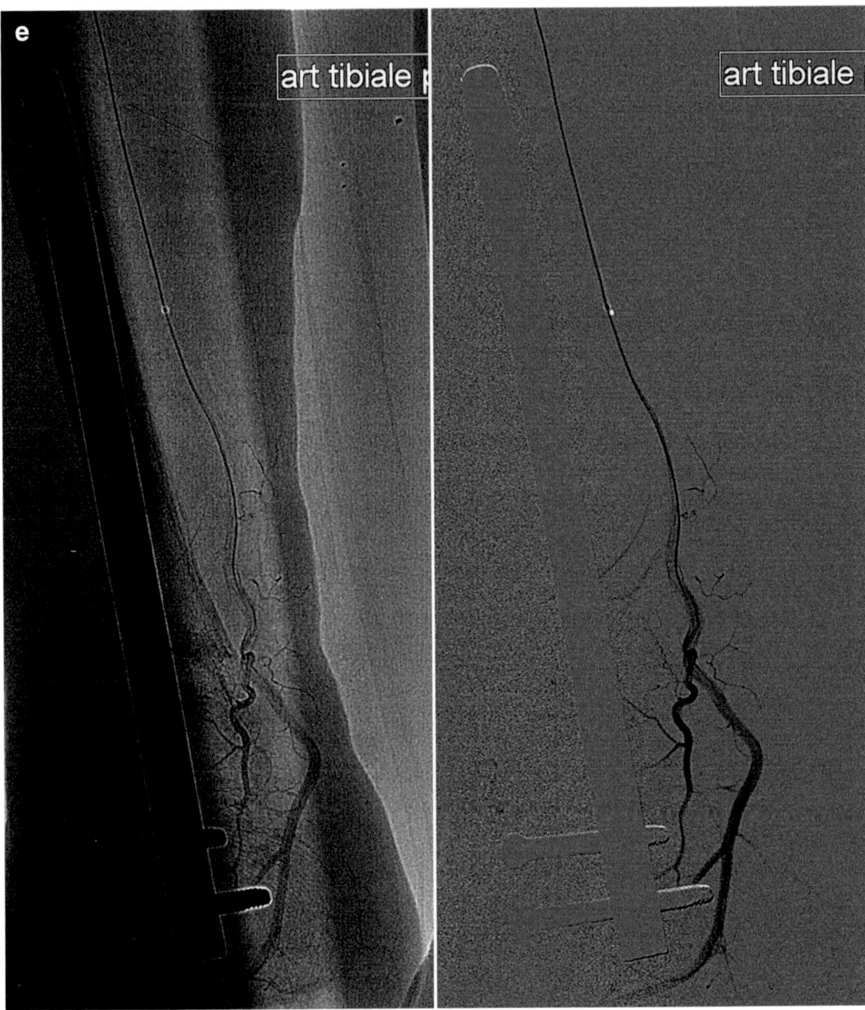

Fig. 22.1 (continued)

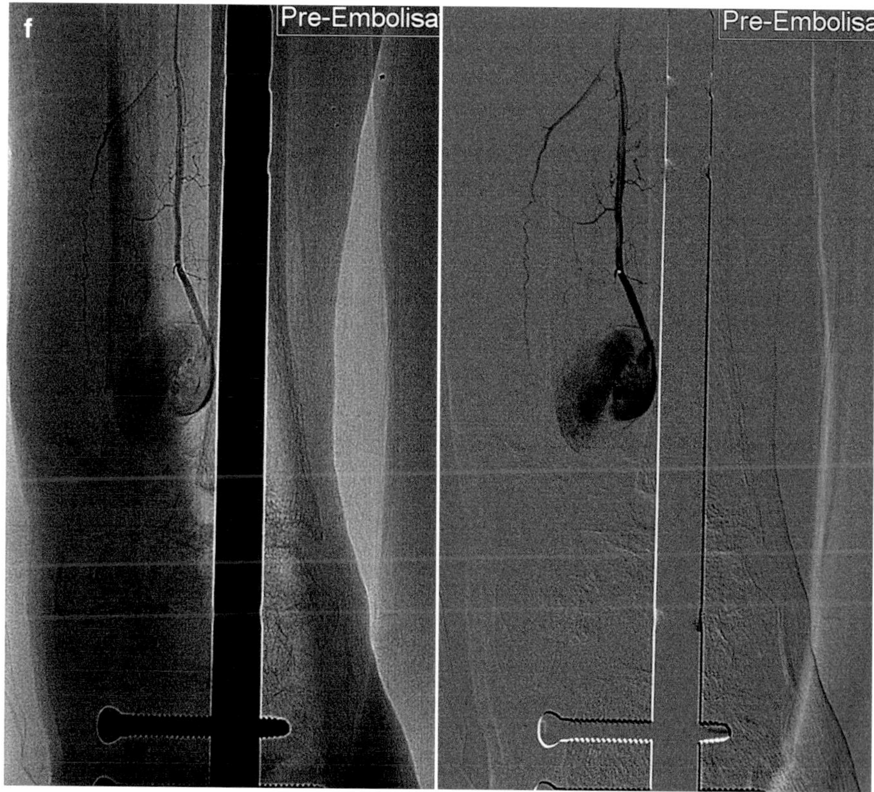

Fig. 22.1 (continued)

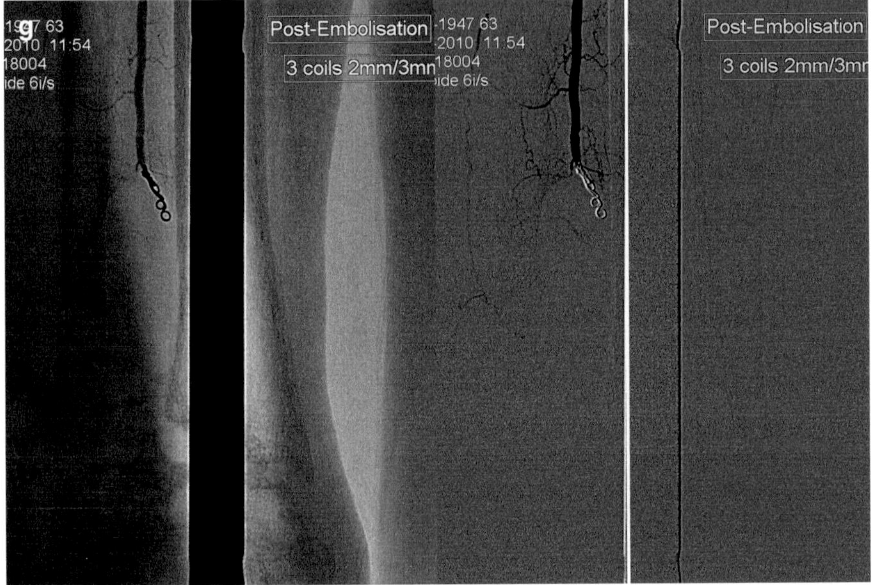

Fig. 22.1 (continued)

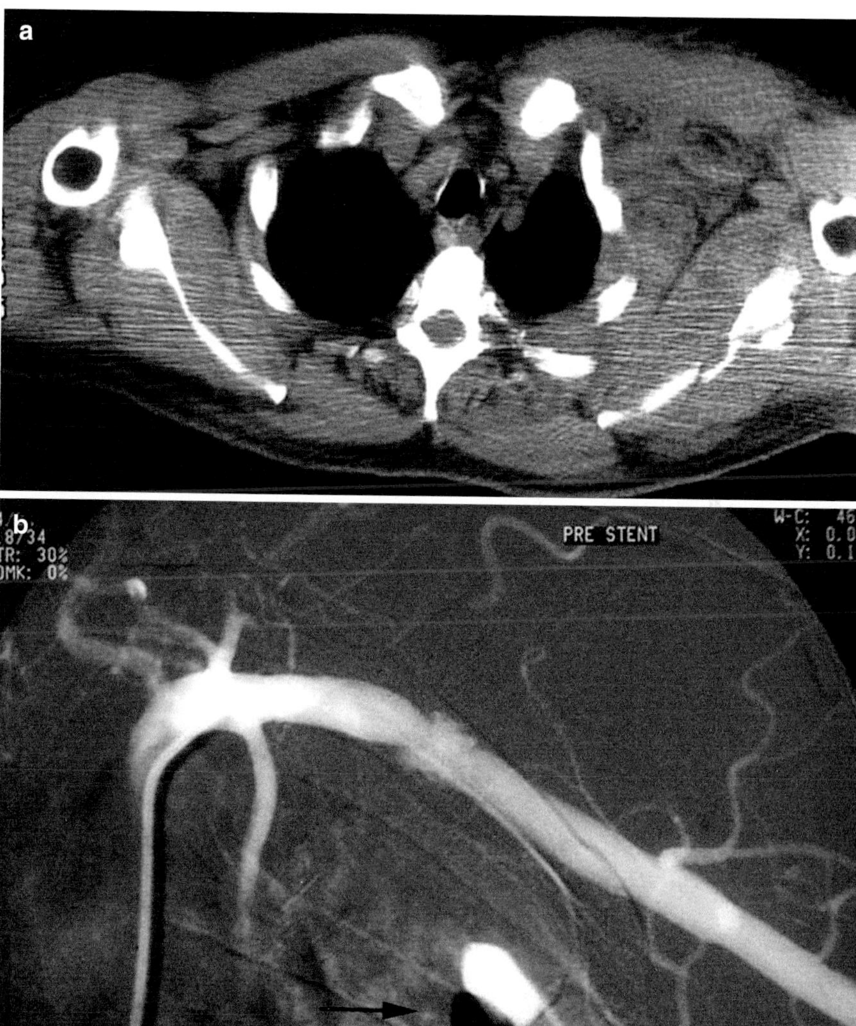

Fig. 22.2 Motorcycle accident: severe trauma to the left shoulder, loss of function, progressive swelling, hypoesthesia, and decreased pulse of the left upper limb. A hemothorax has been drained. (**a**) CT scan passing through the hilum of the upper limb: fracture of the scapula and scapulothoracic disjunction, soft tissue asymmetry and blush suggesting an active bleeding. An arterial wound of the axillo-subclavian arterial segment is suspected. (**b**) Selective injection of the left subclavian artery: stretching-laceration injury of the left subclavian artery. This lesion, in the context of a brachial plexus injury, made the endovascular treatment preferable to surgical repair (chest tube: *arrow*). (**c**) After a careful catheterization, a translesional guide wire was implemented, allowing the use of a stent graft: intermediate opacification during deployment, using a pigtail catheter in the aortic ach (contralateral femoral access). (**d**) Left subclavian artery selective control injection after deployment of the stent graft, which ensures the restoration of arterial patency and continuity, with the coverage of all the traumatic segment

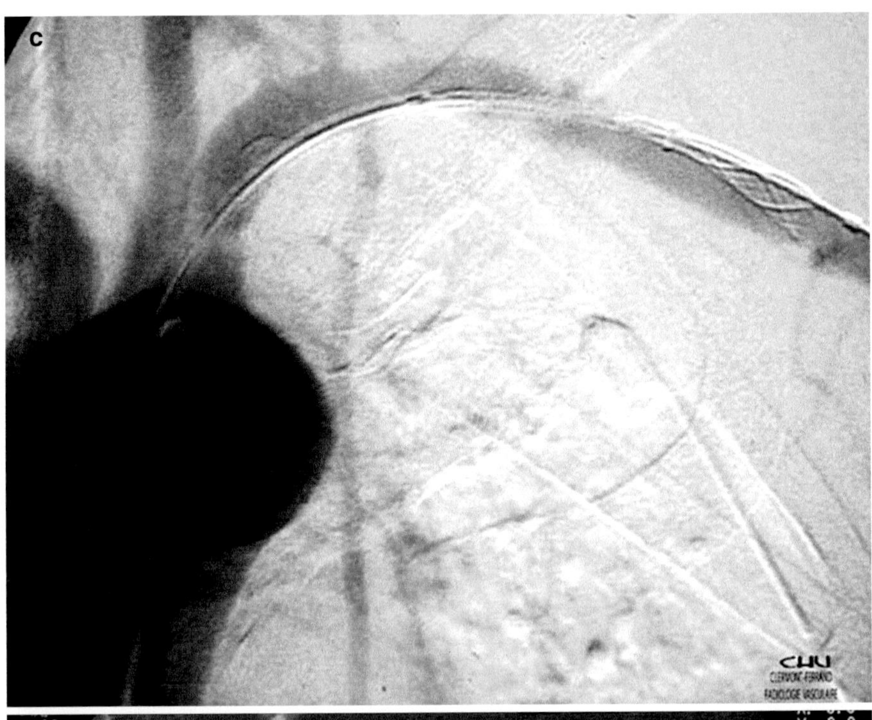

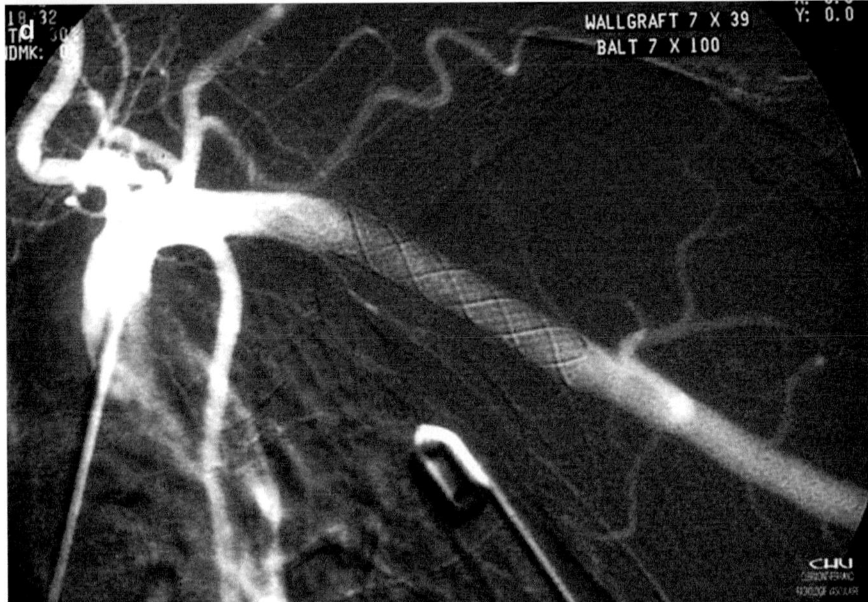

Fig. 22.2 (continued)

Suggested Reading

Carrafiello G, Lagana D, Mangini M, et al. Percutaneous treatment of traumatic upper-extremity arterial injuries: a single-center experience. J Vasc Interv Radiol. 2011;22:34–9.

Mavili C, Donmez H, Ozcan N, Akcali Y. Endovascular treatment of lower limb penetrating arterial traumas. Cardiovasc Intervent Radiol. 2007;30:1124–9.

White R, Krajcer Z, Johnson M, et al. Results of a multicenter trial for the treatment of traumatic vascular injury with a covered stent. J Trauma. 2006;60(6):1189–95.

Chapter 23
Management of Vascular Malformations

Gilles Soulez and Josée Dubois

23.1 Background

Vascular anomalies are classified in vascular tumors and vascular malformations. Regarding vascular tumor, the most frequent is the infantile hemangioma that usually regresses spontaneously before 8 years old.

Vascular malformations are congenital but can sometime be diagnosed in teenager or adult patients. They are classified according to the flow and type of vessel involved in the malformation (classification of Mulliken). Arteriovenous malformations (AVM) and arteriovenous fistulas (AVF) are high-flow malformations with a potential for expansion leading to hemorrhagic or ischemic complications and sometimes cardiac failure. Slow-flow malformations are more quiescent and include venous malformations (VM), capillary malformations (CM), and lymphatic malformations (LM). Complications of slow-flow malformations are related to their mass effect on adjacent structures, occurrence of phlebitis, and esthetic prejudice. However, hemorrhagic complications can be sometimes observed in VM or CM.

There are several syndromes associated with vascular malformations. The Parkes-Weber syndrome associates limb hypertrophy occurring during teenage with a CM (port-wine stain) and multiple AVMs. The Klippel-Trenaunay syndrome associates a limb hypertrophy or hypotrophy present at birth with a CM, multiple VMs, venous dysplasia, and sometimes LM. Significant advancements have been made in the field of vascular malformation genetics; however, only a few clinical entities have been linked to an autosomal transmission even though the vast majority of vascular malformations are congenital.

G. Soulez, MD, MSc (✉)
Department of Radiology, University Hospital Notre Dame, Montréal, QC, Canada
e-mail: gilles.soulez.chcm@ssss.gouv.qc.ca

J. Dubois, MD, MSc
Department of Radiology, University Hospital Sainte Justine, Montréal, QC, Canada

P. Chabrot, L. Boyer (eds.), *Embolization*,
DOI 10.1007/978-1-4471-5182-1_23, © Springer-Verlag London 2014

Interventional radiology is now pivotal in the management of vascular malformations as either a single therapeutic option or in combination with surgery. However, the physician must classify adequately the vascular malformation, evaluate the associated symptoms, and establish a prognosis before proceeding to invasive therapy. Recurrences are frequently observed regardless of the therapeutic approach and iatrogenic complication can be observed. A vascular malformation can rarely be cured. The goal of the treatment is to alleviate symptoms and improve patient's quality of life.

In this setting, the interventional radiologist must be involved in patient's clinical evaluation and work with a multidisciplinary team to manage advanced cases.

23.2 Preprocedural Imaging

Following clinical examination, Doppler ultrasound is the first-line imaging modality to discriminate high- and low-flow malformations. Then MRI is the best examination to assess the extension of the malformation and plan interventional treatment. Catheter angiography is now essentially performed before AVM embolization.

VMs are the most frequent vascular malformations. They appear as a compressible soft tissue mass with a bluish coloration and sometimes dysplastic veins. Their anatomic distribution is head and neck (40 %), trunk (20 %), limbs (40 %). On grayscale ultrasound, they show as a compressible hypoechoic or iso-echoic lesion infiltrating soft tissue with a slow flow on Doppler examination (Fig. 23.1). Hyperechoic areas with acoustic shadowing related to phleboliths can be observed. Phleboliths can also be seen on plain film and are pathognomonic of VM.

On MRI, VMs are characterized by as soft tissue mass with a hypo- or isosignal on T1-weighted sequence. Delayed contrast enhancement is observed after gadolinium injection. On T2-weighted sequence, VMs show a characteristic bright hypersignal (Fig. 23.1).

LMs are characterized by a firm mass involving mostly head and neck or cervicothoracic area the trunk being less frequently involved. They are divided in to macrocystic LM made of uni- or multiloculate cysts easily seen on ultrasound and microcystic LM more infiltrative made of microcysts difficult to distinguish on ultrasound. On Doppler ultrasound, no flow is observed inside the cyst of macrocystic LM, whereas small vessels with high-resistance arterial flow can be seen in the septations (Fig. 23.2). Microcystic LMs are very infiltrative and show frequently a hyperechoic heterogeneous structure. On MRI, both macro- and microcystic LMs display a bright hypersignal; however, macrocysts are observed in macrocystic LM (Figs. 23.2 and 23.3). There is no enhancement after contrast injection in the cysts, but cyst wall can display post-contrast enhancement. Mixed forms of LM combining macro- and microcystic components can be frequently observed.

AVMs are characterized by a pulsatile mass involving frequently head and neck and peripheral limbs. Truncular AVMs are less frequent and involve mainly the pelvis. On Doppler ultrasound, AVMs are made of multiple hypoechoic serpiginous structures displaying a high flow with a high diastolic component on the arterial side and congestive dilated veins with a systolic modulation on the venous side (Fig. 23.4). On MRI, a flow void is typically seen on both T1- and T2-weighted sequences indicating high flow (Fig. 23.5). Magnetic resonance angiography (MRA) with 3D gadolinium-enhanced acquisition or time-resolved angiography (4D angiography) is helpful to detect the nidus of the malformation and identify feeding arteries and draining veins (Fig. 23.5). Selective catheter angiography still remains the best examination to evaluate the architecture of the malformation (nidus, feeder, and draining vessels) and the feasibility of therapeutic embolization (Fig. 23.5).

23.3 Sclerotherapy and Embolization Techniques

23.3.1 Venous Malformations

Symptomatic VMs respond well to sclerotherapy especially in cavernous malformation. Sclerotherapy is usually performed under ultrasound and fluoroscopic guidance.

The puncture is usually performed under ultrasound guidance with 21–23 needle or Jelco. The needle is progressively pulled back while applying a negative pressure via a syringe connected with small flexible tubing. Once blood reflux is obtained, a percutaneous phlebography is performed to assess the positioning of the needle within the malformation and the absence or presence of central venous drainage connected.

Sclerotherapy is usually performed with foam made of sodium tetradecyl sulfate (STS) 3 % mixed 1 ml de LIPIODOL 1 ml and air 3 ml. Foam injection is performed under negative roadmap technique to assess foam diffusion and eventual drainage in central vein. Control of the drainage veins when needed can be achieved with direct pressure (manual or with a clamp) or by using a tourniquet. Tourniquet should be inflated for a short period (typically a few minutes) so it does not cause unnecessary stagnation and accumulation of sclerotherapy by-products in the deep veins and deflated progressively to avoid fast release of sclerosing agent in the systemic circulation. Then foam diffusion inside the malformation is assessed on Doppler ultrasound. If needed, additional punctures are performed to complete sclerosis of the entire VM. The maximum dosage of STS is of 300 mg per session (five vials of 3 % STS). Sclerotherapy with absolute ethanol is very effective, but it is more painful and can lead to cardiorespiratory arrest when large volumes are injected in a short period of time. Sclerotherapy sessions should be resumed every 6–8 weeks until the entire malformation has been injected and also depending on clinical improvement. C-arm CT acquisition at the end of the procedure can be useful to assess foam diffusion in deep VMs or VMs that cannot be imaged properly on ultrasound (Fig. 23.6).

23.3.2 Lymphatic Malformations

LMs are also treated under ultrasound and fluoroscopic guidance. The larger cyst must be punctured first, then a pigtail catheter is inserted to evacuate it completely. If residual cysts are still observed on ultrasound, they will be punctured successively until the whole malformation is emptied. The different cystic components are injected with doxycycline (10 mg/ml, maximal dose 1,000 mg or 20 mg/kg per session) or bleomycin (1 mg/ml, maximal dose, 15 mg per session) diluted with 20 % of iodine contrast (Fig. 23.7). Catheters are retrieved 1 hour following sclerosant injection.

Ethanol, Ethibloc, and OK 432 have also been used with success.

23.3.3 Arteriovenous Malformations

AVM embolization is a complex procedure requiring an appropriate training. General anesthesia is necessary to obtain patient immobility and inject sclerosant agent that can be painful during intra-arterial injection such as ethanol.

The nidus must be embolized hyperselectively with a liquid agent (ethanol, Onyx, glue) to obtain a good filling of AVM nidus and minimize injection of healthy arteries supplying surrounding structures and also embolization proximal to the nidus.

Embolization can be performed through an arterial endovascular approach following hyperselective catheterization of arterial feeders (Fig. 23.8).

Utilization of a coaxial microcatheter is recommended. If the flow is too fast, an occlusion balloon can be inflated (on the arterial or venous side) to slow down the arterial flow. If the malformation presents multiple arterial feeders with a single venous drainage, embolization of the draining vein with coil or an Amplatzer (AVP) plug followed by retrograde sclerotherapy of the nidus with ethanol or sclerosing foam through a microcatheter positioned beyond the coils mass or the amplatzer plug can be the preferred approach. Retrograde injection of sclerosant agent on the venous side can also be performed through a micro-catheter inserted through the lumen of an occlusion balloon. Finally, direct puncture of AVM nidus under ultrasound and fluoroscopic guidance followed by ethanol or glue embolization is also a very good alternative when the arterial and venous routes are no more possible.

Absolute ethanol is a very good agent since it induces an endothelial ablation, thus reducing the risk of recanalization. However, it can be dangerous because of the occurrence of systemic side effects such as pulmonary hypertension or cardiac arrest if large boluses of ethanol are injected too fast. It can also induce local complications like cutaneous necrosis and peripheral nerve injury. Since ethanol is not radio-opaque, the volume and speed of injection should be estimated on a DSA or roadmap fluoroscopic acquisition acquired just before the embolization with the microcatheter positioned exactly at the same position.

Bolus injection should not exceed 5 ml per bolus, and a minimal delay of 5 min must be given between each injection. The total volume of ethanol should not exceed 50 ml (0.5 ml/kg). Continuous monitoring of pulmonary pressure is recommended when large ethanol volume need to be injected in fast-flow AVMs.

Tissular glue is diluted with LIPIODOL to make it radio-opaque and slow down the polymerization process. It is crucial to optimize glue dilution with LIPIODOL according to the flow of the AVM in order to fill the AVM nidus and avoid a proximal embolization (in the feeding artery before the nidus) or glue migration in the draining vein and systemic circulation.

Dilution varying between ½ (33 %) and ¼ (20 %) are usually recommended. All catheters must be flushed with 5 % dextrose and no blood should be in contact with the catheter or the syringe to prevent catheter occlusion

Onyx is an expensive agent that has the advantage of combing an excellent radio-opacity and control during injection. It is useful when injecting dangerous arterial feeders with potential dangerous anastomosis or in the vicinity of peripheral nerves. Its high radio-opacity can impair fluoroscopic visualization when multiple embolization procedures are required and also imaging follow-up by CT scanner. Onyx need to be injected after filling the catheter with a solvent called DMSO. Microcatheters compatible with DMSO must be used when Onyx injection is anticipated.

Onyx injection is performed very slowly under fluoroscopic control. The goal is to create a plug at the tip of the catheter to prevent retrograde reflux and obtain a slow antegrade filling of the nidus of the malformation. When Onyx does not migrate inside the nidus, the injection is stopped for several minutes to create another occlusion area and then resumed to divert Onyx toward the nidus and its arterial feeders. Onyx injection requires long fluoroscopic exposure that can be a drawback in patients with complex AVMs requiring multiple embolization sessions.

As a rule and whenever the type of embolizing agent used, it is recommended to avoid performing extensive AVM embolization in one session since this will increase the risk of complication especially the risk of skin necrosis or nerve injury. Thus, embolization sessions must be fragmented and repeated every 6–8 weeks.

23.4 Results

- For VMS, success rates varying between 70 and 80 % have been reported, but recurrences are frequent requiring re-interventions. Surgery can be indicated following failure of sclerotherapy, if patient symptoms are not alleviated by anti-inflammatory and analgesic medication or if a significant residual mass effect is present.
- For macrocystic LM, success rates between 70 and 95 % have been reported for the different sclerosing agents. Microcystic LM does not respond as well to sclerotherapy and should be treated conservatively or by surgery if symptoms are not controlled by medication. Sclerotherapy with bleomycin could be more efficient in microcystic LM.

- Regarding AVM, the best results are obtained in low-grade and localized AVMs where embolization can be combined with surgery. However, in large AVMs that cannot be resected, palliative embolization is successful in controlling bleeding, ischemic, or congestive symptoms in 70 % of the cases.
- Following embolization, a swelling of the malformation associated with pain exacerbation and fever is frequently observed (post-embolization syndrome). This can be controlled by anti-inflammatory (steroids or nonsteroidal anti-inflammatory drugs) combined with analgesic medications. Corticosteroids are more frequently used in head and neck malformation especially of there is a risk of airway compromise.
- The most frequently observed complications are skin necrosis and nerve injury with sensorial or motricity loss. Skin necrosis healed spontaneously in most cases after adequate dressing, whereas most nerve injuries can also recover slowly.
- Regarding VMs, deep vein thrombosis (DVT) and pulmonary emboli (PE) are rare complications that can be fatal. A compressive stocking must be wear in all VM involving a limb.
- In large VMs, a coagulation profile (fibrinogen, D-dimer, platelets, NRI) must be requested to detect a localized intravascular coagulopathy. If positive, a preventive treatment with low molecular weight heparin can be indicated before sclerotherapy to minimize the risk of DVT or PE.
- Cardiac arrest secondary to acute pulmonary hypertension have been reported with ethanol injection in AVMs and VMs.
- Finally, bleomycin injection can induce in oncology patients a pulmonary fibrosis. However, this is almost impossible in patient treated for vascular anomalies if the cumulative dosage does not exceed 100 UI since the lower threshold for pulmonary toxicity has been estimated at 400 UI. Furthermore, most of the bleomycin injected in LM does not reach the systemic circulation.

23.5 Indications

A multidisciplinary approach is mandatory (interventional radiology, dermatology, plastic surgery, internal medicine) especially in complex cases. The patient must be seen at the interventional radiology clinic before performing any invasive treatment to ensure proper diagnosis and evaluate symptoms' magnitude and preprocedural imaging.

Regarding VMs, sclerotherapy will be indicated after failure of medical therapy: compressive stocking and anti-inflammatory medication. The goal of the sclerotherapy is not to eradicate the malformation but to alleviate patient symptoms. Thus, it should be directed in the area causing clinical symptoms.

For LM, sclerotherapy will be mainly indicated in macrocystic LM with a significant mass effect.

A small asymptomatic AVM does not require invasive treatment. Compressive stocking for limb AVM and patient follow-up to document eventual AVM progression is sufficient.

Invasive treatment is required in case of bleeding or worsening pain, if the malformation is growing (expansion stage), or if it is advanced at a destructive stage with apparition of ulceration, venous congestion, skin atrophy, or high-flow cardiac failure.

Key Points

- Implication of the interventional radiologist in clinical evaluation before indicating the intervention.
- Access to a multidisciplinary team (interventional radiology, dermatology, plastic surgery, internal medicine, nursing).
- Perform a Doppler ultrasound examination in all vascular malformations to characterize them in low- and fast-flow malformation.
- Treat only symptomatic VM and LM after a failure of medical treatment (especially for VM).
- Sclerotherapy is the first-line invasive therapy for VMs and macrocystic LM.
- Symptomatic AVMs are approached first by embolization, but it can be completed by surgery if the malformation is localized and can be entirely resected.
- The nidus of AVM must be injected with liquid agent and proximal embolization must be avoided.
- Avoid extensive embolization in one session. Embolization can be fragmented in several sessions every 6–8 weeks to minimize post-embolization syndrome and complications.

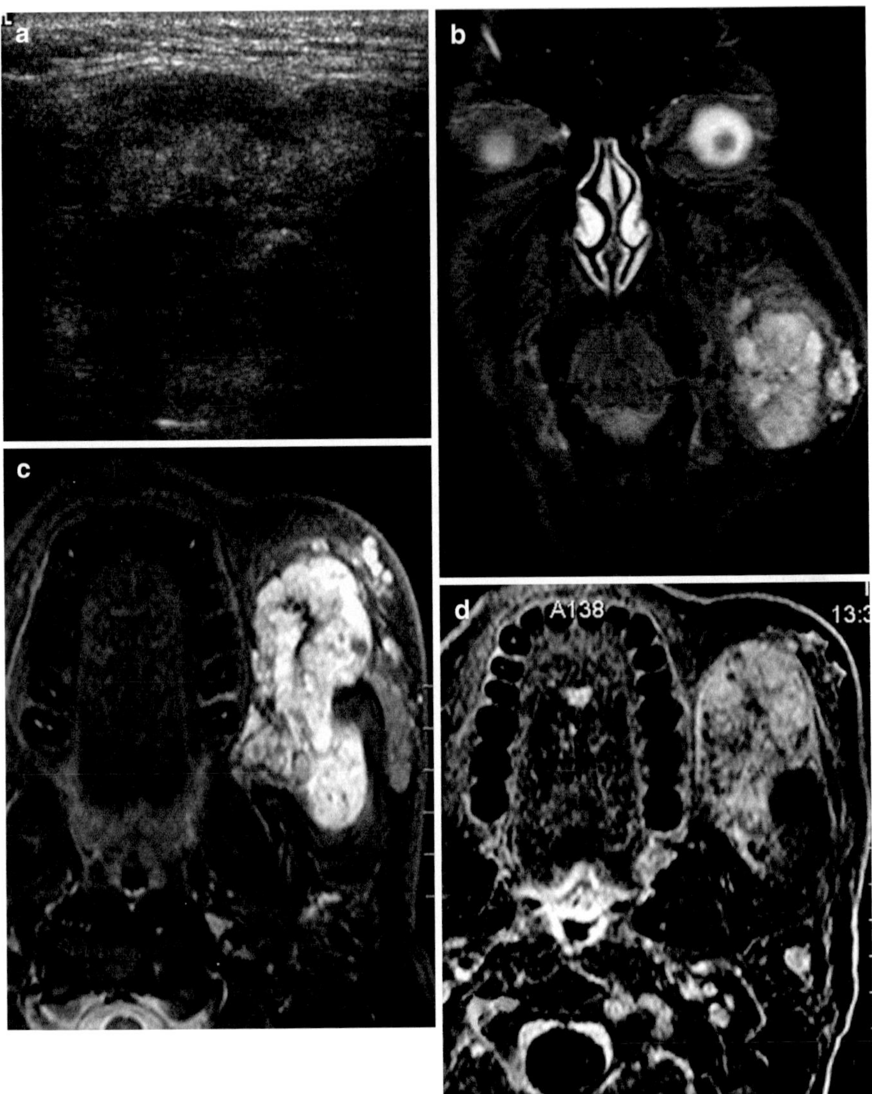

Fig. 23.1 Patient with a large venous malformation (VM) of the left hemiface. (**a**) B-mode ultrasound showing the VM as an infiltrating, hypoechoic, and compressible mass. (**b**, **c**) MRI examination: T2-weighted short TI inversion recovery (STIR) sequences acquired in coronal (**b**) and axial planes (**c**). The VM appears with a bright hypersignal, and its extension is easily delineated in adjacent soft tissues. (**d**) MRI examination: T1-weighted axial volumetric interpolated breath-hold examination (VIBE) MRI acquisition after gadolinium injection (MultiHance) and subtraction with baseline acquisition. The perfused area of the VM is well delineated. Several areas without perfusion are seen corresponding to phleboliths or thrombosed portions of the VM

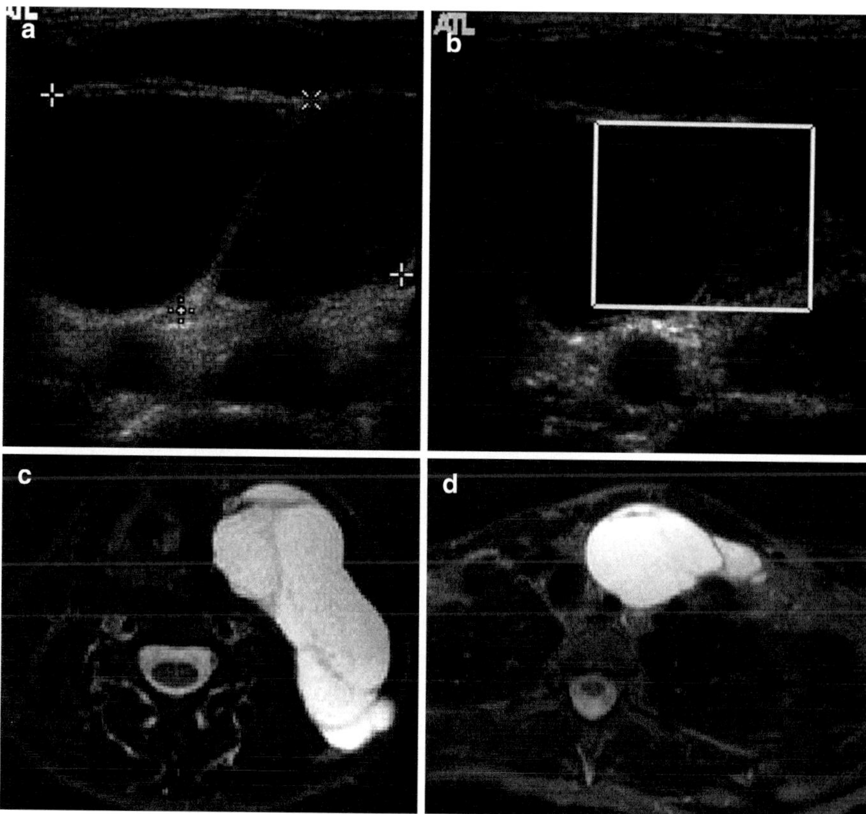

Fig. 23.2 Patient with a voluminous macrocystic lymphangioma of the left portion of the neck. (**a**) B-mode ultrasound showing multiple cysts with septations. (**b**) Color Doppler study showing a vessel with high-resistance flow in a septa. (**c**, **d**) MRI examination: T2-weighted axial (STIR) acquisitions showing the presence of fluid compatible with a macrocystic lymphatic malformation. (**e**) MRI examination: T1-weighted coronal acquisition after gadolinium injection showing contrast enhancement in the septations

Fig. 23.2 (continued)

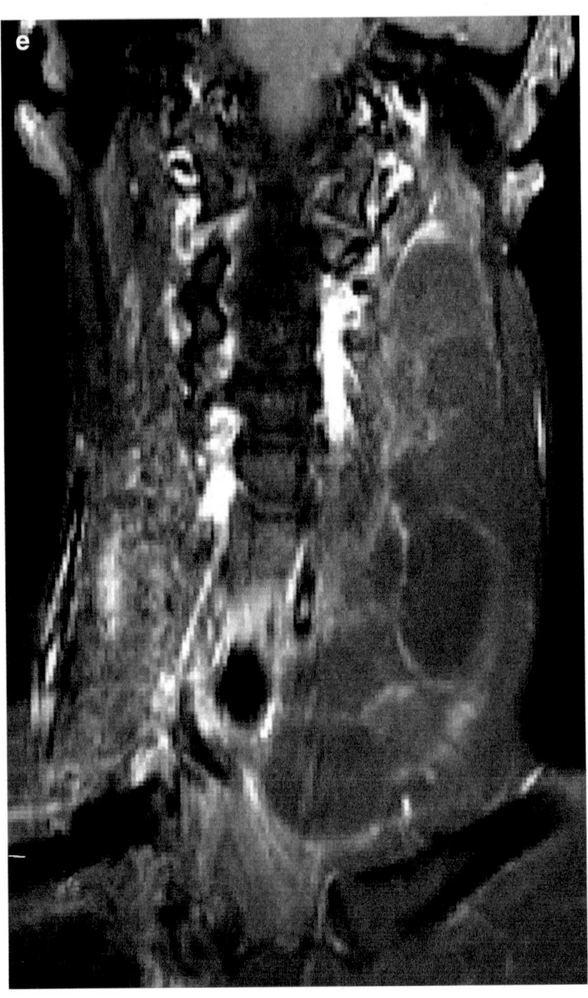

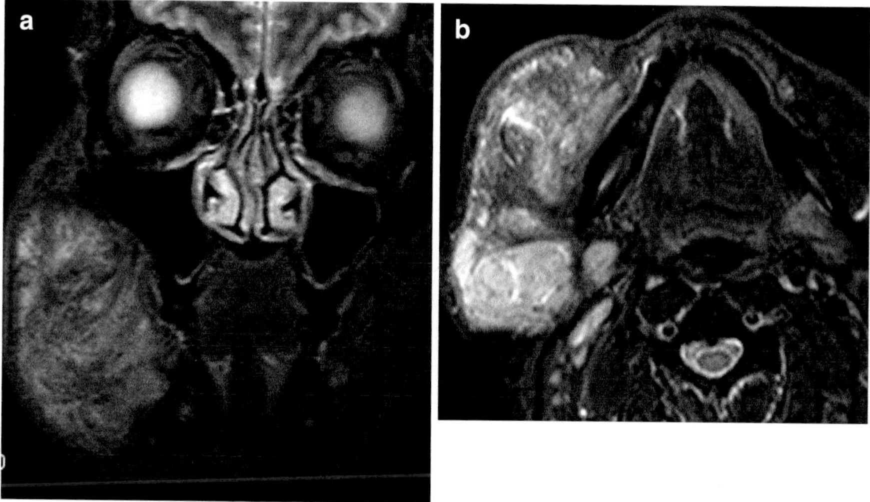

Fig. 23.3 Patient with a large microcystic lymphangioma of the right hemiface. (**a**, **b**) MRI examination: T2-weighted coronal and axial acquisitions showing a hyperintense soft tissue mass made of tiny microcysts infiltrating the cheek and masticator space

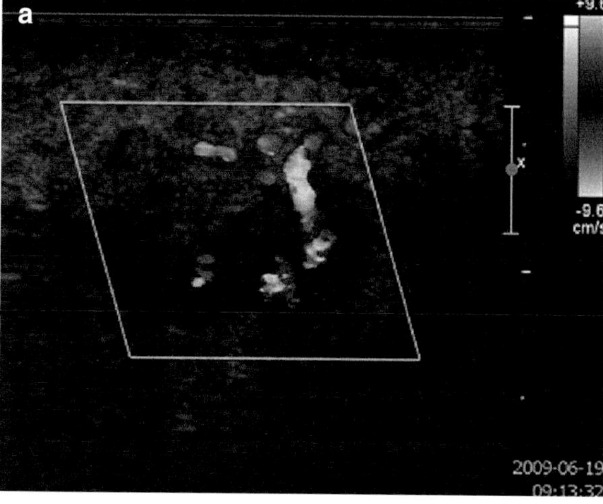

Fig. 23.4 Patient with an AVM of the lip. (**a**) Color Doppler ultrasound showing a high-flow malformation. (**b**) Pulsed Doppler ultrasound showing a high diastolic flow in the feeding artery characteristic of an arteriovenous shunt. (**c**) Pulsed Doppler ultrasound of a draining vein showing a systolic modulation of the flow confirming the presence of an arteriovenous shunt

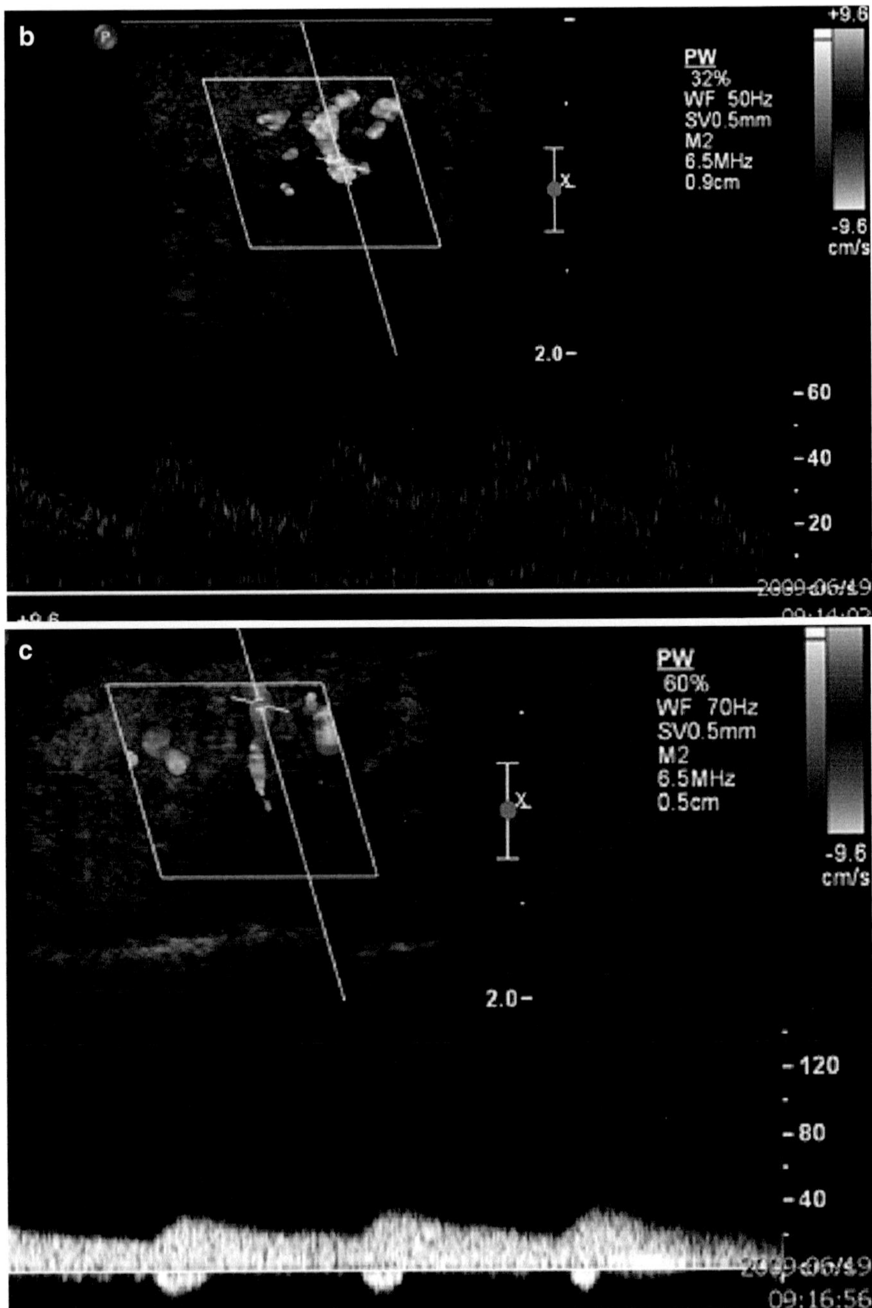

Fig. 23.4 (continued)

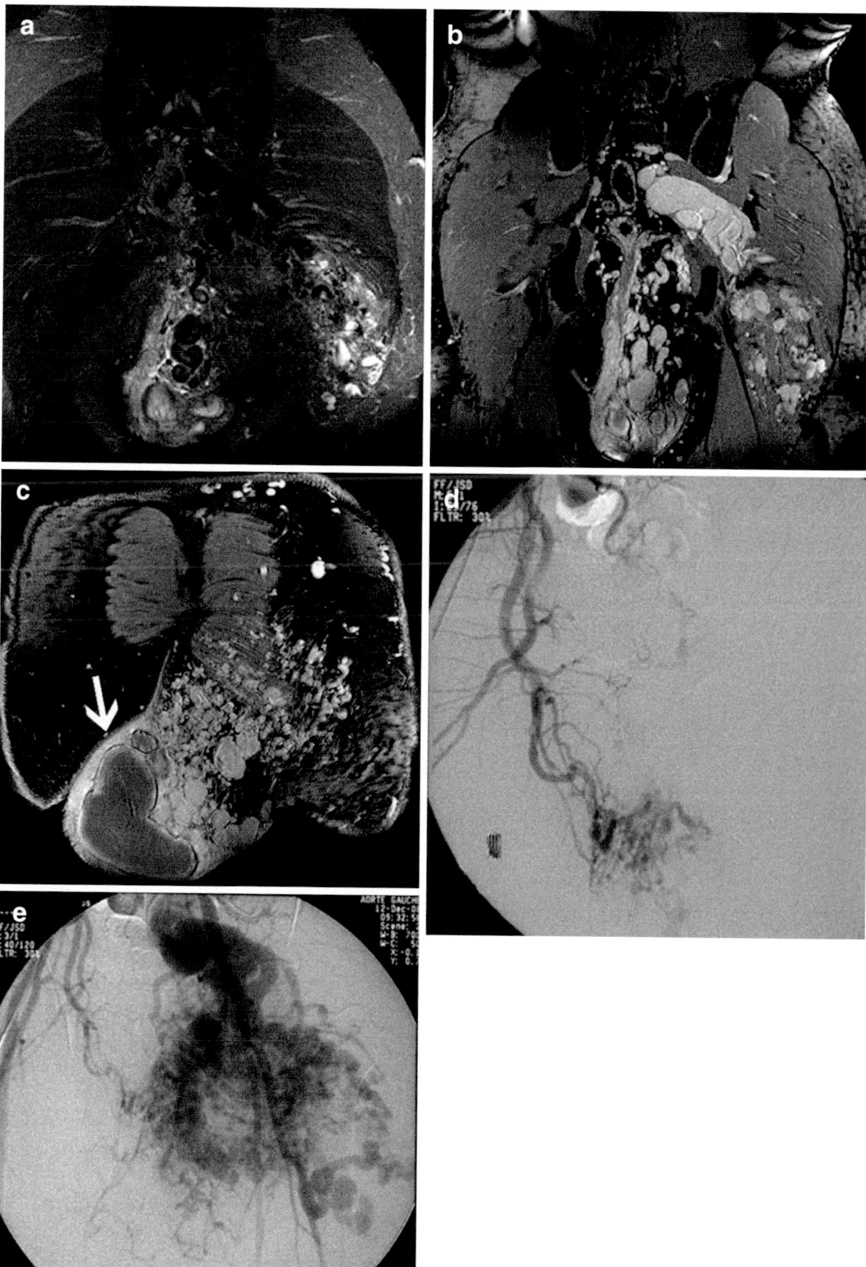

Fig. 23.5 Patient with a voluminous perineal AVM. (**a**) MRI examination. T2-weighted (STIR) coronal acquisition showing feeding arteries originating from the anterior and posterior trunk of the left internal iliac artery with multiple flow voids and areas of hyperintense signal suggesting a venous thrombosis. (**b**, **c**) MRI examination: T1-weighted (balanced fast field echo (FFE)) coronal acquisition after gadolinium (MultiHance) injection in steady state confirming the recruitment of multiple branches of the internal iliac artery and a thrombosis of the main draining vein (*arrow*). (**d**, **e**) Selective angiography of the right and left internal iliac arteries showing the recruitment of the right pudendal and inferior gluteal arteries and a participation of almost all branches of the left internal iliac artery

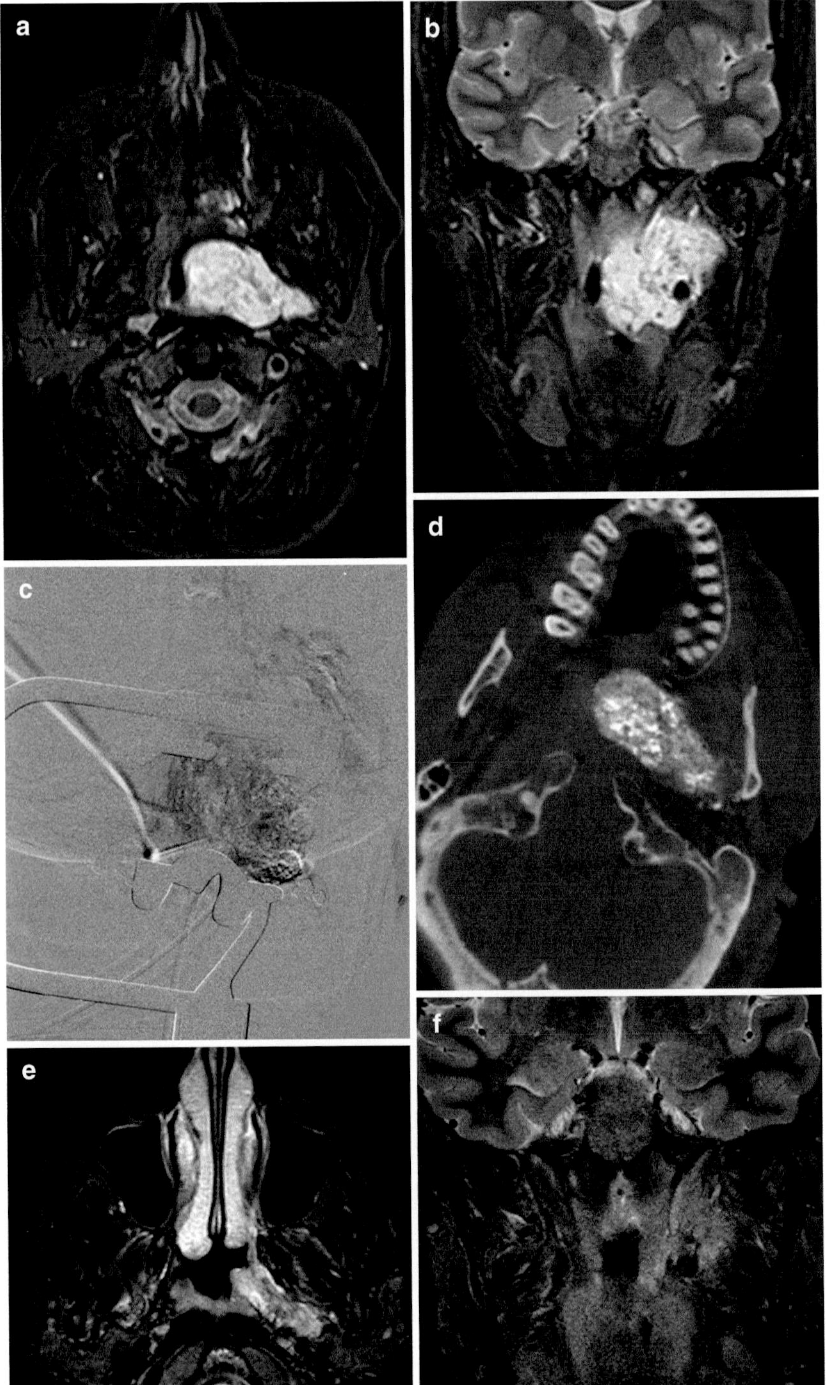

Fig. 23.6 Patient with venous malformation of the rhinopharynx. (**a**, **b**) MRI examination: T2-weighted (STIR) axial and coronal acquisitions showing the voluminous malformation. (**c**) Sclerotherapy session with foam made of 3 % STS and LIPIODOL and air injected under fluoroscopic and endoscopic guidance. (**d**) C-Arm CT acquired in the angio suite showing the diffusion of the foam within the malformation. (**e**, **f**) Control MRI after sclerotherapy showing a significant regression of the malformation

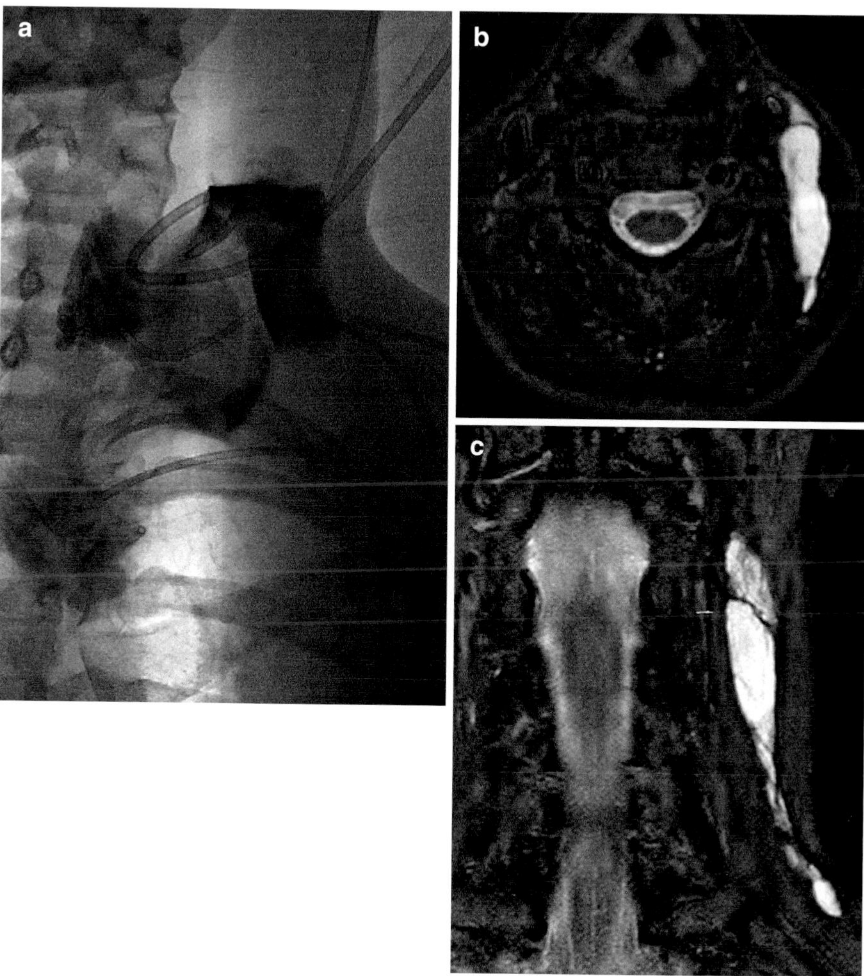

Fig. 23.7 Same patient shown in Fig. 23.3. (**a**) Drainage of multiple cystic components with four different drainage catheters. After fluid evacuation, sclerotherapy with injection of 15 UI bleomycin mixed with 20 % iodine contrast. The bleomycin solution will be macerated for 3 h before being aspirated. (**b**, **c**) Control MRI post-sclerotherapy showing a significant regression of the malformation 6-month post-sclerotherapy

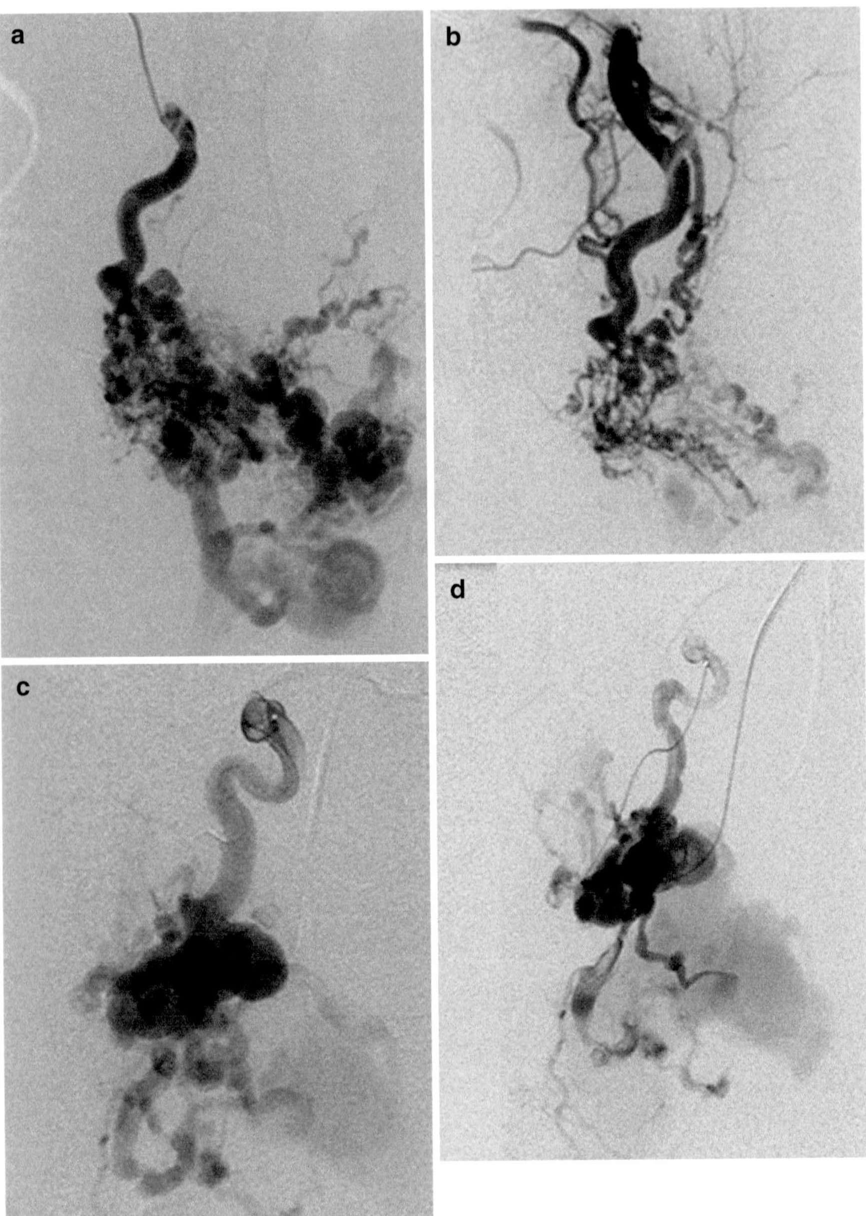

Fig. 23.8 Same patient as Fig. 23.5. (**a**, **b**) Selective angiography of the middle sacral artery (**a**), an important stagnation is observed after embolization with ethanol on (**b**). (**c**, **d**) Selective angiography of the obturator artery before (**c**) and after ethanol embolization (**d**). (**e**) Angiographic acquisition after 13 embolization sessions of the AVM showing almost a complete devascularization of the AVM. (**f**) T2-weighted control MRI showing an important size reduction of the AVM without residual flow void. The residual perineal mass was surgically resected with a good clinical success

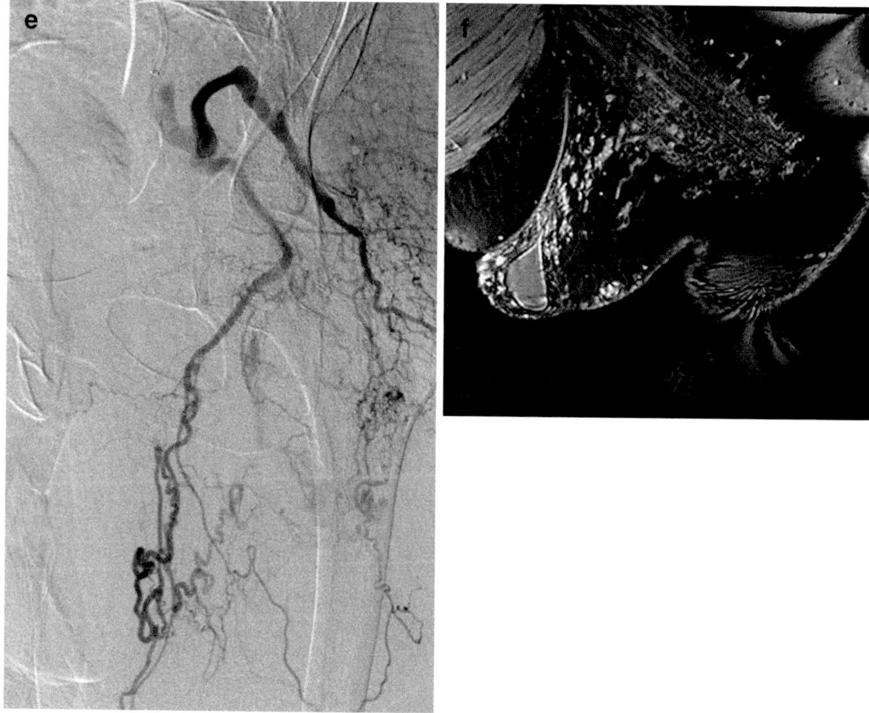

Fig. 23.8 (continued)

Suggested Reading

Dubois J, Soulez G, Oliva VL, Berthiaume MJ, Lapierre C, Thérasse E. Soft tissue venous malformations in adult patients: imaging and therapeutic issues. Radiographics. 2001;21(6):1519–31.

Legiehn GM, Heran MKS. Classification, diagnosis, and interventional radiologic management of vascular malformations. Orthop Clin North Am. 2006;37:435–74.

Mulliken JB, Fishman SJ, Burrows PE. Vascular anomalies. Curr Probl Surg. 2000;37:517–84.

Soulez G, Dubois J, Oliva VL. Soft-tissue vascular malformations. In: Comprehensive vascular and endovascular surgery, vol. 48. 2nd ed. London: Elsevier Science; 2008. p. 842–61.

Chapter 24
Miscellaneous/Marginal/Evolving Indications (Other Abdominopelvic Tumors, Portal Hypertension-Related Varicose Veins, Osteoarticular Pathologies)

Louis Boyer, Agaïcha Alfidja Lankoande, Mickaël Fontarensky, and Pascal Chabrot

24.1 Other Abdominopelvic Tumors

24.1.1 Adrenal Tumors

Corticosurrenalomas are rare. In approximately half of the cases, their diagnosis is based on their hormonal and metabolic consequences; other diagnostic circumstances are a mass syndrome or remote metastatic localizations in patients of 30–50 years old. Adrenal metastases are on the other hand frequent mostly due to lung and breast cancers as well as melanoma. They are often bilateral, with an adrenal insufficiency in 20–30 % of the cases.

The adrenal gland is classically fed by three arteries: the upper artery, arising from the lower diaphragmatic artery, the middle artery from the aorta, and the lower artery from the renal artery.

Embolization has been advocated to treat a retroperitoneal hematoma induced by adrenal tumor bleeding and as a palliative treatment to reduce tumor volume or hormone hypersecretion or to deal with pain [1].

Acute hypertension can complicate the procedure.

We have gathered in this chapter miscellaneous and/or marginal or evolving indications.

L. Boyer, MD, PhD (✉) • A. Alfidja Lankoande, MD • M. Fontarensky
P. Chabrot, MD, PhD
Department of Radiology,
University Hospital of Clermont-Ferrand,
Clermont-Ferrand, France
e-mail: lboyer@chu-clermontferrand.fr; pchabrot@chu-clermontferrand.fr

P. Chabrot, L. Boyer (eds.), *Embolization*,
DOI 10.1007/978-1-4471-5182-1_24,

24.1.2 Pelvic Tumors

The arterial access to the hypogastric artery is carried out via an ipsi- or contralateral (crossover) puncture site.

In 70 % of the cases, the internal iliac artery (IIA) ends in two principal trunks: anterior and posterior in 14 % of the cases, in three trunks, or in more than three trunks in 3 %, and in one trunk in 4 % of the cases [2].

To selectively catheterize the branches feeding the pelvic organs, an aortography depicting the aortoiliac bifurcation on frontal and oblique views is needed. Selective injections of the hypogastric trunk and of its anterior trunk are helpful in identifying the visceral pelvic branches. The use of a micro-catheter is sometimes necessary. The catheterization of the posterior branches can be necessary when a tumor extension to the pelvic wall is the target of the embolization.

The terminal branches of the posterior trunk are the iliolumbar artery, the lateral sacral, and the superior gluteal arteries. The distribution of the anterior trunk is less systematic, with three branches feeding the pelvic wall (obturator, inferior gluteal, and internal pudendal arteries) and three visceral branches (vesical, uterovaginal/vesicoprostatic, and middle hemorrhoidal arteries). The origin of these arteries and their branches is best depicted on an anterior oblique contralateral view (20°–30°) [2]. The left-right symmetry of this distribution has been observed by Pelage in 91 % of the cases.

When intra-arterial chemotherapy for pelvic tumors is carried out so as to increase intra-tumor drug concentration and to decrease the general toxicity of drugs in normal tissues, the upper and lower gluteal arteries can be occluded by coils and Gelfoam.

24.1.2.1 Genitourinary Hemorrhages and Pelvic Tumors

An embolization can be carried out as a palliative treatment of acute or chronic bleeding, due to the pelvic tumors (bladder, uterus, prostate) or consecutive to radiation therapy (especially radiocystitis), to pelvic surgery (prostatectomy), or prostate biopsies [3].

A bilateral embolization is necessary. We prefer using small diameter microparticles.

Rebleedings are however possible and are often retreatable with embolization. A hyperselective micro-catheterization helps in limiting ischemic complications.

24.1.2.2 Bladder Tumors

Intra-arterial chemotherapy infusion has been proposed to deal with T2–T4 bladder cancers, in association with and/or as an alternative to intravenous chemotherapy and radiation therapy [4]. But to our knowledge this technique has yet to be formally recommended.

24.1.2.3 Uterine Cancers

Stages 3 and 4 cervix cancers extending to the pelvic side wall, the vagina, the bladder, as well as lymph nodes have been treated by intra-arterial chemotherapy via the hypogastric anterior trunk and sometimes via the branches of the hypogastric posterior trunk.

But these techniques are no longer used because of their morbidity and limited results in these advanced cancers.

24.1.2.4 Benign Prostatic Hyperplasia

Experimental work in pigs and dogs has shown that a significant reduction of the prostatic volume was obtained with an arterial embolization, without alteration of the sexual and erectile functions. Some patients presenting with drained acute retention have been treated with embolization while awaiting surgery [5] or prospectively in case of benign symptomatic hyperplasia unresponsive to medical treatment [6].

The volume of the prostate could thus be reduced by almost 30 %, with few adverse side effects and without sexual dysfunction.

Embolization could then constitute an alternative to the medical and surgical treatment for symptomatic benign prostate hypertrophy. But the long-term effectiveness and the lack of collateral effect on erection, that would distinguish it from current treatments, has yet to be proven [7].

24.2 Embolization of Portal Hypertension Related to Varicose Veins

Complementary embolization of esophageal varices can be performed after TIPS (transjugular intrahepatic portacaval shunt) to treat bleedings, either immediately after the procedure or in case of a recurrent bleeding with patent shunt. Catheterization is carried out then via a jugular or brachial access, through the shunt, by selecting the branches feeding the varicose veins (left gastric vein above all). Various agents have been used: sclerosing agents, coils, and glues.

Embolization can also constitute a complement or an alternative to the endoscopic sclerosis and to TIPS for the management of *varicose veins*, when access is possible via a spontaneous portacaval gastrorenal shunt (balloon-occluded retrograde transvenous obliteration (BRTO)).

A femoral venous access and catheterization of the left renal vein allow the deployment of an occlusion balloon and the injection of sclerosing agents directly into the varicose vein: the occlusion balloon avoids reflux in the portal and caval circulations. Additional temporary occlusion of the splenic artery by a balloon for a better control of the portal pressure gradient and to ensure a better filling of the varicose veins by the sclerosing agent has been proposed [8]. Coils can be positioned beforehand in the collateral networks (lower phrenic veins, paravertebral veins) to avoid out-of-target embolizations.

During the procedure, CT-like images (cone beam CT) are helpful to follow up the repletion of the varicose veins.

Ethanolamine oleate (Neosclerol, Ethamolin) was up to now mostly used, usually diluted to 5 % and associated with an equivalent quantity of contrast agent. But this agent can induce, via a hemolysis, an acute tubular renal insufficiency. Cardiogenic shock, pulmonary edema, and DIC have also been described. More recently the emulsified 3 % diluted sodium tetradecyl sulfates ((STS) Sotradecol, Trombovar) has been used (3 volumes of air or CO_2, 2 volumes of 3 % STS, 1 volume of Lipiodol). This embolization agent has up to now been used for the treatment of varicoceles, venous pelvic congestion syndrome, and venous malformations. Sabri [9] was able to obtain a technical success in 20 cirrhotic patients out of 22 (the average dosage of STS: 300 mg), with a persistent complete obliteration in 89 % at 3 months, and no clinical recurrence after more than 4 months follow-up. Polidocanol (Aethoxysklerol) has also been used, which has the advantage of not inducing any general effect.

The evaluation of these BRTO was carried out by Hong [10], who found a more constant immediate success rate by endoscopy (100 % versus 77 %), but a rebleeding rate of 77 % after endoscopic sclerosis versus 15 % BRTO.

After TIPS, the rebleeding rate of the gastric varices is more important than with the esophageal varicose veins: in fact the bleeding of the gastric varices occurs with lower portal vein-vena cava gradients than for bleeding of the esophageal varicose veins, because of their larger diameter, which induces a higher wall pressure.

Finally it should be noted that this embolization technique is possible among patients for whom the implementation of a TIPS (hepatic function, encephalopathy) would be difficult.

The occlusion of portacaval shunts between the inferior mesenteric vein and the hypogastric vein or the renal vein by BRTO, to try to limit a portacaval encephalopathy, has been proposed [11]. The risks are extensive thromboses and/or the aggravation of esophageal varicose veins.

Conversely, chronic low GI tract hemorrhages caused by an association of cava-mesenteric anastomosis + chronic caval obstruction have been described and effectively treated with angioplasty and stenting of the caval obstruction [12].

24.3 Embolization in Musculoskeletal Pathologies

Embolization can be used for the devascularization of primary and secondary tumors as a palliative or preoperative treatment or to carry out intra-arterial chemotherapy and chemoembolization.

24.3.1 *Bone Metastases* [13, 14]

Many years ago *embolization* was introduced in order to decrease blood losses during surgery. This indication remains valuable in the preoperative management of hypervascular tumors: embolization is in these cases carried out generally 24–48 h before surgery. Embolization can also take place in addition to radiation therapy. The technique helps in reducing pain induced by inoperable tumors that are inaccessible to radiofrequency ablation or cementoplasty. These palliative embolizations can be repeated.

For these preoperative or palliative procedures, various embolization agents can be used: Gelfoam, coils, particles, alcohols, glues, and collagen. *Chemoembolizations* allow faster and more sustainable pain control than with bland embolization, except for lesions that are not sensitive to the chemotherapy agents (thyroid and renal primitive tumors). The choice of the chemotherapy agent depends on the primary tumor and on previous treatments. A relation between the degree of the devascularization and pain control has been suggested.

Complications are rare:

- Tumor necrosis, which causes pain and fever, is observed in case of large tumors and when small diameter particles or direct alcohol injection have been used.
- Neurotoxicity of certain antimitotics, especially carboplatin, which can induce radicular pain or neurological deficit when the embolized arteries supply nerves: larger particles should then be preferred.
- Skin necrosis that must notably be anticipated in case of associated radiation therapy treatment.

Palliative embolizations can improve the quality of life by attenuating pain and by reducing the size of the tumors. Chemoembolization, when it can be carried out, also adds an antimitotic effect depending on the sensitivity of the tumor.

24.3.2 *Primary Tumors*

24.3.2.1 Osteosarcomas

Occur most frequently in teenager males; these tumors are most often located on the distal femoral, the proximal tibial, or the distal humeral metaphysis. Before chemotherapy was implemented, about 80 % of the patients died from metastases within 2 years. Progress in recent years has allowed the control the micrometastases by adjuvant chemotherapy coupled with surgical resection.

The intra-arterial chemotherapy must be carried out by using thin multi-hole catheters (4 F), whose proximal end must be placed upstream of the multiple branches, including the hypertrophied periosteal/cortical arteries which usually feed the osteosarcoma. The administration of the chemotherapy via a pulsatile pump is recommended.

The goal of these intra-arterial preoperative infusions is the local control of the tumor in order to facilitate the surgical resection and to increase the odds of limb conservation. It also contributes in identifying the most effective drug for the adjuvant chemotherapy according to the degree of necrosis observed on to the resected tissue. Surgery with limb conservation is possible today in about 80 % of the patients who have a mature skeleton.

The limb-isolated perfusion technique reduces the systemic toxicity; when used in inoperable patients, it authorizes the administration of high doses which were not conceivable with the intravenous administration.

24.3.2.2 Giant-Cell Tumors

Women are more frequently concerned, with a peak during the third decade. These benign but locally aggressive tumors have nevertheless a high incidence of local recurrence after surgery; in rare cases, remote metastases are associated. Surgery is the first-choice treatment. The axial skeleton is rarely involved: it most often affects the sacrum, where the surgical resection is difficult and incomplete, with a high recurrence rate.

The therapeutic alternatives for non-resectable tumors include radiation therapy and embolization. Embolization was initially proposed prior to surgical resection for hypervascular tumors. It was secondarily used as a palliative therapy, with good results concerning pain control and a favorable local tumor control.

24.3.2.3 Aneurysmal Cysts

They are fast-growing benign tumors, occurring most frequently in children; the metaphysis of long bones and to a lesser degree the axial skeleton is concerned.

Embolization has been used as a complement to surgery, but has also been proposed alone.

24.3.3 Recurrent Hemarthrosis After Knee Arthroplasty

Spontaneous recurrent hemarthrosis of the knee is frequent, and its cause is often obvious. Hemarthrosis after a knee arthroplasty is rare (0.5 %); its etiology is often not found even after synovectomy. Apart from hemophilia, it can be due to a synovial hyperplasia, a villonodular synovitis, an anticoagulant treatment, or more rarely an articular or extra-articular vascular lesion. In most cases, it concerns cemented arthroplasties for arthrosis, rheumatoid arthritis, or osteonecrosis. Hemarthrosis occurs at least 24 months after surgery with an interval between each bleeding ranging from a few days to 1 year.

Their treatment is not codified. Classically, conservative management is the first-line treatment (voiding puncture, rest, ice, raising the limb), with good results without recurrence in 30 % of the cases. If it fails, a synovectomy via arthroscopy or surgical access is considered. Otherwise if the joint is hypervascularized, we perform [15] a selective arteriography, which helps in ruling out a vascular cause and secondarily exclude the periarticular hypervascularization by particles. We have thus obtained an excellent functional result after a rehabilitation which is much shorter than after surgery.

Key Points

- Embolization can be used to treat bleeding adrenal tumors responsible of retroperitoneal hematoma, so as to reduce the tumor volume, hypersecretion, or pain.
- Bilateral pelvic embolization can be carried out as a palliative treatment of acute or chronic tumor bleeding, or consecutive to radiation therapy (especially radiocystitis), or to pelvic surgery or biopsies.
- Embolization can be an alternative to mini-invasive surgery to treat benign prostrate hypertrophy refractory to the medical treatment.
- Esophageal variceal embolization can be performed in addition to portacaval shunt via the TIPS itself to treat hemorrhagic complication of portal hypertension.
- Embolization of gastric varices via a spontaneous gastrorenal portacaval shunt (balloon-occluded retrograde transvenous obliteration) is an interesting alternative to the TIPS and to endoscopic sclerosis.
- Embolization is a valuable palliative or preoperative technique for the devascularization of primary or secondary bone tumors or to carry out intra-arterial chemotherapy and chemoembolization.
- Embolization of periarticular hypervascularization to treat refractory recurrent hemarthrosis complicating of total knee arthroplasty.

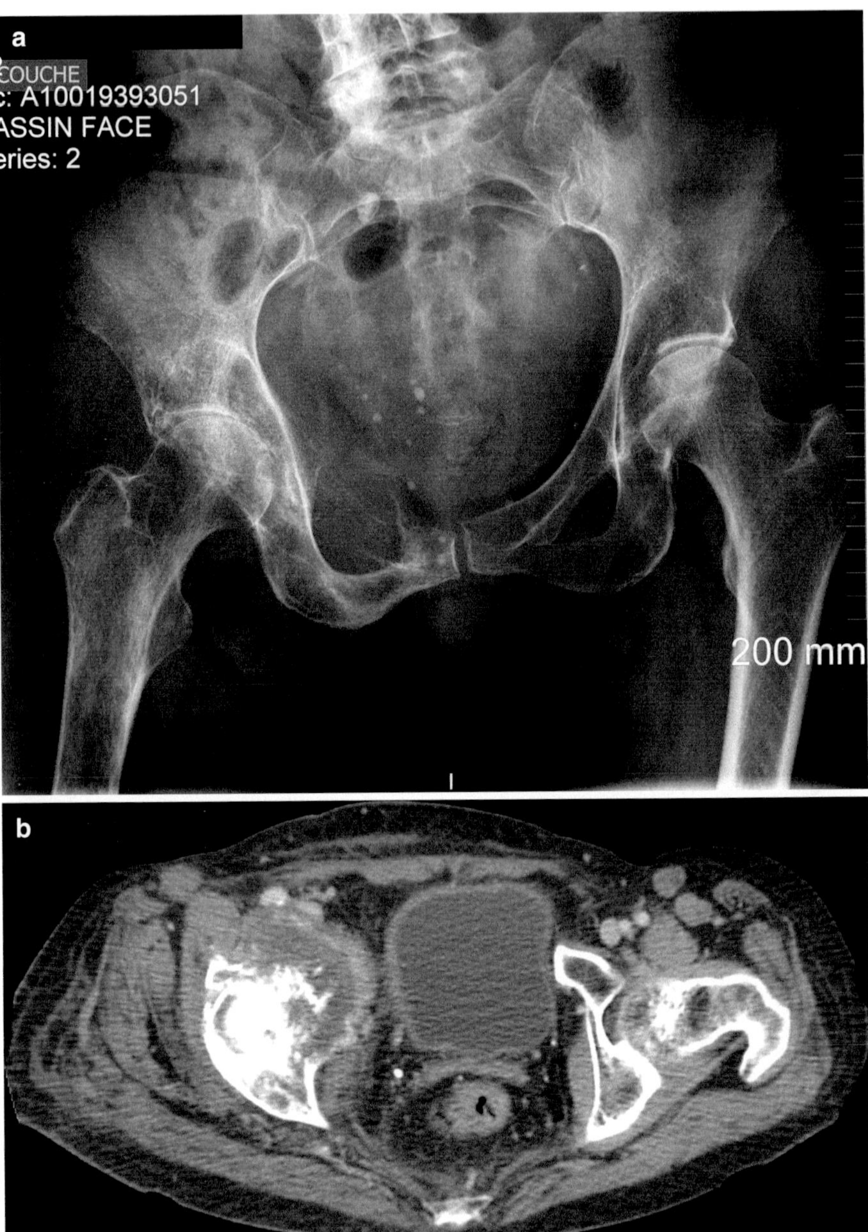

Fig. 24.1 A 63-year-old, osteolytic metastases of the right ischiopubic branch and the right acetabular roof, complicating a thyroid cancer. A total hip replacement was planned, after a preoperative embolization to reduce the risk of bleeding complication. (**a**: standard view) and (**b–e**: CT) Large lytic metastasis, partially necrotic but hypervascular. (**f, g**) Aortoiliac bifurcation injection, to identify the iliofemoral arterial network; late phase: heterogeneous enhancement of metastatic areas. (**h, i**) Selective catheterization of the right hypogastric artery from a left femoral puncture (early phase, late phase). (**j–l**) Hyperselective catheterization of the obturator artery. (**m**) Exclusion by microparticles and then coils. (**n**) Selective catheterization of an enlarged branch of the common femoral artery involved in tumor vascularization: this artery was excluded by coils + particles. (**o**) Ultimate control after devascularization by particles + coils of collateral branches involved in tumor vascularization

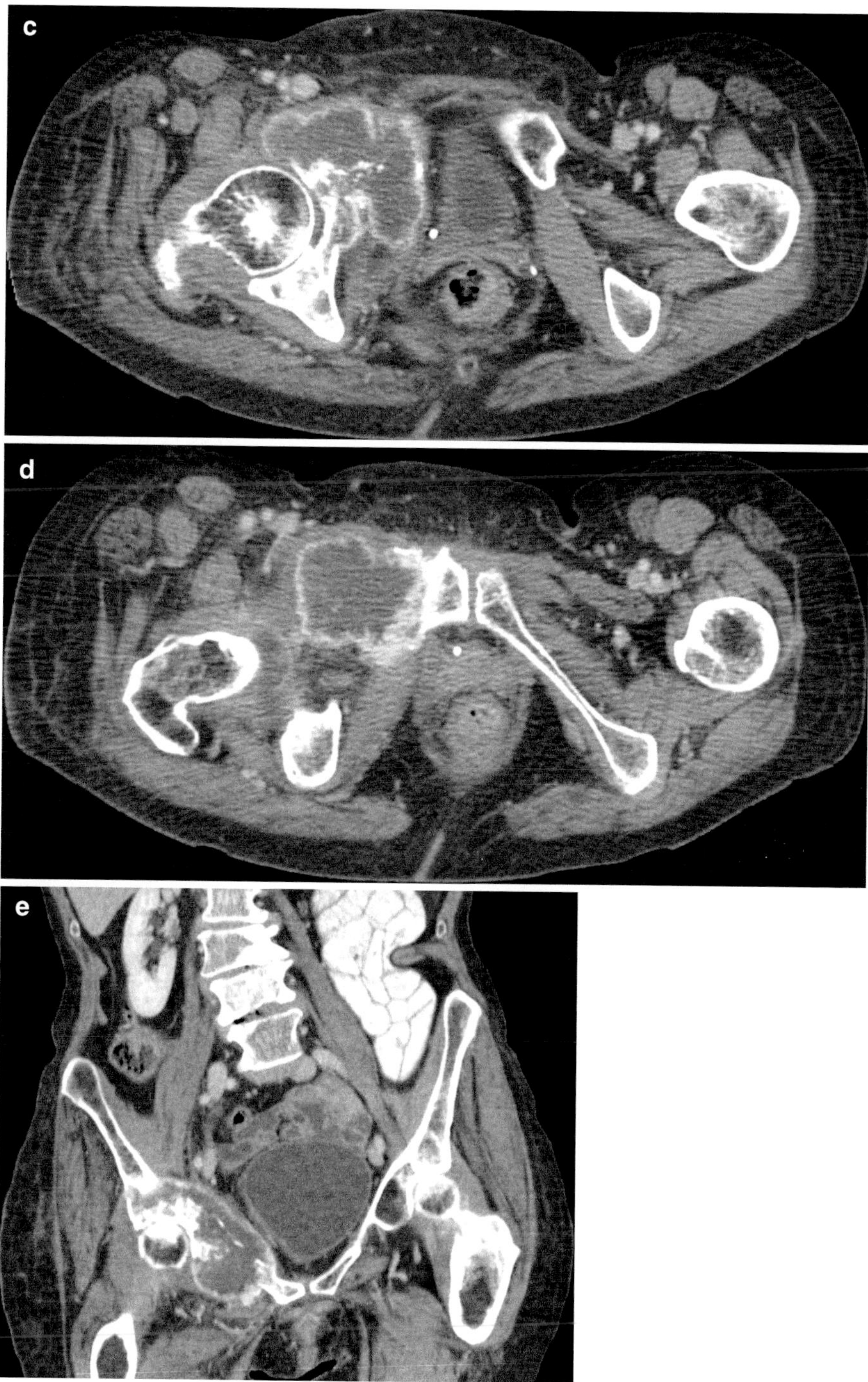

Fig. 24.1 (continued)

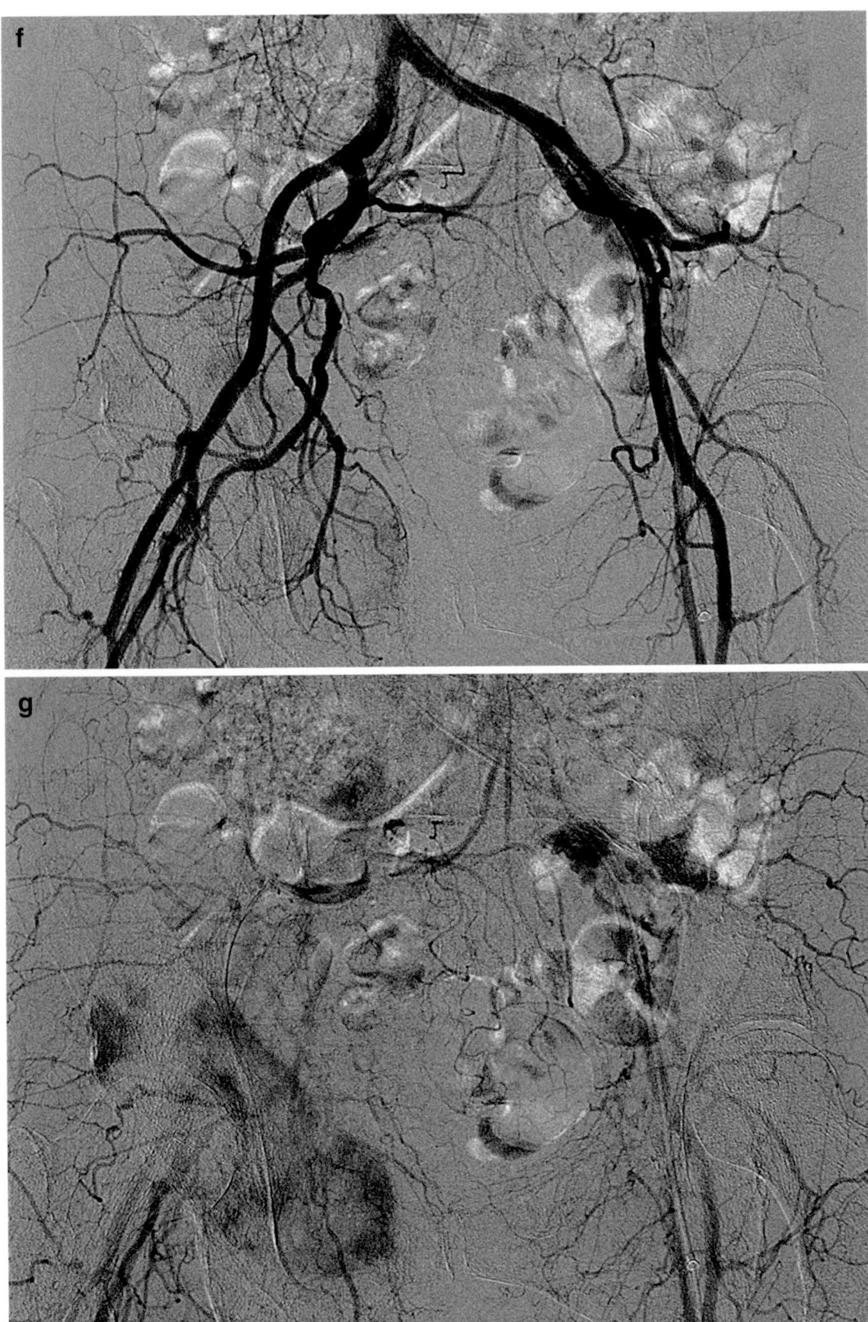

Fig. 24.1 (continued)

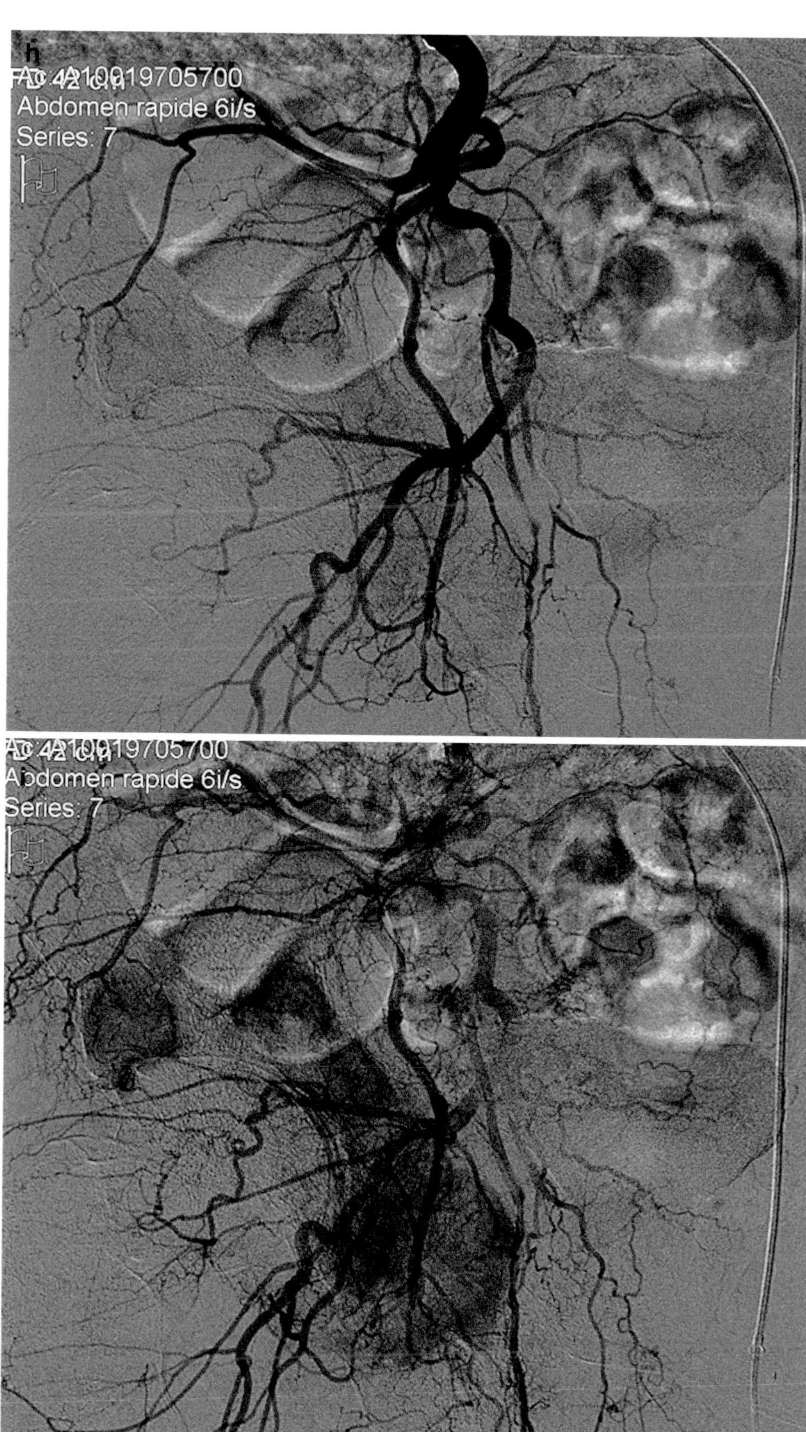

Fig. 24.1 (continued)

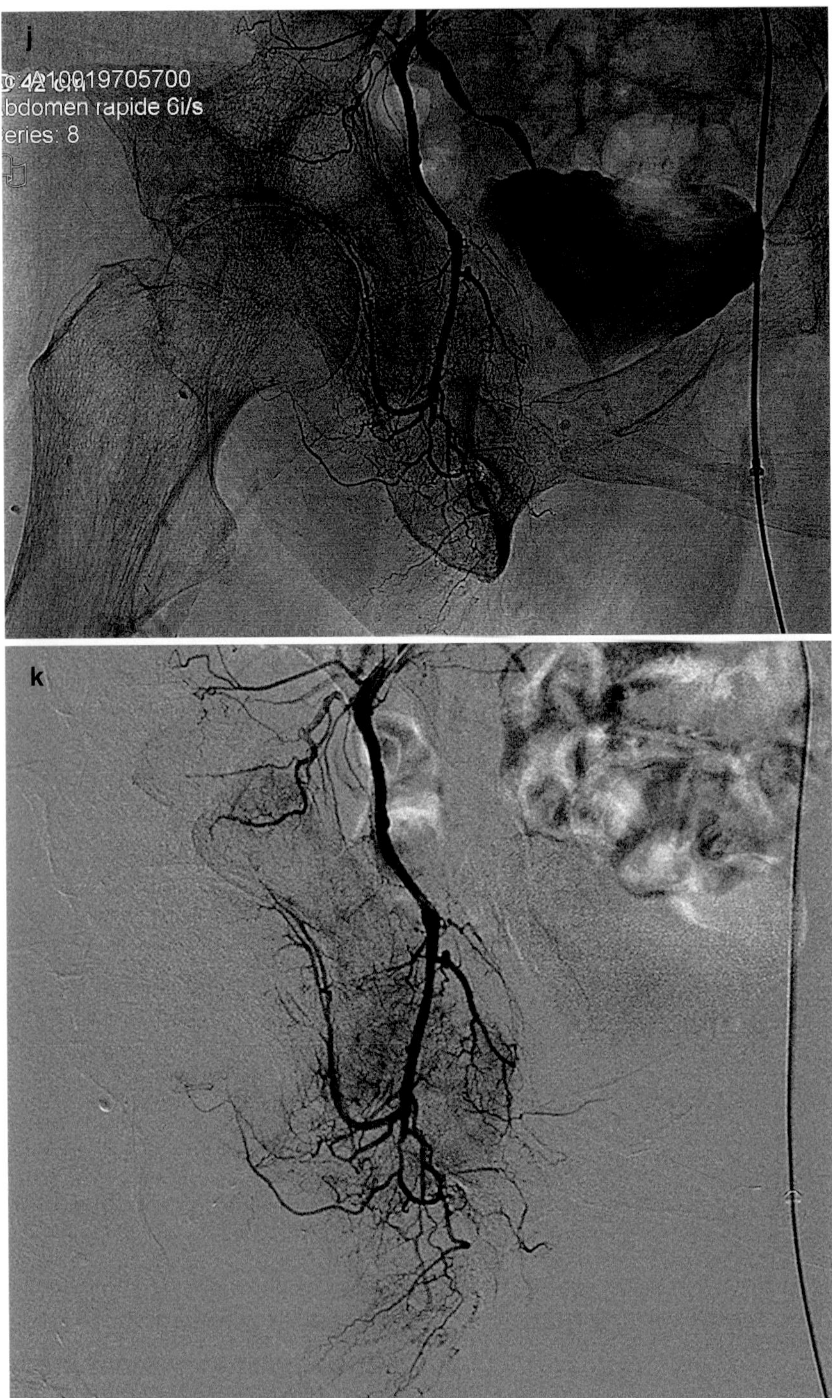

Fig. 24.1 (continued)

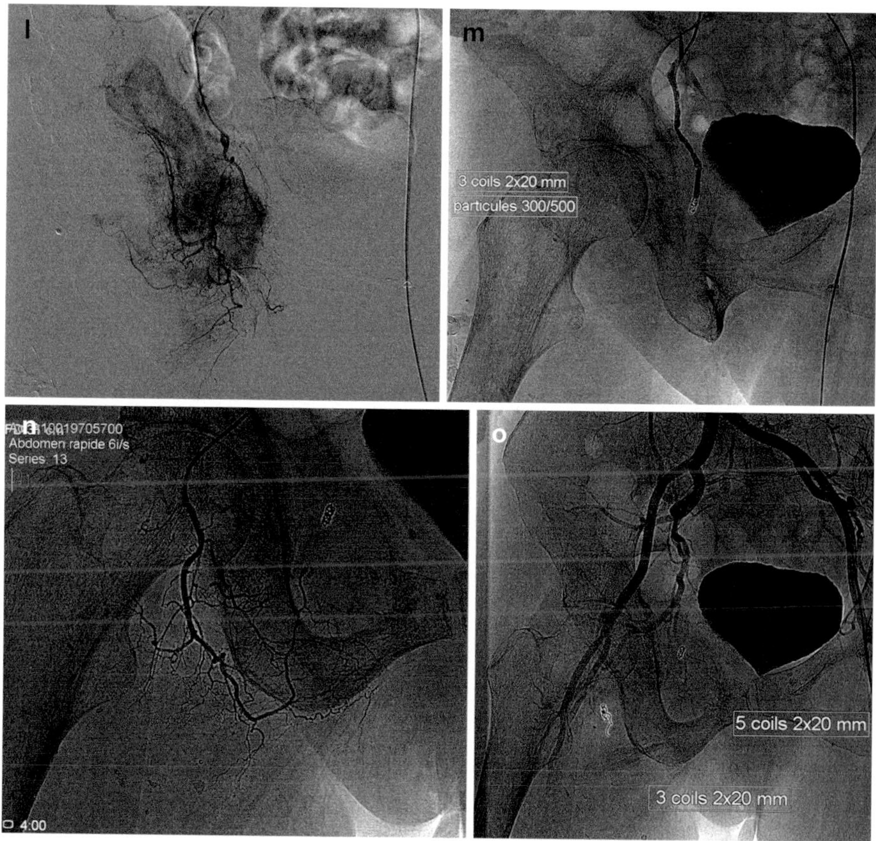

Fig. 24.1 (continued)

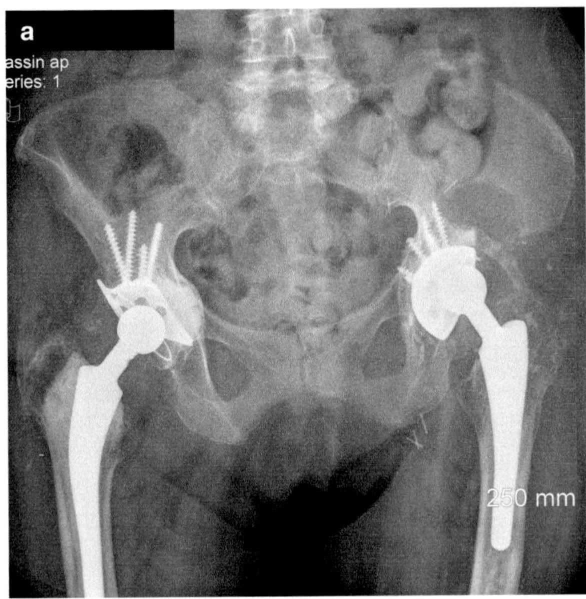

Fig. 24.2 A 74-year-old, pelvic lytic bony metastases of a renal tumor, complicated by the dislocation of a total left hip replacement with fracture of the roof of the acetabulum: a preoperative embolization was requested before osteosynthesis. (**a**) Standard pelvic view: lytic lesions of the iliac wing, left acetabular roof, and left sacral ala. (**b**) Opacification of the aortoiliac bifurcation (right femoral access). Late phase: moderate hypervascularization of the acetabular roof; intense enhancement of a bifocal tumoral hypervascularization, fed by the lateral sacral artery for the larger lesion, and by the gluteal artery for the other. (**c**) Hyperselective catheterization of the inferior gluteal artery (Blush: *arrows*). (**d**) Selective control after exclusion with particles of the territory of the gluteal artery (frontal view). (**e–h**) Frontal and RAO views: identification of the left hypogastric artery, followed by selective catheterization and embolization by particles of the lateral sacral artery, which abundantly vascularize the metastatic lesion. (**i**) Aortoiliac control opacification at the end of the procedure showing the arterial exclusion of the two metastases, allowing reconstructive surgery with less bleeding

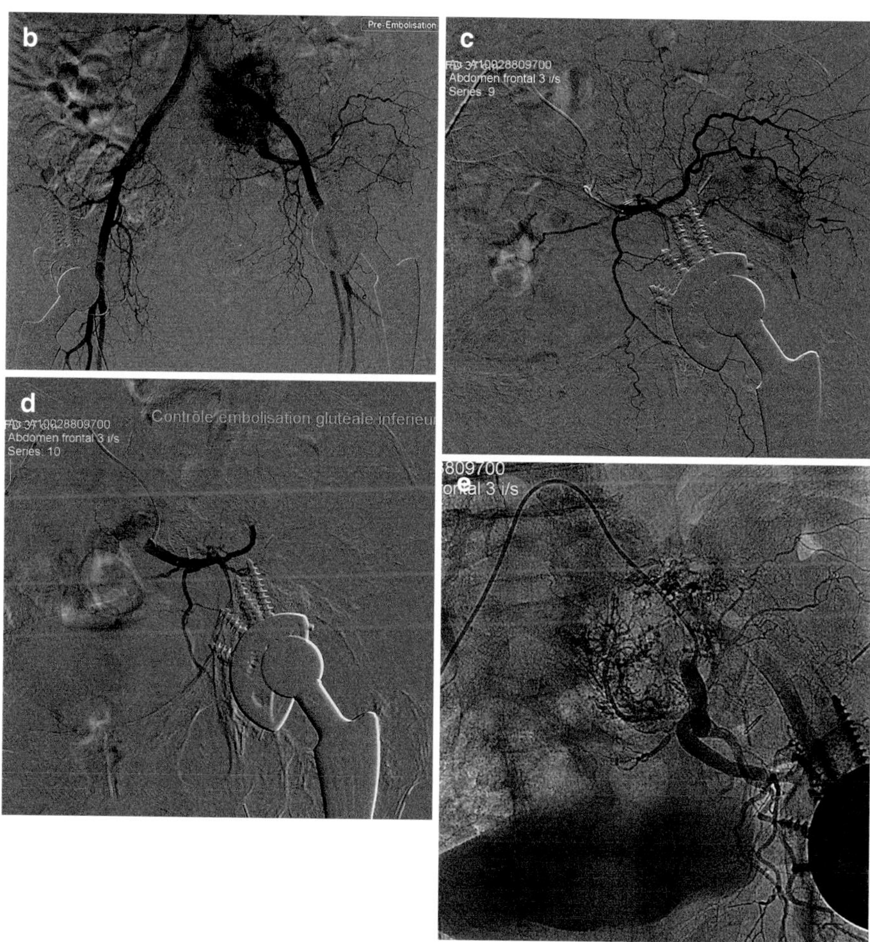

Fig. 24.2 (continued)

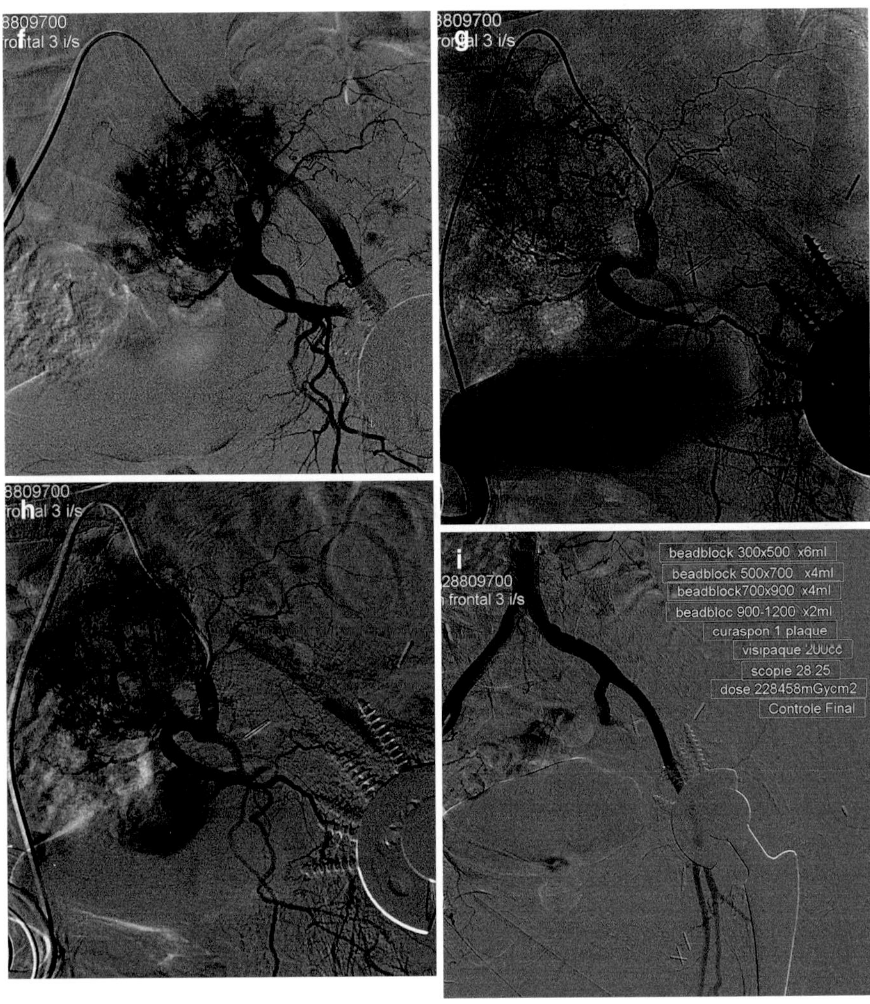

Fig. 24.2 (continued)

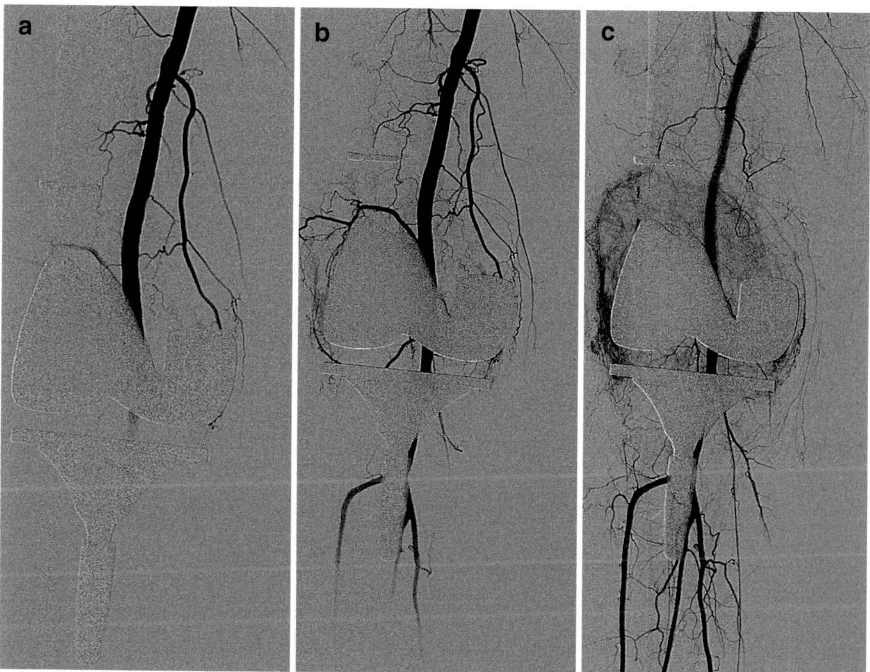

Fig. 24.3 A 62-year-old active patient who was operated 9 months ago of a total knee replacement to a multi operated left knee. After uneventful few weeks, a swelling of the left knee, without biological anomaly, has led to three successive punctures, finding hemarthrosis. There was not any disorder of hemostasis. (**a**–**d**) Antegrade groin puncture of the right common femoral artery, injection on the knee level, early and late phases: articular hyperemia in internal and external compartments. (**e**–**i**) This hypervascularization was essentially provided by two collateral arteries belonging to the periarticular circle of the knee: one emerging anteriorly from the popliteal artery above the prosthesis, which vascularize the outer compartment (**e** and **f**: selective injection in lateral view) and the other arising from the internal lateral edge of the distal SFA, supplying the inner compartment (**g**, **h**, and **i**: frontal view). These both two arteries were embolized by microparticles (diameter: 100–300 μm and then 500–700 μm). (**j**) Final angio control

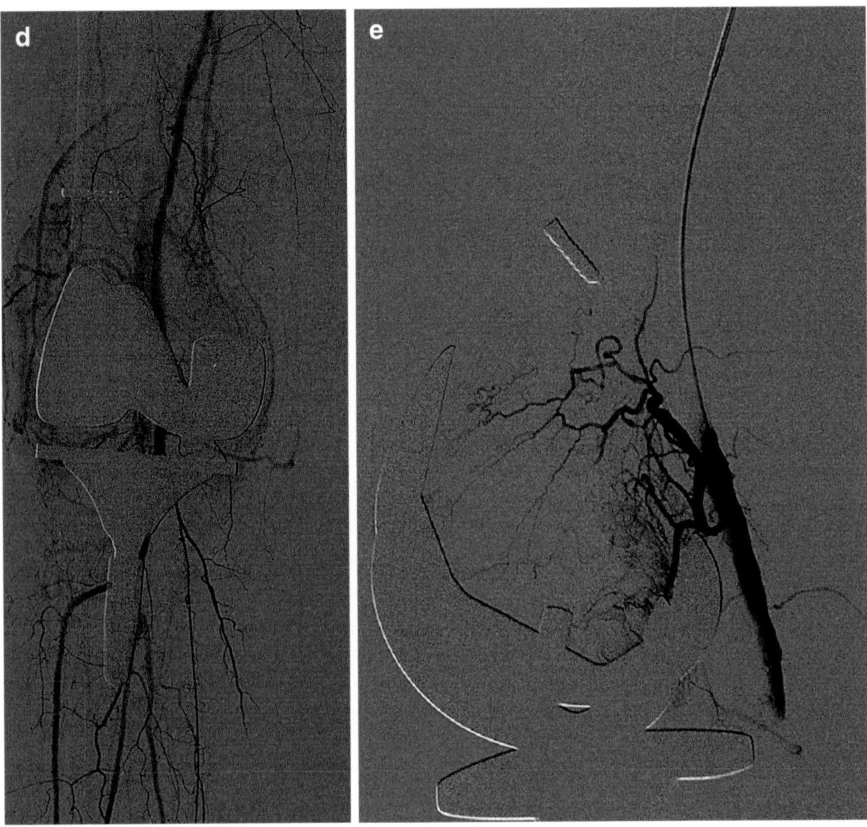

Fig. 24.3 (continued)

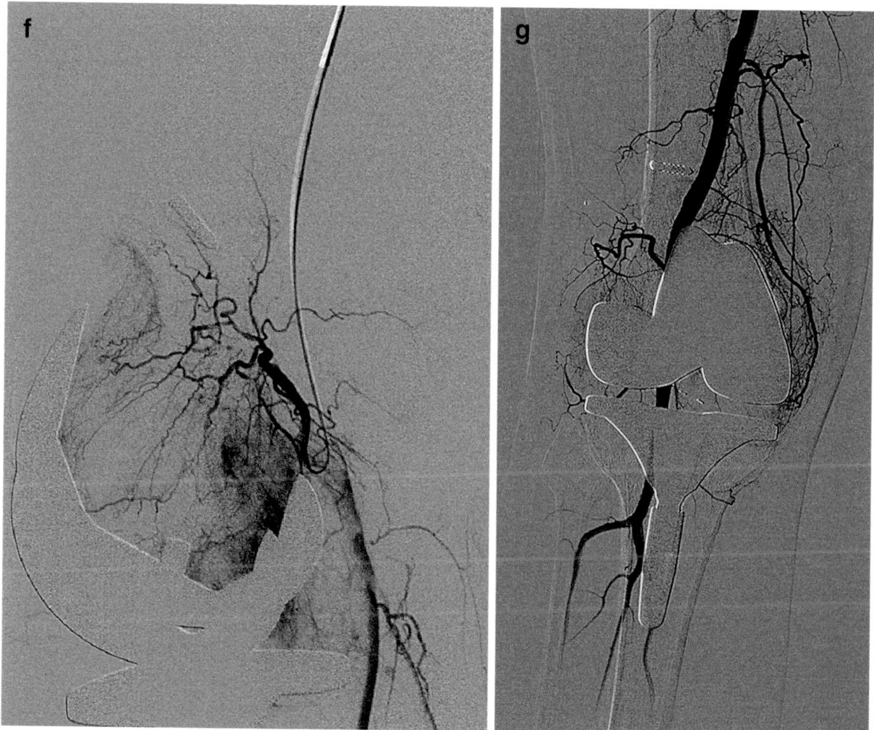

Fig. 24.3 (continued)

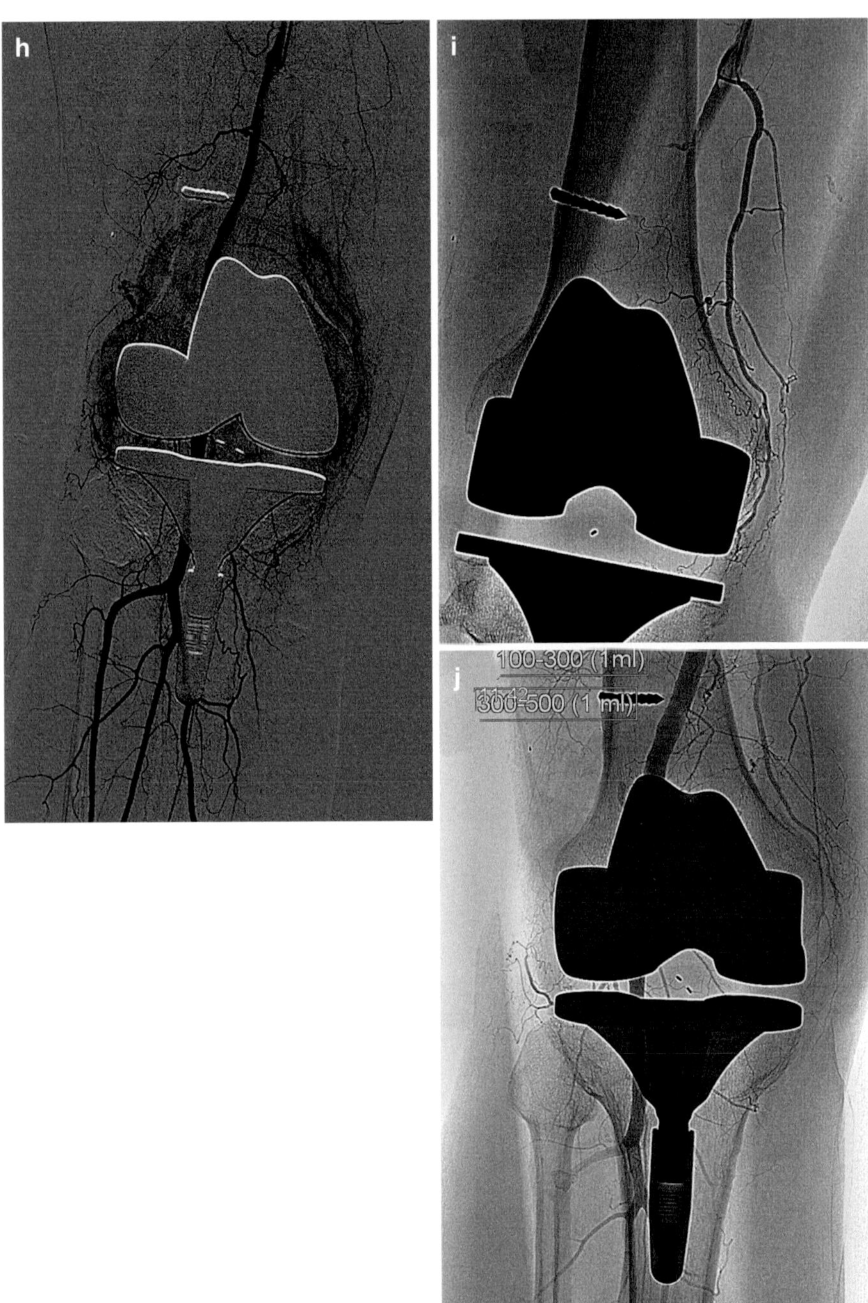

Fig. 24.3 (continued)

References

1. Bourlet P, Dumousset E, Nasser S. P Chabrot and Al Embolization off hepatic and adrenal metastasis to treat Cushing' S syndrome associated with medullary thyroid carcinoma: box carryforward has. Cardiovasc Intervent Radiol. 2007;30:1052–5.
2. Pelage JP, Le Dref O, Soyer P, et al. Arterial anatomy of the female genital tract: variations and relevance to transcatheter embolization of the uterus. AJR Am J Roentgenol. 1999; 172:989–94.
3. Delgal A, Cercueil JP, Koutlidis N, et al. Outcome of transcatheter arterial embolization for bladder and prostate hemorrhage. J Urol. 2010;183:1947–53.
4. Mokarim A, et al. Combined intraarterial chemotherapy and radiotherapy in the treatment of bladder carcinoma. Cancer. 1997;80:1776–85.
5. Carnevale FC, Antunes AA, Motta-Leal-Filho JM, et al. Prostatic artery embolization as a primary treatment for benign prostatic hyperplasia: preliminary results in two patients. Cardiovasc Intervent Radiol. 2010;33(2):355–61.
6. Pisco JM, Pinheiro LC, Bilhim T, et al. Prostatic arterial embolization to treat benign prostatic hyperplasia. J Vasc Interv Radiol. 2011;22:11–9.
7. Mauro MA. Can hyperplastic prostate follow uterine fibroids and be managed with transcatheter arterial embolization? Radiology. 2008;246(3):657–8.
8. Kiyosue H, Tanoue S, Kondo Y, et al. Balloon-occluded retrograde transvenous obliteration of complex gastric varices assisted by temporary balloon occlusion of the splenic artery. J Vasc Interv Radiol. 2011;22:1045–8.
9. Sabri SS, Swee W, Turba UC, et al. Bleeding gastric varices obliteration with balloon-occluded retrograde transvenous obliteration using sodium tetradecyl sulfate foam. J Vasc Interv Radiol. 2011;22:309–16.
10. Hong CH, Kim HJ, Park JH, et al. Treatment of patients with gastric variceal hemorrhage: endoscopic N-butyl-2-cyanoacrylate injection versus balloon-occluded retrograde transvenous obliteration. J Gastroenterol Hepatol. 2009;24:372–8.
11. Minamiguchi H, Kawai N, Sato M, et al. Balloon occlusion retrograde transvenous obliteration for inferior mesenteric vein-systemic shunt. J Vasc Interv Radiol. 2011;22:1039–44.
12. Arabi M, Vellody R, Cwikiel WB, Gemmete JJ. Endovascular treatment of lower gastrointestinal bleeding from systemic-to-mesenteric venous collateral vessels caused by inferior vena cava occlusion: report of two cases. J Vasc Interv Radiol. 2011;22:1035–8.
13. Rossi G, Mavrogenis AF, Rimondi E, et al. Selective embolization with N-butyl cyanoacrylate for metastatic bone disease. J Vasc Interv Radiol. 2011;22:462–70.
14. Koike Y, Takizawa K, Ogawa Y, et al. Transcatheter arterial chemoembolization (TACE) or embolization (TAE) for symptomatic bone metastases as a palliative treatment. Cardiovasc Intervent Radiol. 2011;34:793–801.
15. Pham TT, Bouloudian S, Moreau PE, et al. Recurrent hemarthrosis following total knee. Report of a case treated with arterial embolization. Joint Bone Spine. 2003;70(1):58–60.

Index

P. Chabrot, L. Boyer (eds.), *Embolization*,
DOI 10.1007/978-1-4471-5182-1, © Springer-Verlag London 2014

K

L

M

N

O

P

Printed in the United States
By Bookmasters